Adult Epilepsy

Adult Epilepsy

Edited by Gregory D. Cascino and Joseph I. Sirven
Mayo Clinic College of Medicine, USA

WILEY-BLACKWELL

A John Wiley & Sons, Ltd., Publication

Library of Congress Cataloging-in-Publication Data

Adult epilepsy / edited by Gregory Cascino and Joseph Sirven.
    p. ; cm.
Includes bibliographical references.
ISBN 978-0-470-74122-1 (cloth)
1. Epilepsy. 2. Adult. I. Cascino, Gregory. II. Sirven, Joseph I.
[DNLM: 1. Epilepsy. 2. Adult. WL 385]
RC372.A44 2010
616.8'53—dc22

                                                    2010037013

A catalogue record for this book is available from the British Library.

This book is published in the following electronic formats: ePDF: 978-0-470-97502-2; Wiley Online Library: 978-0-470-97503-9; ePub: 978-0-470-97619-7

Set in 10.5/13pt Times Roman by Laserwords Private Limited, Chennai, India
Printed and bound in Singapore by Markono Print Media Pte Ltd

First Impression   2011

This book is dedicated to our spouses Teresa Griffin Cascino and Joan Sirven who have been so gracious of their efforts and remarkable talents to support our personal and professional careers.

Contents

List of contributors

Eduardo Benarroch, MD
Department of Neurology
Division of Autonomic Disorders
Mayo Clinic
200 First Street SW
Rochester, MN 55905
USA

Jeffrey W. Britton, MD
Department of Neurology
Divisions of Clinical
   Neurophysiology-EEG
   and Epilepsy
Mayo Clinic
200 First Street SW
Rochester, MN 55905
USA

Gregory D. Cascino, MD, FAAN
Professor of Neurology, Mayo
   Clinic College of Medicine, and
Chair, Division of Epilepsy,
Mayo Clinic and Mayo Foundation
200 First Street SW
Rochester, MN 55905
USA

Julie Cunningham, Pharm D
Department of Pharmacy
Mayo Clinic
200 First Street SW
Rochester, MN 55905
USA

Joseph F. Drazkowski, MD
Division of Epilepsy
Mayo Clinic Arizona
5777 East Mayo Boulevard
Phoenix, AZ 85054
USA

Matthew Hoerth, MD
Division of Epilepsy
Mayo Clinic Arizona
5777 East Mayo Boulevard
Phoenix, AZ 85054
USA

Terrence D. Lagerlund, MD
Consultant, Department of
  Neurology,
Division of Clinical
  Neurophysiology
Mayo Clinic, and
Associate Professor of Neurology,
Mayo Clinic College of Medicine,
200 First Street SW
Rochester, MN 55905
USA

Katherine C. Nickels, MD
Child and Adolescent Neurology
  and Epilepsy
Mayo Clinic
200 First Street SW
Rochester, MN 55905
USA

Katherine H. Noe, MD, PhD
Assistant Professor of Neurology
Mayo Clinic College of
  Medicine, and
Consultant, Department of
  Neurology
Division of Epilepsy
Mayo Clinic Arizona
5777 East Mayo Boulevard
Phoenix, AZ 85054
USA

Raj D. Sheth, MD
Professor of Neurology
Mayo Medical School, and
Department of Neurology
Division of Epilepsy
Mayo Clinic
4500 San Pablo Road
Jacksonville, FL 32224;
Chief of Neurology
Division of Pediatric Neurology
Nemours Children's Clinic
807 Children's Way
Jacksonville, FL 32207
USA

Jerry J. Shih, MD
Department of Neurology
Division of Epilepsy
Mayo Clinic
4500 San Pablo Road
Jacksonville, FL 32224
USA

Cheolsu Shin
Department of Neurology
Division of Epilepsy
Mayo Clinic
200 First Street SW
Rochester, MN 55905
USA

Joseph I. Sirven, MD
Professor of Neurology, Mayo
  Clinic College of Medicine,
Chairman of Education, Mayo
  Clinic Arizona, and
Department of Neurology,
  Division of Epilepsy
Mayo Clinic Hospital, 5 East
5777 East Mayo Boulevard
Phoenix, AZ 85054
USA

Elson L. So, MD
Professor of Neurology
Director, Section of
  Electroencephalography
Mayo Clinic College of Medicine
200 First Street SW
Rochester, MN 55905
USA

Korwyn Williams
Department of Pediatrics
  University of Arizona College
  of Medicine
Phoenix, AZ 85004;
Division of Neurology Children's
  Neuroscience Institute
Phoenix Children's Hospital
Phoenix, AZ 85004
USA

Elaine Wirrell
Professor of Neurology
Divisions of Epilepsy and
Child and Adolescent Neurology
Mayo Clinic
200 First Street SW
Rochester, MN 55905
USA

Gregory A. Worrell, MD, PhD
Department of Neurology
Divisions of Epilepsy and Clinical
  Neurophysiology
Mayo Systems Electrophysiology
  Laboratory
Mayo Clinic
Rochester, MN 55905
USA

William O. Tatum IV, DO
Professor Department of
  Neurology
Division of Epilepsy
Mayo College of Medicine
Mayo Clinic
4500 San Pablo Road
Jacksonville, FL 32224
USA

Tarek M. Zakaria, MD
Director, Epilepsy Monitoring
  Unit
Co Director Epilepsy surgery
  program
Norton Neuroscience Institute
Louisville, KY 40241
USA

Preface

The idea for this book came from a Mayo Clinic Clinical Neurophysiology course that is held annually in January or February. Colleagues from the Division of Epilepsy participate as course faculty in the EEG and Epilepsy didactic sections and workshops for the attendees. We are fortunate to have three Mayo Clinic comprehensive epilepsy programs in Jacksonville, FL, Scottsdale/Phoenix, AZ, and Rochester, MN. All authors of this monograph are actively involved in patient care and clinical research, are members of the Mayo Clinic Division of Epilepsy, and have academic appointments at the Mayo Clinic College of Medicine. Similar to our Mayo Clinic educational program, the target audiences for this textbook are health care professionals involved in the diagnostic evaluation or management, or both, of patients with seizure disorders. Our goal is provide a contemporary and concise review of information pertinent to the management of individuals with epilepsy.

Greg Cascino
Rochester, MN

Joe Sirven
Phoenix, AZ

July 2010

1 Introduction: epilepsy

Gregory D. Cascino

Department of Neurology, Division of Epilepsy, Mayo Clinic, Rochester, MN, USA

1.1 Epilepsy care: beginnings of observation and recognition

Epilepsy historically has been one of the most commonly recognized and distinct neurological disorders [1, 2]. In fifth-century BC Greece, Hippocrates, the father of medicine, made several profound observations regarding epilepsy that have survived many centuries [1]. He was a follower of the Greek god of medicine Asclepius whose symbol of a serpent-entwined staff has been representative of medical practice to the present. On the island of Cos in the Aegean Sea, Hippocrates observed patients with a malady referred to as the "sacred disease." He indicated that seizures appeared no more *divine* or spiritual than any other illness. Hippocrates also implicated the brain as the site of seizure onset and recognized the genetic predisposition in selected patients. Galen was another outstanding physician of Greek origin who was born in 129 AD and was influenced by the teachings of Hippocrates. Upon traveling to Rome he made several seminal observations in medicine and introduced the term "aura" to describe the patients' symptoms that recognized the onset of a seizure. Initially Galen recognized the abdominal complaints that may occur in patients prior to the impairment in consciousness. The aura was compared to a "breeze" that may indicate an oncoming weather storm.

Adult Epilepsy, First Edition. Edited by Gregory D. Cascino and Joseph I. Sirven.
© 2011 John Wiley & Sons, Ltd. Published 2011 by John Wiley & Sons, Ltd.

Epilepsy in the Middle Ages was considered to be emblematic of the *absence* of a spiritual or divine presence [1, 2]. The paroxysmal behavior was thought to be related to an external evil force that was possessing the soul of the unfortunate individual. The removal of "demons" was necessary to control the "convulsions" that gripped the patient. Later, patients were often isolated from the general population and placed in institutions or epilepsy colonies. The segregation of people with epilepsy had a profoundly negative impact on the ability of these individuals to successfully integrate and live in "normal" society.

1.2   Epilepsy care: initial understanding and treatment

The contemporary care of patients with seizure disorders began with the pivotal observations and writings of John Hughlings Jackson (1835–1911), the father of epilepsy, at the National Hospital for Diseases of the Nervous System including Paralysis and Epilepsy in Queen Square, London [1–4]. Jackson influenced the Scottish neurologist Sir David Ferrier working in London to confirm the relationship between nervous system physiology and structure to better elucidate the pathophysiology associated with seizures [4]. Ferrier performed electrical stimulation of the motor cortex in the dog providing evidence that focal motor seizures were associated with excitation of the precentral gyrus [1–4]. Prior to the works of Jackson in the mid nineteenth century, there was considered to be only one prominent seizure type, the generalized tonic-clonic seizure. There was a broad consensus that the "grand mal seizure" involved the lower brainstem or upper cervical cord, or both structures. Jackson postulated that the cerebral cortex was the site of seizure onset and that the ictal behavior correlated with the region of functional anatomy. A focal or lateralized neurological abnormality may indicate the region of hemisphere of seizure onset. Further, he introduced the concept of partial epilepsy indicating that *"part"* of the cerebral cortex was involved in seizure onset [3]. This area of cerebral cortex was considered to be abnormal resulting in a focal neurological deficit and seizure activity. The potential therapeutic importance of Jackson's brilliant conclusions was that surgical treatment may be effective as an underlying pathology or structural lesion was presumed to be associated with the site of epileptogenesis [4]. Resection of the lesional pathology was entertained as an effective means of rendering the patient seizure-free [4]. These seminal observations occurred prior to the development of electroencephalography (EEG), neuroimaging, or use of antiepileptic drug therapy. Subsequently, beginning in 1886 Dr. Victor Horsley, a young surgical colleague of Hughlings Jackson, performed neurosurgical procedures for epilepsy in patients at the National Hospital [4]. The localization of the epileptogenic brain tissue was based on the ictal semiology, the neurological examination, and knowledge of functional neuroanatomy. The efforts of Jackson and colleagues began the rewarding and productive relationship between neurology and neurosurgery in the management of patients with intractable epilepsy [4].

1.3 Epilepsy care: the Mayo Clinic

Dr. Willam J. Mayo and Dr. Charles H. Mayo, the brothers who founded the group practice in Rochester, Minnesota, were close colleagues of the "fathers" of contemporary neurosurgery, Dr. Harvey Cushing of Johns Hopkins University and later Harvard University, and Dr. Charles H. Frazier of the University of Pennsylvania [5, 6]. The strong relationship between Dr. Cushing and the Mayos lasted until the time of the brothers' deaths in 1939 [6, 7]. Dr. C. Mayo published his initial experience with neurosurgery in 1891 [8]. The importance of seizures as a diagnostic symptom of neurological disease and the effect of neurosurgery on seizure tendency were recognized. Ultimately, in 1917, Dr. Alfred W. Adson became the first full-time neurosurgeon at the Mayo Clinic [5]. The growth of neurology and neurosurgery at this institution were forever intertwined during this period as Dr. Walter D. Shelden had come to the Mayo Clinic in 1913 and founded the neurology section. Perhaps most importantly, Dr. Adson had insisted that neurosurgery should be a separate department from surgery and a unique subspecialty at the Mayo Clinic. Advances in diagnostic technology would be necessary to expand the care of patients with epilepsy.

The first EEG study at the Mayo Clinic was performed by Dr. E.J. Baldes, a biophysicist, on Dr. Charles LeVant Yeager who was a Mayo neurology fellow in 1936 [9]. Dr. Yeager was an amateur radio operator who became interested in the works of Hans Berger when the first publication of EEG appeared in 1929. He personally translated the 10 works of Berger on EEG into English. Dr. Frederick Moersch, one of the pioneers in neurology at the Mayo Clinic, had visited Nobel Laureate Lord Edgar Douglas Adrian's laboratory working on EEG at the University of Cambridge in 1935, and encouraged development of this innovation in Rochester, MN [9]. The initial EEG recordings were performed at the Rochester State Hospital and the laboratory was subsequently moved to Saint Marys Hospital. The development of EEG at the Mayo Clinic was selected by Dr. Henry Woltman, the section head of neurology, as Dr. Yeager's "research project." Working closely with Dr. Adson the diagnostic utility of EEG was analyzed in patients with known intracranial lesions. Dr. Adson had insisted that only the ages of the patients and not the clinical information be made available to the EEG readers. The results of EEG studies in a series of patients demonstrated the favorable diagnostic importance of the "new" technique for structural localization compared to other studies, for example, ventriculography and pneumoencephalography. EEG was also demonstrated to assess the seizure tendency in these individuals and indicate the likely site of seizure onset.

After World War II the clinical and basic research activities of the EEG laboratory were expanded. The recruitment in 1948 of Dr. Reginald G. Bickford from the University of Cambridge increased the research interests of EEG to include the evaluation of patients with seizure disorders [9]. Dr. Bickford had worked with E.D. Adrian and EEG pioneer Dr. W. Grey Walter during the war and had had the opportunity to perform intracranial EEG recordings in patients with penetrating head injuries undergoing neurosurgical treatment [9, 10]. He brought to the Mayo Clinic his interest in reflex epilepsy and intracranial EEG recordings. Therefore, Rochester, MN was one of the earliest centers in North America performing these depth electrode recordings in patients with seizure disorders. A symposium on "intracerebral electrography" was held in 1953 summarizing the outcome of these studies in patients with epilepsy [10]. Beginning in 1948, Dr. Bickford and colleagues also performed motion picture recordings for diagnostic classification of seizures and nonepileptic events. Dr. Donald W. Klass started as neurology resident at the Mayo Clinic in 1953 and went on to become head of the EEG section in 1967 [11]. Dr. Klass had described the epileptogenic potential of several paroxysmal EEG patterns and recognized the benign nature of selected discharges. Importantly, he also educated a generation of neurologists in EEG interpretation [9].

In 1968, Dr. Frank W. Sharbrough joined the staff at the Mayo Clinic after completing his training at the University of Michigan and serving in the military. His interests included routine EEG, intraoperative EEG monitoring during cerebrovascular surgery and epilepsy surgery, evoked potentials, and use of computer applications to monitor neurophysiological techniques. Focal cortical resections for patients with epilepsy and excisions of potentially epileptogenic lesions were performed by several neurosurgeons including Dr. Ross H. Miller who served as chair of the department of neurosurgery (1975–1980) and performed over 4000 operations for intracranial tumors [5]. Surgical treatment for intractable partial epilepsy achieved a significant advance with the arrival of Dr. Edward P. Laws, Jr. at the Mayo Clinic in 1972 [5]. Dr. Laws was trained in neurosurgery at the Johns Hopkins University by the renowned neurosurgeon Dr. A. Earl Walker and collaborated with famed electroencephalographer, Dr. Ernst Niedermeyer. At the Mayo Clinic he was a prominent academic neurosurgeon and educator actively involved in epilepsy surgery as well as resection of pituitary tumors and craniopharyngiomas [12, 13].

In 1973 the Mayo Clinic was the first institution in the United States to have an x-ray computed tomography (CT) scanner installed [14]. The use of CT and the subsequent development of magnetic resonance imaging (MRI) had a profound effect on the evaluation of patients with epilepsy. The pivotal importance of MRI in identifying structural abnormalities and the potential for performance of intraoperative imaging to guide surgical procedures and implantation of intracranial electrodes had an enormous impact on the care and management of epilepsy.

In 1984, Dr. Patrick J. Kelly joined the staff in neurosurgery [5]. After his neurosurgery residency he completed training at the Hospital Sainte Anne in Paris with the founder of stereotactic neurosurgery, Dr. Jean Talairach. The emergence of the new imaging technology and Dr. Kelly's experience combined for the use of stereotactic neurosurgical procedures to resect epileptogenic lesions and for computer-assisted placement of intracranial depth electrodes [15, 16]. Stereotactic "lesionectomy" was particularly useful for intra-axial lesions involving functional cerebral cortex [15].

The last decade of the twentieth century was remarkable for major advances in neuroimaging at the Mayo Clinic that significantly improved the ability to care for patients with intractable seizure disorders. Colleagues in neuroradiology, neurology, neurosurgery, and nuclear medicine were critical for the development of MRI hippocampal formation volumetry and subtraction ictal single photon emission computed tomography (SISCOM) [17, 18]. The former structural neuroimaging study has proven beneficial in correlating quantitative hippocampal atrophy with neuronal cell loss, neuropsychometric studies, and seizure outcome in patients undergoing temporal lobe surgery for intractable epilepsy [17]. The latter functional neuroimaging procedure has been adapted to the evaluation of patients with nonlesional partial epilepsy or if the preoperative evaluation has conflicting findings regarding the localization of the epileptogenic zone [18].

The practice of epileptology at the Mayo Clinic is predicated on the motto for medical care since the pioneer practice of Dr. William W. Mayo in the nineteenth century: "The needs of the patient always come first." At the three Mayo Clinic sites in Arizona, Florida, and Minnesota the goals of epilepsy treatment are to reduce seizure tendency and improve the quality of life enabling the individual to become a participating and productive member of our society.

References

1. Temkin, O. (1994) *The Falling Sickness: A History of Epilepsy from the Greeks to the Beginnings of Modern Neurology*, 2nd edn, Johns Hopkins University Press, Baltimore.
2. Eadie, M.J. and Bladin, P.F. (2001) *A Disease Once Sacred: A History of the Medical Understanding of Epilepsy*, John Libbey, Eastleigh.
3. Jackson, J.H. (1931) On epilepsy and epileptiform convulsions, in *Selected Writings of John Hughlings Jackson*, vol. 1 (ed. J. Taylor), Hodder and Stoughton, London.
4. Taylor, D.C. (1987) One hundred years of epilepsy surgery: Sir Victor Horsley's contribution, in *Surgical Treatment of the Epilepsies*, (ed. J. Engel Jr.), Raven Press, New York, pp. 7–11.
5. Spinner, R.J., Al-Rodhan, N.R., and Piepgras, D.G. (2001) 100 years of neurological surgery at the Mayo Clinic. *Neurosurgery*, **49**, 438–446.
6. Cohen-Gadol, A.A., Homan, J.M., Laws, E.R. *et al.* (2005) Historical vignette. The Mayo brothers and Harvey Cushing: a review of their 39-year friendship through their personal letters. *J Neurosurg*, **102**, 391–396.
7. Cushing, H. (1939) The Mayo brothers and their clinic. *(Obituary) Science*, **90**, 225–226.

8. Mayo, C.H. (1891) A contribution to cerebral surgery: Part I—Cerebral abscess; operation; recovery. Part II—Arteriovenous aneurism in cavernous sinus; operation; recovery. *Northwest Lancet*, **11**, 59–60.

9. Klass, D.W. and Bickford, R.G. (1992) Reflections on the birth and early development of EEG at the Mayo Clinic. *J Clin Neurophysiol*, **9**, 2–20.

10. (1953) Symposium on intracerebral electrography. *Proc Staff Meet Mayo Clinic*, **28**, 145–192.

11. Thomas, J.E., Reagan, T.J., and Klass, D.W. (1977) Epilepsia partialis continua. A review of 32 cases. *Arch Neurol*, **34**, 266–275.

12. Niedermeyer, E., Laws, E.R. Jr., and Walker, E.A. (1969) Depth EEG findings in epileptics with generalized spike-wave complexes. *Arch Neurol*, **21**, 51–58.

13. Meyer, F.B., Marsh, W.R., Laws, E.R. Jr., and Sharbrough, F.W. (1986) Temporal lobectomy in children with epilepsy. *J Neurosurg*, **64**, 371–376.

14. Baker, H.I. Jr. and Houser, O.W. (1976) Computed tomography in the diagnosis of posterior fossa lesions. *Radiol Clin North Am*, **14**, 129–147.

15. Cascino, G.D., Kelly, P.J., Hirschorn, K.A. *et al.* (1990) Stereotactic resection of intra-axial cerebral lesions in partial epilepsy. *Mayo Clin Proc*, **65**, 1053–1060.

16. Cascino, G.D., Kelly, P.J., Sharbrough, F.W. *et al.* (1992) Long-term follow-up of stereotactic lesionectomy in partial epilepsy: predictive factors and electroencephalographic results. *Epilepsia*, **33**, 639–644.

17. Jack, C.R. Jr., Sharbrough, F.W., Twomey, C.K. *et al.* (1990) Temporal lobe seizures: lateralization with MR volume measurements of the hippocampal formation. *Radiology*, **17**, 423–429.

18. O'Brien, T.J., So, E.L., Mullan, B.P. *et al.* (1998) Subtraction ictal SPECT co-registered to MRI improves clinical usefulness of SPECT in localizing the surgical seizure focus. *Neurology*, **50**, 445–454.

Section 1

Pathophysiology and epidemiology of seizures and epilepsy

2 Seizure and epilepsy syndromes classification

Jerry J. Shih

Department of Neurology, Division of Epilepsy, Mayo Clinic, Jacksonville, FL, USA

2.1 Introduction

Understanding the classification of epileptic seizures is the first step towards the correct diagnosis, treatment, and prognostication of the condition. The initial management of a patient with seizures begins with an understanding of the patient's seizure type and, if pertinent, epilepsy syndrome. The classification of epileptic seizures is still largely based on clinical observation and expert opinions. The International League Against Epilepsy (ILAE) first published a classification system in 1960. The last official update for seizures was published in 1981 [1], and the last official update for the epilepsies was in 1989 [2]. These updates form the officially accepted classification system, although there is a new proposal to amend the current system [3].

2.2 The classification of epileptic seizures

By definition, epilepsy is diagnosed after a patient has two or more unprovoked seizures.

Adult Epilepsy, First Edition. Edited by Gregory D. Cascino and Joseph I. Sirven.
© 2011 John Wiley & Sons, Ltd. Published 2011 by John Wiley & Sons, Ltd.

Partial seizures

Partial or focal seizures comprise one of the two main classes of epileptic seizures, with generalized seizures being the other. Partial seizures are subdivided between simple and complex partial seizures, which are distinguished by the presence or absence of impairment of consciousness. Simple partial seizures are defined as seizures without impairment of consciousness while complex partial seizures are defined as seizures with impairment of consciousness. Partial seizures manifest themselves in many different forms, depending on which area of the cortex is involved in the onset and spread of the ictal discharge. Partial seizures originate from a focal area of cerebral cortex and may spread to other cortical regions either unilaterally or bilaterally. A partial seizure may manifest with motor signs, autonomic symptoms, somatosensory or special sensory symptoms, or psychic symptoms. The term aura is synonymous with a simple partial sensory or psychic seizure. An aura often reflects the location of the seizure onset zone.

Simple partial motor seizures can cause clonic activity in the contralateral hand, arm, shoulder, face, and leg. Focal seizures originating from the language area may cause speech arrest or vocalization. Epilepsia partialis continua (EPC) is defined as a continuous focal motor seizure which remains confined to a specific body part and usually consists of clonic movements which can persist for up to months with preserved consciousness. After a focal motor seizure, postictal weakness (Todd's paralysis) can last for minutes to hours.

Simple partial seizures can also have autonomic symptoms such as vomiting, sweating, piloerection, pupil dilation, pallor, flushing, boborygmi, and incontinence. Simple partial seizures originating from the postcentral gyrus may include feelings of focal paresthesias, numbness, warmth, or electrical sensations. Sensory seizures from the insular cortex often manifest with throat paresthesias, warmth, or a sense of strangulation or suffocation [4]. Visual seizures may present with primary visual hallucinations such as flashing lights, or more complex visual hallucinations such as persons or scenes. Auditory seizures arise from the lateral temporal region, and manifest as sensations of buzzing, hyper- or hypoacusis, sound distortion, or hearing words or music. Olfactory seizures originating from the uncinate gyrus or mesial temporal region typically involve smelling unpleasant odors. Gustatory sensations originating from the temporal lobe, insula, or parietal operculum can be pleasant or unpleasant and usually are described as a metallic taste but can also be bitter or sweet.

Simple partial seizures with psychic symptoms indicate a disturbance of higher cortical function. Symptoms involve a distortion of memory and include *déjà vu*, *jamais vu*, dreamy states, distorted time sense, derealization, or a sense of unreality. Psychic auras often originate from the temporal lobe.

Complex partial seizures are partial seizures with impairment of consciousness. They may start as simple partial seizures (auras) and progress to complex partial seizures or may begin as complex partial seizures with impairment of consciousness at the onset of the seizure. They may or may not involve automatisms. The clinical features of the complex partial seizure depend on the region affected by abnormal electrical activity. Complex partial seizures usually originate in the frontal or temporal lobes but can occur in parietal or occipital lobe.

Generalized seizures

Absence seizures are characterized by a sudden onset behavioral arrest, a blank stare, unresponsiveness, and sometimes a brief upward rotation of the eyes. The duration is typically a few seconds to half a minute. There is little to no postictal confusion, and the patient typically resumes the activity he/she was doing prior to the seizures. The ILAE 1981 classification also recognizes five subtypes of absence seizures: absence with impairment of consciousness only, with mild clonic components, with atonic components, with tonic components, and with automatisms. The ictal EEG pattern in absence seizures is a 3 Hz generalized monomorphic spike and wave with abrupt onset and termination.

Atypical absence seizures are usually seen in patients with symptomatic generalized epilepsy. They are similar to absence seizures in that they have both simple and complex presentations. One distinguishing feature is that they are less abrupt in onset clinically. The seizures are usually less than 10 seconds but may be prolonged and result in absence status. They also are not usually induced by hyperventilation or photic stimulation.

Tonic-clonic seizures, also known as grand mal seizures, are characterized by abrupt loss of consciousness followed by tonic contraction of the muscles. This often leads to the ictal cry, where air is forcefully expired against a closed glottis. The upper extremities often symmetrically abduct and flex at the elbows while the lower extremities may briefly flex and then extend and adduct with the toes pointed. Clonic activity then ensues which is initially rapid and then slows. The patient may become cyanotic. Tongue biting and urinary incontinence may occur. The patient is usually postictally disoriented and fatigued. Tonic-clonic seizures may occur independently, may arise from other generalized seizures, or may occur during secondary generalization of a partial onset seizure.

Myoclonic seizures are generalized seizures characterized by brief, irregular, shock-like jerks of the head, trunk, or limbs. They can be symmetric or asymmetric and involve the whole body, regions of the body, or focal areas. They tend to occur close to sleep onset and upon awakening from sleep. Myoclonic seizures can be a feature of some idiopathic generalized epilepsies (juvenile myoclonic epilepsy, JME), symptomatic generalized epilepsies (myoclonic-astatic epilepsy), the progressive myoclonic epilepsies (Lafora disease), and infantile spasms. Myoclonic seizures can occur in clusters and evolve into clonic-tonic-clonic seizures, with resultant loss of consciousness and postictal confusion. The ictal EEG pattern is characterized by brief generalized polyspike or polyspike and wave discharges which correspond to the myoclonic jerk.

Tonic seizures are seizures which involve tonic contraction of the face, neck, axial, or appendicular musculature lasting from 10 seconds to 1 minute. They can involve extension or flexion of the muscles and often lead to falls and head injuries. They are usually seen in patients with symptomatic generalized epilepsy such as Lennox-Gastaut syndrome (LGS). They can also occur in epilepsy with myoclonic-astatic seizures. The ictal EEG usually shows a brief generalized attenuation of cerebral activity followed by generalized paroxysmal fast activity in the beta frequency range. *Clonic seizures* are generalized seizures that are characterized by repetitive rhythmic clonic jerks (1–2 Hz) with impairment of consciousness and a short postictal phase. They can lead into a clonic-tonic-clonic seizure.

Atonic seizures are characterized by a sudden loss of muscle tone which can lead to a head drop, a limb drop, or a drop of the whole body (a.k.a. drop attack). A brief loss of consciousness and injuries, particularly to the face, may occur [1]. Atonic seizures may be preceded by a brief myoclonic jerk or tonic component. Atonic seizures are usually seen in the symptomatic generalized epilepsies such as LGS.

The classification of epilepsies and epileptic syndromes

An epileptic disorder can be symptomatic, idiopathic, or cryptogenic. Symptomatic indicates the etiology is known—usually a structural lesion within the brain. Idiopathic refers to an epilepsy of presumed genetic etiology without a structural brain lesion or other neurological signs or symptoms. Cryptogenic refers to an epilepsy that is presumed to be symptomatic but the etiology is unknown [2]. The term cryptogenic has been replaced by "probably symptomatic" [5]. The currently used 1989 classification system is divided into four main categories: localization-related (focal, local, or partial), generalized, epilepsies and syndromes undetermined whether focal or generalized, and special syndromes (see Table 2.1).

An epilepsy syndrome is defined as "a complex of signs and symptoms that define a unique epilepsy condition" [5]. The groups of syndromes are: idiopathic focal epilepsies of infancy and childhood, familial (autosomal dominant) focal epilepsies, symptomatic (or probably symptomatic) focal epilepsies, idiopathic generalized epilepsies, reflex epilepsies, epileptic encephalopathies, progressive myoclonus epilepsies, and seizures not necessarily requiring a diagnosis of epilepsy (see Table 2.1). There are over 25 specific syndromes in the 1989 ILAE report. A discussion regarding a few of the more common syndromes affecting adolescents and adults follows.

Temporal lobe epilepsies

Temporal lobe seizures are the most common type of partial epilepsy. Temporal lobe seizures often begin with an aura [6]. Auras may include viscerosensory

Table 2.1   ILAE's 1989 international classification of epilepsies and epileptic syndromes

1 Localization-related epilepsies and syndromes
   1.1 Idiopathic
      Benign childhood epilepsy with centrotemporal spikes
      Childhood epilepsy with occipital paroxysms
      Primary reading epilepsy
   1.2 Symptomatic
      Chronic progressive epilepsia partialis continua of childhood (Kojewnikow's
        syndrome)
      Syndromes characterized by seizures with specific modes of precipitation
      Temporal lobe epilepsies
      Frontal lobe epilepsies
      Parietal lobe epilepsies
      Occipital lobe epilepsies
   1.3 Cryptogenic
2 Generalized epilepsies and syndromes
   2.1 Idiopathic
      Benign neonatal familial convulsions
      Benign neonatal convulsions
      Benign myoclonic epilepsy in infancy
      Childhood absence epilepsy
      Juvenile absence epilepsy
      Juvenile myoclonic epilepsy
      Epilepsy with GTCS on awakening
      Other generalized idiopathic epilepsies not defined above
      Epilepsies with seizures precipitated by specific modes of activation
   2.2 Cryptogenic or symptomatic
      West syndrome
      Lennox-Gastaut syndrome
      Epilepsy with myoclonic-astatic seizures
      Epilepsy with myoclonic absences
   2.3 Symptomatic
      2.3.1 Nonspecific etiology
         Early myoclonic encephalopathy
         Early infantile epileptic encephalopathy with suppression burst
         Other symptomatic generalized epilepsies not defined above
      2.3.2 Specific syndromes
         Diseases in which seizures are a presenting or predominant feature
3 Epilepsies and syndromes undetermined whether focal or generalized
   3.1 With both generalized and focal seizures
      Neonatal seizures
      Severe myoclonic epilepsy in infancy
      Epilepsy with continuous spike-waves during slow wave sleep
      Acquired epileptic aphasia (Landau-Kleffner syndrome)
      Other undetermined epilepsies not defined above
   3.2 Without unequivocal generalized or focal features (i.e., sleep-related GTCS; when the
      EEG shows both focal and generalized ictal or interictal discharges, and when focal or
      generalized onset cannot be determined clinically)

(Continued)

Table 2.1   *(Continued)*

4 Special syndromes
   4.1 Situation-related seizures
        Febrile convulsions
        Isolated seizures or isolated status epilepticus
        Seizures occurring only when there is an acute metabolic or toxic event (alcohol,
            drugs, eclampsia, nonketotic hyperglycemia)

Source: Reproduced from "Proposal for revised classification of epilepsies and epileptic syndromes." Commission on Classification and Terminology of the International League Against Epilepsy [2], with permission from John Wiley & Sons Ltd.

symptoms or sensory illusions or hallucinations. The ictal event is usually characterized by a blank stare, loss of contact with the environment, oroalimentary automatisms, hand automatisms, upper limb tonic or dystonic posturing, early head or eye deviation. Oroalimentary automatisms often have the appearance of chewing or lip-smacking. Hand automatisms are repetitive, purposeless movements of the hands including grasping, fumbling, and searching movements. Unilateral automatisms are typically ipsilateral to region of seizure onset, and postictal dysphasia lateralizes to the dominant hemisphere [7]. Mesial temporal lobe seizures (MTLEs) are often characterized by an initial epigastric sensation or viscerosensory sensation, longer seizure duration, delayed loss of contact, and delayed oroalimentary and upper limb automatisms while lateral temporal lobe seizures are characterized by an initial sensory illusion or hallucination (mainly auditory), an initial loss of contact, a shorter duration (<1 minute), and frequent secondary generalizations. Distinguishing between mesial (limbic) and lateral (neocortical) temporal lobe epilepsy is important because prognosis after epilepsy surgery differs. Hippocampal sclerosis is the most common pathological substrate found in patients with medial temporal lobe epilepsy who undergo surgical resection. The majority of patients who undergo surgical resection for MTLE become seizure-free [8].

Frontal lobe epilepsies

Frontal lobe seizures are the second most common type of focal epilepsy and occur in approximately 30% of patients with partial epilepsy [9]. Frontal lobe seizures are often confused with pseudoseizures due to the bizarre clinical semiology [10]. Frontal lobe seizures are usually brief (less than 30 seconds), tend to occur in clusters, can occur multiple times per day, and often have minimal or no postictal confusion. The clinical semiology includes an abrupt onset of stereotyped hypermotor behavior and may include vocalizations, gestural or sexual automatisms, and bilateral leg automatisms consisting of pedaling or bicycling movements. The seizure semiology of frontal lobe seizures depends on what region of the frontal lobe is involved. Because of the extensive inter-regional connectivity within the frontal lobe and rapid seizure propagation, frontal lobe seizures are difficult to localize on the basis of clinical semiology.

Juvenile absence epilepsy

Juvenile absence epilepsy (JAE) is classified as an idiopathic generalized epilepsy. The age of onset is typically at or after puberty between the ages of 10 and 17. Unlike in childhood absence epilepsy (CAE) where absence seizures can occur many times per day, absence seizures in JAE may only occur sporadically. There is less impairment of consciousness with absence seizures in JAE compared to absences in CAE. Patients with JAE can have generalized tonic-clonic seizures (GTCS) (usually upon awakening), myoclonic seizures, and even absence status epilepticus. There is a strong genetic component with linkage to chromosomes 5, 8, 18, and 21. The response to antiepileptic medication is usually excellent [11].

Juvenile myoclonic epilepsy

JME is also classified as an idiopathic generalized epilepsy. The age of onset is usually mid-teens. Patients may present with myoclonic jerks upon awakening in the morning. The myoclonus usually involves the neck, shoulders, arms, or legs with the upper extremities being more frequently affected. Consciousness is usually not impaired during the myoclonic seizures. Generalized tonic-clonic and absence seizures are also seen. The ictal EEG consists of generalized polyspike and wave discharges >3 Hz. There is a strong genetic component with linkage to chromosomes 2, 3, 5, 6, and 15. The response to antiepileptic drug (AED) treatment is excellent but needs to be continued lifelong in most patients due to a high rate of relapse [11].

Lennox-Gastaut syndrome

Lennox-Gastaut syndrome (LGS) is classified as an epileptic encephalopathy. The age of onset is usually before eight with a peak age of onset between three and five years of age. The syndrome is characterized by a triad of multiple seizure types (tonic and atypical absence are the most common), slow spike and wave on EEG (1–2.5 Hz), and some degree of mental retardation. The etiology can be symptomatic or cryptogenic. Tonic seizures are considered a prerequisite for the diagnosis. The interictal EEG is characterized by slow spike and wave complexes (<2.5 Hz) and activation of generalized paroxysmal fast activity during sleep. The seizures in LGS are typically refractory to medical treatment [12].

2.3 Conclusion

The current ILAE classification system for seizures and the epilepsies has formed the basis for a worldwide standardized approach to diagnosing, treating, and studying seizure disorders. The seizure classification system is primarily based on clinical semiology and EEG correlation, with a major distinction made between focal and generalized seizures. Focal seizures are further subdivided into simple and complex partial seizures, with the presence or absence of impairment of consciousness distinguishing the two. Generalized seizures are divided into absence, tonic, tonic-clonic, myoclonic, or atonic seizures. The epilepsy classification system highlights specific syndromes defined from anatomic-pathological bases (mesial temporal lobe epilepsy with hippocampal sclerosis) to electroclinical bases (LGS). This system has been useful for both clinicians and researchers over the past 20 years, but new data from modern neuroimaging techniques, molecular biology studies, and genetics research will likely lead to a substantive revision of the current classification system in the near future. However, until that time arrives, the current classification system for seizures and the epilepsies provides a common language for clinicians and researchers worldwide.

References

1. Commission on Classification and Terminology of the International League Against Epilepsy (1981) Proposal for revised clinical and electroencephalographic classification of epileptic seizures. *Epilepsia*, **22** (4), 489–501.
2. Commission on Classification and Terminology of the International League Against Epilepsy (1989) Proposal for revised classification of epilepsies and epileptic syndromes. *Epilepsia*, **30** (4), 389–399.
3. Berg, A.T. (2009) Report of the Commission on Classification and Terminology: Update and Recommendations. Available from: http://www.ilae-epilepsy.org/Visitors/Documents/CandTSummaryReportFINAL.pdf [accessed November 15, 2009].
4. Nguyen, D.K., Nguyen, D.B., Malak, R. *et al.* (2009) Revisiting the role of the insula in refractory partial epilepsy. *Epilepsia*, **50** (3), 510–520.
5. Engel, J. Jr. (2001) A proposed diagnostic scheme for people with epileptic seizures and with epilepsy: report of the ILAE task force on classification and terminology. *Epilepsia*, **42** (6), 796–803.
6. Quesney, L.F. (1986) Clinical and EEG features of complex partial seizures of temporal lobe origin. *Epilepsia*, **27** (Suppl 2), S27–S45.
7. Chee, M.W., Kotagal, P., van Ness, P.C. *et al.* (1993) Lateralizing signs in intractable partial epilepsy: blinded multiple-observer analysis. *Neurology*, **43** (12), 2519–2525.
8. Ozkara, C., Uzan, M., Benbir, G. *et al.* (2008) Surgical outcome of patients with mesial temporal lobe epilepsy related to hippocampal sclerosis. *Epilepsia*, **49** (4), 696–699.
9. Bancaud, J. and Talairach, J. (1992) Clinical semiology of frontal lobe seizures. *Adv Neurol*, **57**, 3–58.

10. Shih, J.J., LeslieMazwi, T., Falcao, G., and Van Gerpen, J. (2009) Directed aggressive behavior in frontal lobe epilepsy: a video-EEG and ictal spect case study. *Neurology*, **73** (21), 1804–1806.

11. Beghi, M., Beghi, E., Cornaggia, C.M., and Gobbi, G. (2006) Idiopathic generalized epilepsies of adolescence. *Epilepsia*, **47** (Suppl 2), 107–110.

12. Arzimanoglou, A., French, J., Blume, W.T. *et al.* (2009) Lennox-Gastaut syndrome: a consensus approach on diagnosis, assessment, management, and trial methodology. *Lancet Neurol*, **8** (1), 82–93.

3 Epidemiology of seizure disorders

Joseph I. Sirven

Department of Neurology, Division of Epilepsy, Mayo Clinic Arizona, Mayo Clinic Hospital, Phoenix, AZ, USA

3.1 Incidence and prevalence of epilepsy

Epilepsy is one of the most common neurological disorders encountered by most physicians. Regardless of whether one resides in an industrialized country or a developing nation, seizures are frequent occurrences and the condition of repeated seizures (epilepsy) is extraordinarily widespread. In order to follow a discussion on the epidemiology of epilepsy, it is important to define the terminology.

A *seizure* is characterized by an abnormal discharge of synchronized neurons in a discrete or generalized portion of the brain. *Acute provoked seizures* [1] are ones that occur in the context of an acute brain insult or systemic disorder such as head trauma, stroke, or metabolic condition. Conversely a seizure that occurs in the absence of an acute provoked event is considered an *unprovoked* [1] event. *Epilepsy* is the occurrence of at least two unprovoked seizures separated by a minimum of 24 hours. The condition of having recurrent, repeated events underlies the definition of an epileptic disorder. Because the diagnosis of epilepsy is a clinical diagnosis and there is not a fixed test or biomarker that conclusively designates an individual as having epilepsy, studies that address the epidemiology of seizures or epilepsy can be fraught with error. This is due to the fact that

Adult Epilepsy, First Edition. Edited by Gregory D. Cascino and Joseph I. Sirven.
© 2011 John Wiley & Sons, Ltd. Published 2011 by John Wiley & Sons, Ltd.

Table 3.1 Incidence and prevalence of epilepsy as reported in various population-based studies around the world

Author	Year	Country	Age groups	Incidence 100 000/year	Prevalence/ 1000
Annegers et al.	1999 [23]	USA	All	35.5	—
Beilmann et al.	1999 [4]	Estonia	0–19	—	3.6
Karaagac et al.	1999 [29]	Turkey	All	—	10.2
Jallon	1997 [30]	Switzerland	All	45.6	—
Camfield et al.	1996 [8]	Canada	<16	41	—
de la Court et al.	1996 [15]	Netherlands	55–95	—	9
Mendizabal & Salguero	1996 [31]	Guatemala	All	—	5.8
Olafsson et al.	1996 [7]	Iceland	All	47	—
Aziz et al.	1994 [32]	Pakistan	All	—	10.1
Snow et al.	1994 [33]	Kenya	All	—	4
Loiseau et al.	1990 [34]	France	All	24–42	—
Li et al.	1985 [35]	China	All	—	4.4
Bharucha et al.	1988 [36]	India	All	—	4.7
Hauser & Kurland	1975 [37]	USA	All	—	5.4

Source: Adapted with permission from Berg [2].

multiple lines of converging data, that is, history and diagnostic tests are the basis to make a diagnosis and there is not one single point that is utilized to confirm the disorder. Therefore it is essential to know the population on which an epidemiologic study is conducted in order to extrapolate accurate incidence and prevalence data.

Table 3.1 [2] provides results displaying the incidence and prevalence of epilepsy as reported in several population-based studies throughout the world. Clearly, the incidence rates for epilepsy are estimated to be typically between 30 and 50 per 100 000 population although some studies have reported higher approximations between 60 and 80 per 100 000 per year [2].

In order to provide context comparing epilepsy incidence rates versus other neurological disorders, the American Academy of Neurology systematically analyzed the incidence and prevalence of common neurological maladies [3]. Their results showed that epilepsy ranks among the top disorders in children, adults, and older adults. In four Class I studies [4–7] and six Class II studies [8–12] of incidence, the median estimate was 46 per 100 000 per year, (range 32–71). The incidence of epilepsy is related to age. Analyzing studies restricted to children and adolescents alone led to a higher median estimate of 57 per 100 000 per year, (range 41–65) [3]. Even higher incidence rates occurred among infants younger than one year and among people older than 60 years [3]. Most studies do not show any gender differences.

Six Class I [4, 13–17] and seven Class II studies [6, 10, 12, 18–21] have addressed the prevalence of epilepsy. Three Class I studies in children and adolescents up to age 19 [4, 14, 16] found the median prevalence value is 3.9 per 1000 and among the Class II studies that included all age groups [6, 7, 12, 20, 21] the median estimate was 7.1 per 1000 population. Observably, seizures and epilepsy have a fairly high incidence and prevalence globally.

3.2 Incidence and prevalence of acute symptomatic seizures

Acute symptomatic seizures differ from epilepsy in that each seizure has a clear, identifiable, proximal cause. Potential etiologies can include metabolic causes such as medications or electrolyte derangements, trauma, stroke, neoplasms, and many other possibilities. The incidence of acute seizures has been provided by several studies. Two often-cited studies based on the population of Rochester, Minnesota reported age-adjusted incidence rates of 39 per 100 000 person years in 1970 [22, 23]. This represents about 40% of all cases of a febrile seizure identified in the community. This result has been replicated in European studies.

The incidence of acute symptomatic seizures tends to be higher in men than in women [22]. Just like epilepsy, the age-specific incidence of acute symptomatic seizures is highest during the first year of life. This is attributed to the high incidence of acute symptomatic seizures associated with metabolic, infectious, and encephalopathic causes during the neonatal and perinatal periods. Incidence declines in childhood and early adult years and reaches a nadir among those between the ages of 25–34 years of age [22]. After 35 years of age the incidence increases progressively, reaching 123/100 000 among those more than 75 years of age [22]. Therefore acute symptomatic seizures have a bimodal age distribution.

The most commonly reported cause of acute symptomatic seizures arises from metabolic conditions. Several conditions can precipitate seizures and this is further discussed in Chapter 7, "Etiologies of Seizures." Common conditions that need to be considered when evaluating a patient presenting with a seizure include hypoglycemia and hyperglycemia which are often reported in patients with diabetes. Hyponatremia, uremia, and hypocalcemia are also well represented in the literature. Abrupt discontinuation of antiepileptic drugs, sedative, and anxiolytic agents is a prominent cause of seizures as well. All barbiturates and benzodiazepines present a risk of withdrawal seizures. The use of medications that lower the seizure threshold is an important cause of acute seizures. Drugs, such as phenothiazines, tricyclic antidepressants, theophylline, bupropion, antibiotics such as new generation quinolones and certain pain medications such as meperidine can cause seizures as well. Recently stimulant agents, such as ephedra often found in over-the-counter herbal/botanicals and weight loss preparations, have been causally implicated in seizures [24].

Central nervous system and systemic infections such as meningitis, pneumonia, and urosepsis can promote seizures. Acute trauma, embolic, and hemorrhagic strokes are also common causes of seizures. It is important to consider all of these risk factors when assessing a patient with an acute symptomatic seizure as this is a relatively common occurrence in any age group.

3.3   Looking beyond epidemiology: the state of epilepsy care in the United States

In 2005, the United States (US) Centers for Disease Control and Prevention (CDC) conducted surveillance work to assess the state of epilepsy and seizure care in the United States based on 19 reporting states [25]. The US CDC worked with the Behavioral Risk Factor Surveillance System (BRFSS) and assessed a number of epilepsy and seizure-related variables to better characterize how well the US healthcare structure was handling epilepsy care. The BRFSS is an ongoing, state-based, random digit dial telephone survey of non-institutionalized US adults over the age of 18. This system collects information on health risk, behaviors, and preventative health services that relate to the leading causes of death and morbidity.

The surveillance system included a total of 2207 adults from 19 states or 1.65% with a reported history of epilepsy [25]. Moreover 0.84% had active epilepsy defined as either a history of epilepsy and currently taking medications, or reporting one or more seizures during the past three months. 0.75% were classified as having inactive epilepsy or a history of epilepsy or seizure disorder but not currently taking medicine to control epilepsy and no seizures in the three months preceding the survey [25]. There were no differences among the states with regards to prevalence of lifetime epilepsy, active epilepsy, or inactive epilepsy. Prevalence estimates for active and inactive epilepsy revealed no significant difference by sex, race, or ethnicity.

However, American adults with a history of epilepsy and active epilepsy were much more likely to report fair or poor health by being unemployed or unable to work [25]. These individuals also lived in households with the lowest annual incomes, had a history of concomitant disorders such as stroke or arthritis. Adults with a history of epilepsy and active epilepsy also reported significantly worse health-related quality of life. Individuals with epilepsy were more likely to be obese, physically inactive, and smoking. In adults with active epilepsy with recent seizures, 16.1% reported not taking their epilepsy medications and 65.1% reported having had more than one seizure in the past month [25]. Among adults with a history of epilepsy almost 24% reported cost as a barrier to seeking care from a physician over the previous year [25]. A total of 35% of adults with active epilepsy with seizures reported not having seen a neurologist or an epilepsy specialist in the previous year [25].

This study showed that the incidence and prevalence rates that are reported by population-based studies as previously outlined are relatively accurate. Seizures and epilepsy are a frequent occurrence among the American population. Yet, the CDC analysis also demonstrated the significant burden of disease that cannot be assessed from epidemiological studies. A number of public health interventions are necessary in order to better educate the public, understand the barriers to care, financing of the care and how to improve quality of life for patients with epilepsy.

3.4 Risk factors for epilepsy

The risk factors for epilepsy in adults are somewhat established and are further discussed in Chapter 7, "Etiologies of Seizures." There are several known risk factors for epilepsy in adults including head trauma, central nervous system infections, strokes, both embolic and hemorrhagic, central nervous system malignancies, particularly cortically based tumors such as gliomas and metastatic lesions, Alzheimer's disease and other neurodegenerative conditions. However, the relationship between epilepsy and other conditions such as subcortical white matter diseases, demyelinating conditions, and certain psychiatric conditions (i.e., depression and schizophrenia) have not been sufficiently characterized.

Of all the various potential risk factors toward epilepsy there are three that merit further review: Alzheimer's disease, head trauma, and neurocysticercosis. The underlying pathology of Alzheimer's disease appears to be associated with a potential increased susceptibility toward seizures. Given that the diagnosis of Alzheimer's disease is confirmed only by autopsy, makes it difficult to establish whether some patients may have concurrent epilepsy because of the overlapping similar presentations. One study found a 10-fold increased risk for unprovoked seizures in Alzheimer's disease [22]. Another reported new onset seizures developed in 16% of patients with probable Alzheimer's disease after they became severely demented [23]. Moreover, a Class I study of geriatric epilepsy in a veterans population found that neurodegenerative conditions accounted for almost 11% of epilepsy disorders in this group [26]. Clearly more investigations are needed to understand this relationship.

Because trauma is a relatively preventable but common condition, its role in epileptogenesis has been evaluated. There are three major categories of traumatic head injury loosely divided as mild, moderate, and severe [27]. Severe head injuries have a significant relative risk (RR) of development of epilepsy over the course of one's life with a commonly reported RR of 29 compared to a normal population of 1 [27]. Moderate head injury has a RR of 4 and a mild head injury is equivocal with regards to seizure risk as compared to a normal-aged population [27].

Neurocysticercosis deserves special mention due to its frequent nature in developing countries. This infection is caused by the taenia solium tapeworm by ingestion of uncooked pork. The tapeworms have a predilection for brain tissue and the ensuing inflammatory response often results in epilepsy. Neurocysticercosis is one of the most common causes of epilepsy in the third world and one that is completely preventable by adequately cooking pork and simple hygiene [28]. Given recent immigration patterns and globalization with easy transport to and from various parts of the world, this condition has become endemic in areas with no previous history of this problem. It is important to understand the highly preventable aspect of this condition and be aware of the increasing regularity of this epilepsy cause.

3.5 Conclusion

This chapter has served to outline the incidence and prevalence of epilepsy in the world. Epilepsy and acute symptomatic seizures are common disorders which can present as an independent condition or can often be associated with other co-morbidities such as cerebrovascular disease, neurodegenerative disorders, and traumatic brain injuries. The disorder is seen in the extremes of age, but can afflict anyone. The plight of individuals with epilepsy in the US based on current public health estimates suggests that there is a significant psychosocial, economic, and quality of life burden for patients who have seizures and epilepsy.

References

1. Commission on Epidemiology and Prognosis, International League Against Epilepsy (1993) Guidelines for epidemiologic studies on epilepsy. *Epilepsia*, **34** (4), 592–596.
2. Berg, A. (2006) Epidemiologic aspects of epilepsy, in *The Treatment of Epilepsy*, 4th edn (eds. E. Wyllie, A. Gupta and D. Lachhwani), Lippincott, Williams & Wilkins, Philadelphia, PA, p. 113.
3. Hirtz, D., Thurman, D.J., Gwinn-Hardy, K. *et al.* (2007) How common are the "common" neurologic disorders? *Neurology*, **68** (5), 326–337.
4. Beilmann, A., Napa, A., Hämarik, M., *et al.* (1999) Prevalence of childhood epilepsy in Estonia. *Brain Dev*, **21** (3), 166–174.
5. Freitag, C.M., May, T.W., Pfäfflin, M. *et al.* (2001) Incidence of epilepsies and epileptic syndromes in children and adolescents: a population-based prospective study in Germany. *Epilepsia*, **42** (8), 979–985.
6. MacDonald, B.K., Cockerell, O.C., Sander, J.W., and Shorvon, S.D. (2000) The incidence and lifetime prevalence of neurological disorders in a prospective community-based study in the UK. *Brain*, **123** (Pt 4), 665–676.
7. Olafsson, E., Hauser, W.A., Ludvigsson, P., and Gudmundsson, G. (1996) Incidence of epilepsy in rural Iceland: a population-based study. *Epilepsia*, **37** (10), 951–955.

8. Camfield, C.S., Camfield, P.R., Gordon, K. *et al.* (1996) Incidence of epilepsy in childhood and adolescence: a population-based study in Nova Scotia from 1977 to 1985. *Epilepsia*, **37** (1), 19–23.

9. Rantala, H. and Ingalsuo, H. (1999) Occurrence and outcome of epilepsy in children younger than 2 years. *J Pediatr*, **135** (6), 761–764.

10. Kurtz, Z., Tookey, P., and Ross, E. (1998) Epilepsy in young people: 23 year follow up of the British national child development study. *Br Med J*, **316** (7128), 339–342.

11. Hauser, W.A., Annegers, J.F., and Kurland, L.T. (1993) Incidence of epilepsy and unprovoked seizures in Rochester, Minnesota: 1935–1984. *Epilepsia*, **34** (3), 453–468.

12. Holden, E.W., Thanh Nguyen, H., Grossman, E. *et al.* (2005) Estimating prevalence, incidence, and disease-related mortality for patients with epilepsy in managed care organizations. *Epilepsia*, **46** (2), 311–319.

13. Oun, A., Haldre, S., and Mägi, M. (2003) Prevalence of adult epilepsy in Estonia. *Epilepsy Res*, **52** (3), 233–242.

14. Eriksson, K.J. and Koivikko, M.J. (1997) Prevalence, classification, and severity of epilepsy and epileptic syndromes in children. *Epilepsia*, **38** (12), 1275–1282.

15. de la Court, A., Breteler, M.M., Meinardi, H. *et al.* (1996) Prevalence of epilepsy in the elderly: the Rotterdam study. *Epilepsia*, **37** (2), 141–147.

16. Waaler, P.E., Blom, B.H., Skeidsvoll, H., and Mykletun, A. (2000) Prevalence, classification, and severity of epilepsy in children in western Norway. *Epilepsia*, **41** (7), 802–810.

17. Luengo, A., Parra, J., Colás, J. *et al.* (2001) Prevalence of epilepsy in northeast Madrid. *J Neurol*, **248** (9), 762–767.

18. Verity, C.M., Ross, E.M., and Golding, J. (1992) Epilepsy in the first 10 years of life: findings of the child health and education study. *Br Med J*, **305** (6858), 857–861.

19. Olafsson, E. and Hauser, W.A. (1999) Prevalence of epilepsy in rural Iceland: a population-based study. *Epilepsia*, **40** (11), 1529–1534.

20. Begley, C.E., Famulari, M., Annegers, J.F. *et al.* (2000) The cost of epilepsy in the United States: an estimate from population-based clinical and survey data. *Epilepsia*, **41** (3), 342–351.

21. Hauser, W.A., Annegers, J.F., and Kurland, L.T. (1991) Prevalence of epilepsy in Rochester, Minnesota: 1940–1980. *Epilepsia*, **32** (4), 429–445.

22. Annegers, J.F., Hauser, W.A., and Lee, J.R. (1995) Incidence of acute symptomatic seizures in Rochester, Minnesota: 1935–1994. *Epilepsia*, **36**, 327–333.

23. Annegers, J.F., Dubinsky, S., Coan, S.P. *et al.* (1999) The incidence of epilepsy and unprovoked seizures in multiethnic, urban health maintenance organizations. *Epilepsia*, **40** (4), 502–506.

24. Sirven, J., Drazkowski, J., Zimmerman, R. *et al.* (2003) CAM for epilepsy in Arizona. *Neurology*, **61**, 576–577.

25. Kobau, R., Zahran, H., Thurman, D. *et al.* (2005) Epilepsy Surveillance Among Adults— 19 states. Behavioral Risk Factors Surveillance Risk System. At http://www.cdc.gov/mmwr /preview/mmwrhtml/ss5706a1.htm [accessed September 4, 2010].

26. Rowan, A., Ramsay, R.E., Collins, J.F. *et al.* (2005) New onset geriatric epilepsy: a randomized study of gabapentin, lamotrigine and carbamazepine. *Neurology*, **64**, 1868–1873.

27. Salazar, A.M., Jabbari, B., and Vance, S.C. (1985) Epilepsy after penetrating head injury. I. Clinical correlates; a report of the Vietnam head injury study. *Neurology*, **35**, 1406–1414.

28. Nash, T., Del Brutto, O., Butman, J., and Corona, T. (2004) Calcific neurocysticercosis and epileptogenesis. *Neurology*, **62**, 1934–1938.

29. Karaagac, N., Yeni, S.N., Senocak, M. *et al.* (1999) Prevalence of epilepsy in Silivri, a rural area of Turkey. *Epilepsia*, **40** (5), 637–642.
30. Jallon, P. (1997) Epilepsy in developing countries. *Epilepsia*, **38** (10), 1143–1151.
31. Mendizabal, J.E. and Salguero, L.F. (1996) Prevalence of epilepsy in a rural community in Guatemala. *Epilepsia*, **37** (4), 373–376.
32. Aziz, H., Ali, S.M., Frances, P., Khan, M.I., and Hasan, K.Z. (1994) Epilepsy in Pakistan: a population-based epidemiologic study. *Epilepsia*, **35** (5), 950–958.
33. Snow, R.W., Williams, R.E., Rogers, J.E., Mung'ala, V.O., and Peshu, N. (1994) The prevalence of epilepsy among a rural Kenyan population. Its association with premature mortality. *Trop Geogr Med*, **46** (3), 175–179.
34. Loiseau, J., Loiseau, P., Duche, B. *et al.* (1990) Survey of seizure disorders in the French Southwest. I. Incidence of epileptic syndromes. *Epilepsia*, **31**, 391–396.
35. Li, S.C., Schoenberg, B.S., Bolis, C.L. *et al.* (1985) Epidemiology of epilepsy in urban regions of the People's Republic of China. *Epilepsia*, **26**, 391–394.
36. Bharucha, N.E., Bharucha, E.P., Bharucha, A.E., Bhise, A.V., and Schoenberg, B.S. (1988) Case-control study of epilepsy in the Parsi community of Bombay: a population-based study. *Neurology*, **38**, 312.
37. Hauser, W.A. and Kurland, L.T. (1975) The epidemiology of epilepsy in Rochester, Minnesota, 1935through 1967. *Epilepsia*, **16**, 1–66.

Section 2

Diagnostic evaluation

4 The role of routine scalp electroencephalography

Terrence D. Lagerlund[1] and Gregory A. Worrell[2]

[1]Department of Neurology, Division of Clinical Neurophysiology, Mayo Clinic, Rochester, MN, USA
[2]Department of Neurology, Division of Epilepsy, Mayo Clinic, Rochester, MN, USA

4.1 Introduction

Routine electroencephalography (EEG) involves the recording of electrical potentials from electrodes applied to the scalp. It continues to be the core technology for the diagnosis and management of epilepsy and seizures. EEG is a unique method because of its ability to directly detect the collective electrical activity generated by cortical neuronal populations with unsurpassed temporal resolution. Because scalp EEG is a noninvasive technique without risk to patients, the characteristics of EEG recordings of normal and pathologic brain activity have been investigated thoroughly and are well established for large populations of healthy control patients and patients with various disease states. The EEG changes associated with most neurologic disorders affecting the central nervous system are

Adult Epilepsy, First Edition. Edited by Gregory D. Cascino and Joseph I. Sirven.

nonspecific. Epilepsy, defined as the spontaneous, recurrent generation of unprovoked seizures, is an exception.

Advanced imaging techniques, such as CT, MRI, functional MRI, positron emission tomography (PET), and single-photon emission computed tomography (SPECT) may offer the best spatial resolution for evaluation of structural and functional abnormalities of the brain in patients with epilepsy. However, EEG still provides the best temporal resolution of cortical function. In particular, interictal epileptiform discharges (IEDs), which are due to the pathologic coordinated activity of epileptogenic neuronal populations and thus represent the electrophysiologic signature of the epileptogenic brain [1], are best identified by their temporal characteristics (i.e., morphologic features and duration). These characteristics include epileptiform spikes, sharp waves, and temporal intermittent rhythmic delta activity. Thus, scalp EEG continues to be an essential tool in the diagnosis and treatment of epilepsy [2, 3] because of the high specificity and high sensitivity of IEDs for seizures [4, 5]. Of note, for patients with known central nervous system disease and no history of epilepsy, the specificity of IEDs may be considerably lower [6].

Although the fundamental concepts of EEG recording have stayed the same for the past 80 years, advances in digital computer technologies have led to tremendous practical improvements in how the EEG is recorded, viewed, and archived. Because of their numerous practical advantages, digital EEG systems have replaced older, analog EEG systems in most clinics and hospitals. These digital advances have led to substantial improvements in EEG over the past few decades and include the extension of the bandwidth beyond the classic Berger bands (1–25 Hz) (Figure 4.1) and computational EEG analysis.

This chapter summarizes the role of routine scalp EEG recordings in the evaluation of suspected seizure disorders, particularly the advantages and limitations of routine scalp EEG in the diagnosis of epilepsy. We describe the morphologic characteristics of IEDs, as well as common benign EEG transients that can be misinterpreted as IEDs, and review the clinical importance and predictive value of IEDs in the diagnosis of epilepsy.

4.2 Clinical application of EEG

The possibility of a seizure disorder is frequently considered for a patient who reports paroxysmal clinical events involving sensory, motor, and psychic phenomena, including alteration of consciousness. The neurological examination often has normal results for patients who have paroxysmal events with neurological manifestations. Only rarely is a clinician able to witness one of the paroxysmal spells in question. Therefore, patient history is of paramount importance (especially a description of the paroxysmal events by the patient and family members).

Following history taking and physical examination, a routine EEG is the most common neurodiagnostic test performed for evaluation of suspected seizures [2].

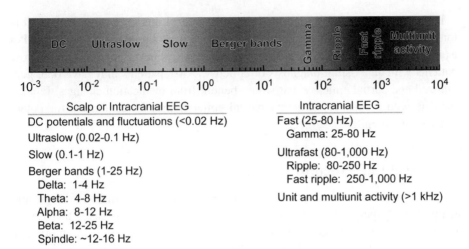

Scalp or Intracranial EEG | Intracranial EEG

DC potentials and fluctuations (<0.02 Hz)
Ultraslow (0.02-0.1 Hz)
Slow (0.1-1 Hz)
Berger bands (1-25 Hz)
  Delta: 1-4 Hz
  Theta: 4-8 Hz
  Alpha: 8-12 Hz
  Beta: 12-25 Hz
  Spindle: ~12-16 Hz

Fast (25-80 Hz)
  Gamma: 25-80 Hz
Ultrafast (80-1,000 Hz)
  Ripple: 80-250 Hz
  Fast ripple: 250-1,000 Hz
Unit and multiunit activity (>1 kHz)

Figure 4.1 The frequency range of human brain electrophysiology. The electrical activity recorded from the scalp is limited to oscillations below approximately 25 Hz. However, the low-frequency end of the spectrum recorded with scalp electroencephalography (EEG) extends well below 1 Hz and, with nonpolarizable electrodes, it is possible to record ultraslow oscillations. The potential clinical applications of wide-bandwidth EEG is an active area of current research.

Definitive proof for the diagnosis of epilepsy can be obtained when a habitual seizure is recorded and the EEG shows a pattern typical for a partial or generalized seizure. However, because of the intermittent nature of a partial or generalized seizure, there is only a small chance of recording the patient's stereotypic events during a routine sleep-and-awake EEG recording [2, 7]. Despite this limitation, a routine scalp EEG often provides important supportive information for the diagnosis of a seizure disorder.

IEDs are highly correlated with the diagnosis of a seizure disorder, and their presence on an EEG performed after a single seizure has been found to be helpful in predicting the risk of seizure recurrence. However, the decision to initiate antiepileptic drug therapy must be made on the basis of the individual clinical scenario. The classification system for epilepsy syndromes incorporates interictal EEG abnormalities with the clinical features [8].

Although the presence of IEDs on a routine EEG is helpful for the appropriate diagnosis of a seizure disorder, patients with epilepsy may have no IEDs, even on repeated EEG studies [7]. Rarely, patients without epilepsy may have IEDs [6, 9]. When a routine EEG fails to show IEDs of a patient with a suspected seizure disorder, repeating the EEG may increase the diagnostic sensitivity. In addition, to obtain an ictal EEG recording, a long-term ambulatory or long-term video-EEG should be considered.

Patients with seizures not eliminated with medical therapies often benefit from long-term video-EEG monitoring to capture their habitual clinical events. For example, patients may have coexisting nonepileptic behavioral events, even those patients with an existing diagnosis of epilepsy. Also, patients may have both generalized and partial epilepsy that would benefit from medication changes. Finally, patients with medically refractory partial epilepsy may be candidates for potentially curative epilepsy surgery.

4.3   Scalp EEG recording methods

Because of the advances in digital computer technologies, digital EEG instruments have largely replaced analog instruments. Digital EEG makes the process of recording, storage, and retrieval of large quantities of EEG data more efficient [10]. Furthermore, with the use of digital systems, it is possible to select the most appropriate montage, filters, sensitivity, and time base at the time the EEG is reviewed. Also, signal processing techniques can be applied, including automated spike and seizure detection algorithms that can increase substantially the efficiency in reviewing long-term video-EEG and ambulatory EEG [11–13]. The ability to remontage the EEG presents an important advantage of digital EEG over analog EEG and has been shown to reduce the variability between electroencephalographers for identifying EEG abnormalities and determining whether these abnormalities are generalized or focal [14].

The bandwidth of the EEG generators is an active area of research [15, 16]. It is widely recognized that the range of cerebral activity extends well beyond Berger bands. Wide-bandwidth EEG presents specific challenges at both the high-frequency (>25 Hz) and the low-frequency (<0.1 Hz) ends of the spectrum. Recording cerebral electrical activity from the scalp in the high-frequency range is difficult for numerous reasons that include (i) electrical activity greater than 25 Hz has low amplitude in scalp recordings, (ii) the generators of gamma and ripple frequency oscillations tend to have a highly localized distribution [17] and the smearing effect of the skull prevents effective conduction of such activity to scalp electrodes, and (iii) scalp muscle artifact frequently obscures EEG activity greater than 25 Hz. Similarly, there are challenges in recording EEG activity in frequencies less than 0.1 Hz, particularly the technical challenge of the polarizability of many electrode materials [18] and the generation of artifacts due to movements and noncerebral sources, such as the galvanic skin response [16].

Standard scalp EEG uses 19 electrodes [19]. Use of greater spatial sampling with high-density scalp electrodes (e.g., 64–256 scalp electrodes) can help localize focal regions of epileptogenic brain when combined with use of sophisticated computational tools to image putative ictal generators by solving the bioelectric inverse solution [20, 21]. These powerful computational methods can be combined with other noninvasive methods, such as structural MRI and functional studies (e.g., interictal and ictal SPECT) [22].

Routine wake-and-sleep EEG

A routine EEG performed for the evaluation of seizures should include a period of wakefulness, as well as sleep. The total recording period is typically 20–40 minutes, although longer recordings may be necessary to adequately assess the presence of IEDs. The guidelines established by the American Clinical Neurophysiology Society should be used for all recordings [23].

Electrodes should be placed according to the International 10–20 System, which usually provides adequate coverage. Sometimes, supplemental electrodes may be added in the anterior temporal head region, which is often a site of IEDs in temporal lobe epilepsy [24]. Sphenoidal electrodes are used by some epilepsy centers to supplement the International 10–20 System [25]. The available data support the improved sensitivity of additional anterior temporal region surface electrodes for recording IEDs—97% of EEGs that use these electrodes have IEDs versus 58% of EEGs that use only the International 10–20 System electrodes—but the advantage of sphenoidal electrodes is less clear [25, 26].

4.4 Activation procedures

Studies have shown the importance of standard activating procedures in increasing the sensitivity of the routine EEG for detection of IEDs. The yield of recording IEDs of patients with seizures can be increased by 30–70% through requiring that the patient be sleep-deprived before the EEG recording [27]. In patients with both absence seizures and complex partial seizures, hyperventilation can activate IEDs and, sometimes, ictal EEG discharges [3, 28].

Generalized IEDs can occur during photic stimulation and may outlast the photic stimulus by one to several seconds. Such a photoparoxysmal response may evolve into a clinical seizure. It is important to distinguish this response from the photomyogenic response. The latter response consists of myogenic and superimposed eye movement artifact induced by photic stimulation, which usually does not outlast the stimulus. Between 70 and 77% of individuals with generalized IEDs activated by photic stimulation have epilepsy [29]. Provocative testing and suggestion may elicit typical spells in patients with nonepileptic events [30]. Nevertheless, ethical questions exist regarding the use of provocative testing in patients with nonepileptic spells [31].

The possibility of noninvasively probing the brain through use of external electrical stimulation or transcranial magnetic stimulation may ultimately prove useful for identifying and localizing epileptogenic brain regions [32]. The concept of interictal activation to localize epileptogenic brain regions is attractive conceptually and would be important clinically. For many patients with medically intractable partial epilepsy, no IEDs are apparent and their seizures are difficult to localize. For patients with normal structural imaging (e.g., MRI, normal interictal EEG, nonlocalized ictal EEG), there is little to guide the epileptologist in localizing the region of the brain that is generating the seizures. These patients generally are poor surgical candidates.

4.5   Interictal discharges correlated with epilepsy

IEDs are seen in a high percentage of patients with epilepsy but are rare in patients without epilepsy. Because of the high sensitivity and high specificity of IEDs for seizure disorders and the high correlation of IED localization with seizure onset localization, IEDs can be interpreted as the electrophysiologic signature of the epileptogenic brain in the appropriate clinical setting. Evidence from simultaneous microelectrode and macroelectrode recordings suggests that IEDs represent the macroscopic field resulting from the summation of potentials from a population of pathologically synchronized bursting neurons.

The common types of IEDs recorded during routine EEG studies are spikes, sharp waves, and spike-and-wave complexes [3, 33, 34], which can be either focal or generalized (Figure 4.2). Spikes and sharp waves are most commonly focal but may be generalized in distribution. Spike-and-wave patterns (including 3-Hz spike and wave, slow spike and wave, atypical spike and wave, and polyspike and wave) and paroxysmal fast activity are frequently generalized but may have a focal or regional distribution [3, 34]. IEDs include the following features, which help distinguish them from normal EEG background activity and other nonepileptiform transients [3, 34].

1 Epileptiform spikes and sharp waves are often followed by a smoothly con-toured slow wave (forming a spike-and-wave complex) (Figure 4.2), which disrupts the ongoing EEG background activity.
2 Epileptiform sharp waves and spikes are transient waveforms that arise abruptly out of the EEG background activity. Sometimes, they occur repetitively in trains. The waveforms have more than one phase (usually two or three) and are characteristically asymmetrical. In contrast, nonepileptiform, sharply contoured transients (such as wicket waves and rhythmic temporal theta of drowsiness) are usually approximately symmetrical (Figure 4.3).
3 The duration of an epileptiform sharp wave is 70–200 ms and the duration of an epileptiform spike is less than 70 ms, although the distinction is of no clinical significance. Waveforms lasting more than 200 ms may be sharply contoured but are not considered potentially epileptogenic, with the exception of such periodic discharges as periodic lateralized epileptiform discharges.

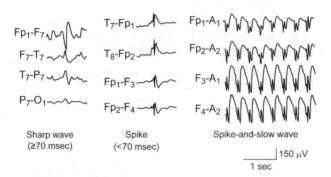

Sharp wave   Spike   Spike-and-slow wave
(≥70 msec)   (<70 msec)

150 μV
1 sec

Figure 4.2 Electroencephalographic tracings of epileptiform sharp waves, spikes, and spike-and-wave discharges. (Adapted from Westmoreland *et al.* (1994) [35]. Used with permission of Mayo Foundation for Medical Education and Research.)

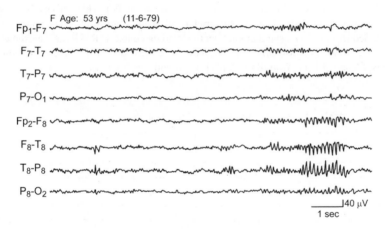

40 μV
1 sec

Figure 4.3 Electroencephalographic tracing of a 53-year-old patient showing wicket waves in the right temporal region. Sometimes called *wicket spikes*, these waves may occur as single, sharply contoured focal transients (left side of figure) or in repetitive trains, usually in the theta frequency range (right side of figure). Wicket waves often occur independently in both temporal regions and are considered a benign pattern of no clinical significance.

4 An epileptiform discharge has a physiologic field and is not confined to a single electrode. Waveforms associated with a single electrode are most often electrode artifacts.

The presence of intermittent rhythmic delta activity in the temporal head region (Figure 4.4) has specificity for temporal lobe epilepsy similar to that of the presence of interictal epileptiform spikes and sharp waves [36, 37].

Periodic IED patterns associated with seizures are also recognized [3]. The patterns include periodic lateralized epileptiform discharges, which are unilateral

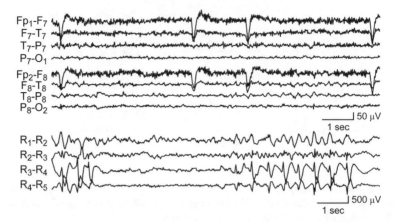

Figure 4.4   Electroencephalographic tracing showing temporal intermittent rhythmic delta activity (TIRDA) in the right temporal region (maximum at F_8). This activity is considered to have the same clinical significance as interictal spikes and sharp waves. The bottom tracings were recorded from right mesial temporal depth electrode contacts (R_1–R_5). They show a train of spike and slow-wave discharges that are correlated with the TIRDA recorded from scalp electrodes. (Adapted from Worrell *et al.* [41]. Used with permission.)

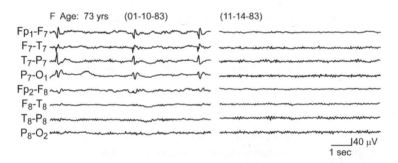

Figure 4.5   Electroencephalographic tracing from a 73-year-old patient with sudden onset of aphasia showing periodic lateralized epileptiform discharges (PLEDs) in left hemisphere. PLEDs are often seen in patients with acute or subacute focal neurological deficits and are often associated with obtundation, as well as partial seizures. Over time, they usually resolve as the neurological deficit improves (shown here), but they may evolve into focal nonperiodic interictal epileptiform discharges.

but hemispheric in extent (Figure 4.5), as well as periodic epileptiform discharges in the midline, generalized periodic epileptiform discharges, bilateral independent periodic lateralized epileptiform discharges, and multifocal independent periodic epileptiform discharges [38–40].

True IEDs often lack some of these characteristic features and some waveforms or patterns of noncerebral origin can have many of these characteristics. The electroencephalographer should review possible IEDs using different montages—for example, bipolar, referential, and Laplacian recording montages—to better distinguish true IEDs from other waveforms that may mimic IEDs [14]. Use of different montages also may help both localize focal discharges and distinguish them from generalized discharges. Of note, the Laplacian montage can make a generalized discharge appear more focal. In addition, when the reference electrode is active, use of a referential montage may make a focal discharge appear generalized [10].

Several types of waveforms seen on EEG may be mistakenly interpreted as epileptiform patterns, including electrode and external interference artifacts, noncerebral physiologic artifacts, and benign transients and patterns of cerebral origin. Artifacts can be produced by electrodes, the recording equipment, and other electrical devices in the vicinity. During recordings performed in the hospital, especially in intensive care units, such artifacts occur frequently and can be particularly difficult to recognize. Artifacts of physiologic origin include those due to eye movements, muscles, swallowing, body movements, sweating, pulse, and electrocardiogram. In addition, various EEG transients and patterns of cerebral origin but not associated with epilepsy can be mistaken for IEDs. Among these transients and patterns are wicket waves (Figure 4.3), small sharp spikes (Figure 4.6), rhythmic midtemporal theta of drowsiness (Figure 4.7), central midline rhythmic theta (Figure 4.8), subclinical rhythmic electrographic discharge of

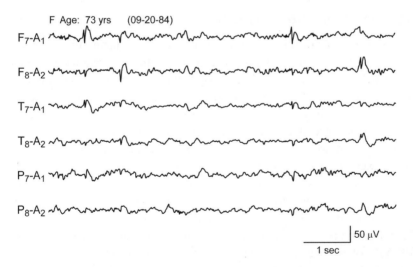

Figure 4.6 Electroencephalographic tracing from a 73-year-old patient that shows small sharp spikes. They are low-amplitude, short-duration spikes that most commonly occur in the temporal regions and often occur independently on both sides. These spikes are seen during drowsiness and light sleep but disappear with deeper sleep.

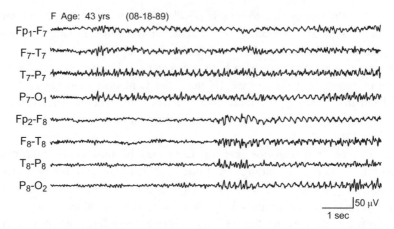

Figure 4.7   Electroencephalographic tracing from a 43-year-old patient that shows rhythmic temporal theta of drowsiness (RTTD) in the left and right temporal regions. RTTD is a common benign rhythmic pattern seen in the temporal regions during drowsiness, often independently on the left and the right. It consists of theta frequency waveforms that frequently have a sharp or notched appearance (shown here).

adults (Figure 4.9), 14&6-Hz positive bursts (Figure 4.10), phantom (6-Hz) spike and wave (Figure 4.11), and paroxysmal hypnagogic hypersynchrony (Figure 4.12) [3, 42, 43].

Evidence for the importance of IEDs

There are methodological problems in many studies evaluating the sensitivity and specificity of IEDs for the diagnosis of epilepsy. Although simultaneous recording of ictal EEG and associated ictal behavior provides the most convincing evidence for a diagnosis of epilepsy, this simultaneous recording is seldom achieved during routine EEG recordings. Thus, epilepsy continues to be a clinical diagnosis in most cases. Consequently, some studies probably include patients with an incorrect diagnosis. In addition, in some studies the EEG findings, including the presence of IEDs, were among the factors leading to a diagnosis of epilepsy and thus introduced a bias. Also, a substantial referral bias is likely toward patients with refractory epilepsy, since the studies were performed by major epilepsy centers using retrospective analysis of patient medical records.

The published retrospective studies show that an initial EEG demonstrated IEDs in 29–55% of patients with a clinical diagnosis of epilepsy. When one or more additional EEGs were performed, the fraction of patients having IEDs on at least one EEG was 80–90% [4, 5, 7, 44]. However, the sensitivity of the initial EEG and subsequent EEGs is expected to be lower for patients with infrequent seizures. In one study, only 12% of patients who had had a single seizure showed IEDs

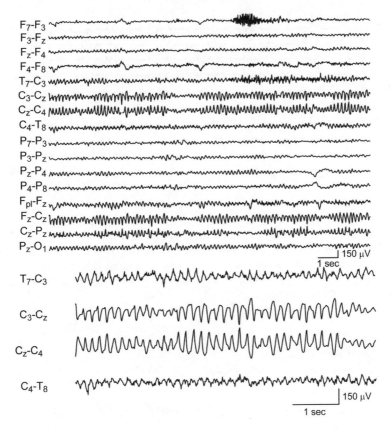

Figure 4.8   Electroencephalographic tracing showing central midline rhythmic theta. This benign rhythmic pattern often occurs in elderly patients during drowsiness. It consists of theta frequency waveforms that typically have an archiform appearance (shown here). (Adapted from Westmoreland and Klass [43]. Used with permission.) Copyright © (1986) American Medical Association. All rights reserved.

on their first EEG, and a second EEG showed IEDs in an additional 14%, giving a cumulative sensitivity of 26% after two EEGs [45]. Even some patients whose epilepsy is refractory have infrequent IEDs (e.g., patients with mesial frontal lobe epilepsy) [5, 45]. Continuous long-term EEG recordings have a substantially greater yield than routine EEG recordings for detection of IEDs. Nevertheless, one study of patients with proven epilepsy found no IEDs in 19% of patients during an average of 6.9 days of prolonged recording [46].

The specificity of IEDs for the diagnosis of epilepsy is highly dependent on the population studied. In a study of 13 658 healthy men who were candidates for aircrew training, only 69 (0.5%) had IEDs on a routine EEG recording [9]. In this study, 43 of the 69 patients with IEDs were observed clinically for between 5 and 29 years, and epilepsy eventually developed in only one of the 43 patients.

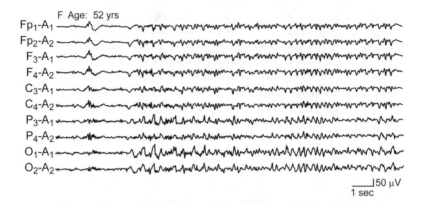

Figure 4.9　Electroencephalographic tracing from a 52-year-old patient that shows subclinical rhythmic electrographic discharge of adults (SREDAs). The discharge often begins abruptly with a sharply contoured waveform or a series of such waveforms. It then evolves to widespread sharply contoured theta frequency activity with some intermixed delta frequencies. The discharge causes no clinical symptoms. SREDA is a rare electrographic pattern seen during wakefulness or light drowsiness.

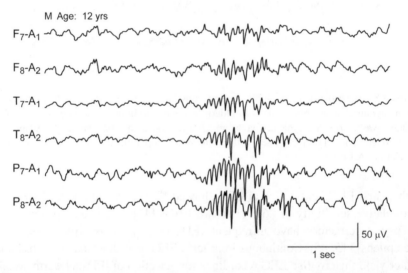

Figure 4.10　Electroencephalographic tracing from a 12-year-old patient that shows 14&6-Hz positive bursts. This benign pattern is seen during sleep or deep drowsiness. It consists of bursts of arch-shaped waves with sharp peaks of positive polarity, with a frequency of approximately 14 Hz (range, 13–17 Hz) or 6 Hz (range, 5–7 Hz), typically maximal in the posterior temporal regions, sometimes unilateral and sometimes bilateral (shown here). Both 6- and 14-Hz frequencies may occur at different times in the same recording. This pattern is most common in children and adolescents.

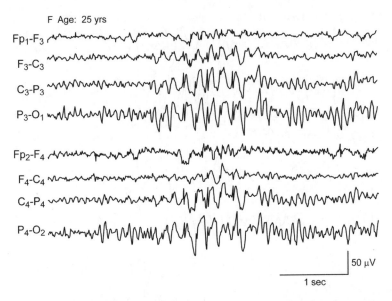

Figure 4.11 Electroencephalographic tracing from a 25-year-old patient that shows 6-Hz spike-and-wave discharges. This uncommon benign pattern is seen during drowsiness, consisting of low-amplitude spikes followed by slow waves repeating at 6 Hz that are widespread but maximal in the occipital regions and without clinical accompaniment. This spike-and-wave pattern must be distinguished from anterior-predominant, 5- to 6-Hz spike-and-wave discharges seen during wakefulness, which usually are a variant of atypical spike and wave with potentially epileptogenic significance.

By comparison, a study of 521 patients with no history of seizures residing in Rochester, Minnesota, found 64 patients (12.3%) with IEDs on a routine EEG performed as part of a neurological evaluation [6]. Not surprisingly, 47 (73.3%) of the 64 patients with IEDs had acute or progressive cerebral disorders at the time the IEDs were detected. During 230.8 patient-years of follow-up, none of these patients subsequently had seizures. These findings emphasize that the presence of IEDs on routine EEG recordings should be interpreted in the context of the clinical history, especially for patients with neurological disorders, structural lesions, or previous craniotomy [6, 47].

In general, the clinical usefulness of a diagnostic test depends on the disease prevalence in the population under consideration. For example, if 55% of patients with epilepsy have IEDs and 4% of patients without epilepsy have IEDs, then the positive predictive value of IEDs for the diagnosis of epilepsy does not exceed 80% until the prevalence of epilepsy in the population tested is greater than 20% [4, 5]. This fact emphasizes the diagnostic complications that can be produced by an inappropriately ordered EEG.

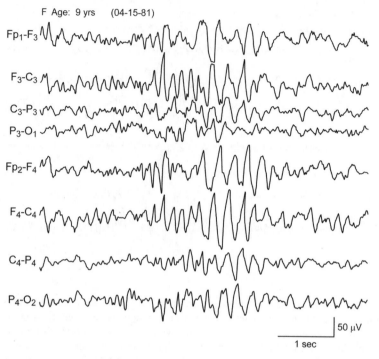

Figure 4.12 Electroencephalographic tracing from a 9-year-old patient that shows the drowsy pattern hypnagogic hypersynchrony. This pattern consists of paroxysmal widespread, high-amplitude bisynchronous activity of 3- to 7-Hz frequency that is usually maximal in the anterior head regions (although in small children, a posterior predominance is commonly seen instead). This normal finding should be distinguished from a similar pattern occurring during wakefulness known as *frontal intermittent rhythmic delta activity* (FIRDA), which is a nonspecific abnormality associated with diffuse cerebral or diencephalic dysfunction, and from paroxysmal atypical spike-and-wave bursts (which are potentially epileptogenic).

4.6   Epileptic syndromes and the role of EEG

The most important distinction from the standpoint of choosing appropriate therapy is between localization-related epilepsy and primary generalized epilepsy. In addition, a diagnosis of a specific epilepsy syndrome may be important for determining prognosis and treatment. For example, it is known that patients with JME typically respond to therapy with sodium valproate.

Focal IEDs are seen most often in localization-related epilepsy, whereas generalized IEDs are typically found in primary generalized epilepsy. However, two relatively common situations make this distinction challenging. Occasionally, patients with partial seizures have generalized-appearing IEDs through a phenomenon known as *secondary bilateral synchrony*. Of note, the generalized IEDs in primary generalized epilepsy are often higher in amplitude in one region (e.g., in a bifrontal distribution) and may sometimes be asymmetrical with a higher amplitude in one hemisphere, especially in patients who have had previous surgery with a resulting skull defect. Also, within a specific spike or sharp wave discharge, a time lag of the peak scalp negativity may exist in one hemisphere compared with the other hemisphere. Yet, in primary generalized epilepsy, the peak of some discharges may occur earlier on the left while the peak of other discharges occurs earlier on the right. Thus, for a reliable diagnosis of secondary bilateral synchrony from a focal region of onset, it is necessary to find evidence that the generalized discharges consistently begin in a specific region and later spread to the contralateral hemisphere (Figure 4.13) or show a consistent time lag on one side

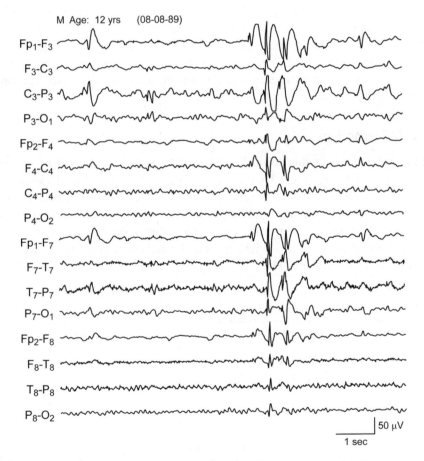

Figure 4.13 Electroencephalographic tracing from a 12-year-old patient with a left porencephalic cyst and partial seizures since age 1 year. Near the beginning of the tracing is a left frontocentrotemporal spike discharge. Later, a focal spike-and-wave discharge is apparent in the left frontocentrotemporal region (with some reflection on the right) and quickly evolves into a generalized spike-and-wave discharge.

compared with the other. Finding such evidence may sometimes be facilitated with examination of the IEDs on an expanded timescale. The occurrence of focal discharges in the region of onset without secondary bilateral synchrony is also helpful.

In addition, regional "fragments" of the generalized IEDs in primary generalized epilepsy are often seen [48, 49]. These fragmentary discharges seen in primary generalized epilepsy are typically maximal in the bifrontal head regions and may at times be higher in amplitude on the left and at other times be higher in amplitude on the right. Especially during drowsiness and sleep, fragments that appear unilateral and relatively focal may be seen. As long as these focal-appearing IEDs have morphologic characteristics similar to the generalized discharges and show no consistent predominance in one location or one hemisphere, it is reasonable to classify them as focal fragments of generalized discharges and not to conclude that the patient has partial, as well as primary, generalized seizures. Nevertheless, in some cases, the distinction between localization-related and primary generalized epilepsy based on the IEDs seen during routine EEG can be inaccurate. Recording the patient's habitual seizures during prolonged video-EEG monitoring may be the best way to make an accurate diagnosis.

Ictal EEG recordings

Partial seizures originating from the temporal lobes have been studied in detail by Ebersole and Pacia [50]. They reviewed 391 scalp-recorded ictal EEGs from 93 patients with temporal lobe epilepsy, and localization was ultimately determined by intracranial monitoring. They identified seven patterns of temporal-onset seizures and proposed that in many cases, the scalp-recorded seizure can be used to determine whether seizures originate from the medial temporal versus temporal neocortical region (Table 4.1).

Table 4.1 Temporal lobe seizure patterns

Seizure type	Earliest ictal rhythms	Likely site of origin
1A	Inferotemporal rhythm of 5–9 Hz that is regular for at least 5 sec and often longer	Hippocampus
1B	Vertex rhythm of 5–9 Hz that is regular for ≥5 sec	Hippocampus
1C	Seizure type 1B followed by type 1A	Hippocampus
2A	Temporal and/or frontocentral rhythm of 2–5 Hz that is irregular or is regular for only brief periods	Temporal neocortex
2B	Seizure type 2A followed by type 1A	Temporal neocortex
2C	Seizure type 2A or 2B preceded by irregular or repetitive sharp or slow waves	Temporal neocortex
3	Nonlateralized or diffuse arrhythmic change in background	Temporal neocortex

Localization of the seizure onset zone from scalp EEG in extratemporal epilepsy can be challenging [51] because of multiple factors that include the large size of the epileptogenic zone, the rapid propagation of the ictal discharge, and the presence of focal or generalized attenuation seen with focal-onset seizures. The presence of a focal beta frequency discharge has been shown to be associated with localized seizure onset from the dorsal lateral convexity [52] and is associated with a good surgical outcome.

4.7 Conclusions

Routine EEG continues to be a cornerstone in the diagnosis and treatment of epilepsy. In the appropriate clinical context, the presence of IEDs is highly specific for the diagnosis of a seizure disorder. The sensitivity for recording IEDs can be increased substantially during a single EEG through the recording of serial EEGs or a prolonged EEG recording. However, the results of EEG should always be interpreted within the entire clinical setting, since the sensitivity and specificity of IEDs depend on the population studied.

References

1. Gloor, P. (1975) Contributions of electroencephalography and electrocorticography to the neurosurgical treatment of the epilepsies. *Adv Neurol*, **8**, 59–105.
2. Daly, D.D. and Pedley, T.A. (eds.) (1990) *Current Practice of Clinical Electroencephalography*, 2nd edn, Raven Press, New York.
3. Fisch, B.J. (1991) *Spehlmann's EEG Primer*, Elsevier, Amsterdam.
4. Goodin, D.S. and Aminoff, M.J. (1984) Does the interictal EEG have a role in the diagnosis of epilepsy? *Lancet*, **1**, 837–839.
5. Walczak, T.S. and Jayakar, P. (1998) Interictal EEG, in *Epilepsy: A Comprehensive Textbook*, vol. **1** (eds. J. Engel Jr. and T.A. Pedley), Lippincott-Raven, Philadelphia, PA, pp. 831–848.
6. Sam, M.C. and So, E.L. (2001) Significance of epileptiform discharges in patients without epilepsy in the community. *Epilepsia*, **42**, 1273–1278.
7. Marsan, C.A. and Zivin, L.S. (1970) Factors related to the occurrence of typical paroxysmal abnormalities in the EEG records of epileptic patients. *Epilepsia*, **11**, 361–381.
8. Wyllie, E. and Luders, H.O. (2001) Classification of the epilepsies, in *Treatment of Epilepsy: Principles and Practice*, 3rd edn (ed. E. Wyllie), Lippincott Williams & Wilkins, Philadelphia, PA, pp. 453–455.
9. Gregory, R.P., Oates, T., and Merry, R.T. (1993) Electroencephalogram epileptiform abnormalities in candidates for aircrew training. *Electroencephalogr Clin Neurophysiol*, **86**, 75–77.
10. Lagerlund, T.D., Cascino, G.D., Cicora, K.M. *et al.* (1996) Long-term electroencephalographic monitoring for diagnosis and management of seizures. *Mayo Clin Proc*, **71**, 1000–1006.
11. Wilson, S.B. and Emerson, R. (2002) Spike detection: a review and comparison of algorithms. *Clin Neurophysiol*, **113**, 1873–1881.

12. Wilson, S.B., Scheuer, M.L., Plummer, C. *et al.* (2003) Seizure detection: correlation of human experts. *Clin Neurophysiol*, **114**, 2156–2164.
13. Gotman, J. (1990) Automatic seizure detection: improvements and evaluation. *Electroencephalogr Clin Neurophysiol*, **76**, 317–324.
14. Levy, S.R., Berg, A.T., Testa, F.M. *et al.* (1998) Comparison of digital and conventional EEG interpretation. *J Clin Neurophysiol*, **15**, 476–480.
15. Miller, J.W., Kim, W., Holmes, M.D. *et al.* (2007) Ictal localization by source analysis of infraslow activity in DC-coupled scalp EEG recordings. *Neuroimage*, **35**, 583–597 [Epub 2006 Dec 23].
16. Vanhatalo, S., Voipio, J., and Kaila, K. (2005) Full-band EEG (FbEEG): an emerging standard in electroencephalography. *Clin Neurophysiol*, **116**, 1–8.
17. Logothetis, N.K., Kayser, C., and Oeltermann, A. (2007) In vivo measurement of cortical impedance spectrum in monkeys: implications for signal propagation. *Neuron*, **55**, 809–823.
18. Tallgren, P., Vanhatalo, S., Kaila, K. *et al.* (2005) Evaluation of commercially available electrodes and gels for recording of slow EEG potentials. *Clin Neurophysiol*, **116**, 799–806 [Epub 2004 Nov 23].
19. Sharbrough, F., Chatrian, G-E., Lesser, R.P. *et al.* (1991) American electroencephalographic society guidelines for standard electrode position nomenclature. *J Clin Neurophysiol*, **8**, 200–202.
20. Michel, C.M., Lantz, G., Spinelli, L. *et al.* (2004) 128-channel EEG source imaging in epilepsy: clinical yield and localization precision. *J Clin Neurophysiol*, **21**, 71–83.
21. Ding, L., Worrell, G.A., Lagerlund, T.D. *et al.* (2007) Ictal source analysis: localization and imaging of causal interactions in humans. *Neuroimage*, **34**, 575–586 [Epub 2006 Nov 16].
22. Worrell, G.A., Lagerlund, T.D., Sharbrough, F.W. *et al.* (2000) Localization of the epileptic focus by low-resolution electromagnetic tomography in patients with a lesion demonstrated by MRI. *Brain Topogr*, **12**, 273–282.
23. American Electroencephalographic Society (1994) Guidelines in electroencephalography, evoked potentials, and polysomnography. *J Clin Neurophysiol*, **11**, 1–147.
24. Sharbrough, F.W. (1990) Electrical fields and recording techniques, in *Current Practice of Clinical Electroencephalography*, 2nd edn, (eds. D.D. Daly and T.A. Pedley), Raven Press, New York, pp. 29–49.
25. Goodin, D.S., Aminoff, M.J., and Laxer, K.D. (1990) Detection of epileptiform activity by different noninvasive EEG methods in complex partial epilepsy. *Ann Neurol*, **27**, 330–334.
26. Marks, D.A., Katz, A., Booke, J. *et al.* (1992) Comparison and correlation of surface and sphenoidal electrodes with simultaneous intracranial recording: an interictal study. *Electroencephalogr Clin Neurophysiol*, **82**, 23–29.
27. Ellingson, R.J., Wilken, K., and Bennett, D.R. (1984) Efficacy of sleep deprivation as an activation procedure in epilepsy patients. *J Clin Neurophysiol*, **1**, 83–101.
28. Miley, C.E. and Forster, F.M. (1977) Activation of partial complex seizures by hyperventilation. *Arch Neurol*, **34**, 371–373.
29. Walter, W.G., Dovey, V.J., and Shipton, H. (1946) Analysis of the electrical response of the human cortex to photic stimulation. *Nature*, **158**, 540–541.
30. Benbadis, S.R. (2001) Provocative techniques should be used for the diagnosis of psychogenic nonepileptic seizures. *Arch Neurol*, **58**, 2063–2065.

31. Gates, J.R. (2001) Provocative testing should not be used for nonepileptic seizures. *Arch Neurol*, **58**, 2065–2066.

32. Valentin, A., Arunachalam, R., Mesquita-Rodrigues, A. *et al.* (2008) Late EEG responses triggered by transcranial magnetic stimulation (TMS) in the evaluation of focal epilepsy. *Epilepsia*, **49**, 470–480 [Epub 2007 Nov 19].

33. Buzsaki, G., Traub, R.D., and Pedley, T.A. (2003) The cellular basis of EEG activity, in *Current Practice of Clinical Electroencephalography*, 3rd edn (eds. J.S. Ebersole and T.A. Pedley), Lippincott Williams & Wilkins, Philadelphia, PA, pp. 1–11.

34. Westmoreland, B.F. (1996) Epileptiform electroencephalographic patterns. *Mayo Clin Proc*, **71**, 501–511.

35. Bennarroch, E.E., Daube, J.R., Flemming, K.D. *et al.* (2008) *Mayo Clinic Medical Neurosciences: Organized by Neurologic Systems and Levels*, 5th edn. Mayo Clinic Scientific Press, Rochester, Minnesota.

36. Reiher, J., Beaudry, M., and Leduc, C.P. (1989) Temporal intermittent rhythmic delta activity (TIRDA) in the diagnosis of complex partial epilepsy: sensitivity, specificity and predictive value. *Can J Neurol Sci*, **16**, 398–401.

37. Geyer, J.D., Bilir, E., Faught, R.E. *et al.* (1999) Significance of interictal temporal lobe delta activity for localization of the primary epileptogenic region. *Neurology*, **52**, 202–205.

38. Chatrian, G.E., Shaw, C.M., and Leffman, H. (1964) The significance of periodic lateralized epileptiform discharges in EEG: an electrographic, clinical and pathological study. *Electroencephalogr Clin Neurophysiol*, **17**, 177–193.

39. de la Paz, D. and Brenner, R.P. (1981) Bilateral independent periodic lateralized epileptiform discharges: clinical significance. *Arch Neurol*, **38**, 713–715.

40. Lawn, N.D., Westmoreland, B.F., and Sharbrough, F.W. (2000) Multifocal periodic lateralized epileptiform discharges (PLEDs): EEG features and clinical correlations. *Clin Neurophysiol*, **111**, 2125–2129.

41. Worrell, G.A., Lagerlund, T.D., and Buchhalter, J.R. (2002) Role and limitations of routine and ambulatory scalp electroencephalography in diagnosing and managing seizures. *Mayo Clin Proc*, **77**, 991–998.

42. Westmoreland, B.F. (1990) Benign EEG variants and patterns of uncertain clinical significance, in *Current Practice of Clinical Electroencephalography*, 2nd edn (eds. D.D. Daly and T.A. Pedley), Raven Press, New York, pp. 243–252.

43. Westmoreland, B.F. and Klass, D.W. (1986) Midline theta rhythm. *Arch Neurol*, **43**, 139–141.

44. Salinsky, M., Kanter, R., and Dasheiff, R.M. (1987) Effectiveness of multiple EEGs in supporting the diagnosis of epilepsy: an operational curve. *Epilepsia*, **28**, 331–334.

45. van Donselaar, C.A., Schimsheimer, R.J., Geerts, A.T. *et al.* (1992) Value of the electroencephalogram in adult patients with untreated idiopathic first seizures. *Arch Neurol*, **49**, 231–237.

46. Walczak, T.S., Scheuer, M.L., Resor, S. *et al.* (1993) Prevalence and features of epilepsy without interictal epileptiform discharges. *Neurology*, **43** (Suppl 2), 287–288 [Abstract].

47. Cobb, W.A., Guiloff, R.J., and Cast, J. (1979) Breach rhythm: the EEG related to skull defects. *Electroencephalogr Clin Neurophysiol*, **47**, 251–271.

48. Kobayashi, K., Ohtsuka, Y., Oka, E. *et al.* (1992) Primary and secondary bilateral synchrony in epilepsy: differentiation by estimation of interhemispheric small time differences during short spike-wave activity. *Electroencephalogr Clin Neurophysiol*, **83**, 93–103.

49. Lombroso, C.T. (1997) Consistent EEG focalities detected in subjects with primary generalized epilepsies monitored for two decades. *Epilepsia*, **38**, 797–812.

50. Ebersole, J.S. and Pacia, S.V. (1996) Localization of temporal lobe foci by ictal EEG patterns. *Epilepsia*, **37**, 386–399.

51. Kutsy, R.L. (1999) Focal extratemporal epilepsy: clinical features, EEG patterns, and surgical approach. *J Neurol Sci*, **166**, 1–15.

52. Worrell, G.A., So, E.L., Kazemi, J. *et al.* (2002) Focal ictal beta discharge on scalp EEG predicts excellent outcome of frontal lobe epilepsy surgery. *Epilepsia*, **43**, 277–282.

5 Neuroimaging in epilepsy

Gregory D. Cascino

Department of Neurology, Division of Epilepsy, Mayo Clinic, Rochester, MN, USA

5.1 Introduction

Partial epilepsy is the most common seizure disorder [1–3]. The most frequently occurring seizure-type in the adult patient is a complex partial seizure of mesial temporal lobe origin [1–3]. Approximately 45% of patients with partial epilepsy will experience medically refractory seizures that may be physically and socially disabling [1]. Patients with intractable epilepsy are at increased risk for serious morbidity and mortality. "New" AEDs do not appear to be more effective than "older" drugs. In add-on trials of patients with refractory epilepsy, new AEDs reduce seizure frequency by 30–50%; complete control is rare [3–7]. Very few patients become seizure-free on new AEDs [5–7]. Patients who "fail" two AED medications used appropriately are likely to have a medically refractory seizure disorder and should be investigated for alternative forms of treatment [3]. The goals of therapy in patients with medically refractory seizures include significantly reducing seizure tendency, avoiding adverse effects, and permitting the individual to become a participating and productive member of society [2]. This chapter will discuss the importance of neuroimaging in the evaluation and treatment of patients with partial seizure disorders [8].

Adult Epilepsy, First Edition. Edited by Gregory D. Cascino and Joseph I. Sirven.
© 2011 John Wiley & Sons, Ltd. Published 2011 by John Wiley & Sons, Ltd.

Epilepsy surgery is an effective and safe alternative form of therapy for selected patients with intractable partial epilepsy [1, 2, 9–16]. Patients with medial temporal lobe epilepsy and substrate-directed epilepsy may be favorable candidates for epilepsy surgery and have a surgically remediable epileptic syndrome [2, 9–14]. The majority of these patients experience a significant reduction in seizure tendency following surgical ablation of the epileptic brain tissue [2, 9–14]. The hallmark pathology of medial temporal lobe epilepsy is mesial temporal sclerosis (MTS) [16–18]. The resected hippocampus in these patients shows focal cell loss and gliosis [13, 14, 16–18]. Patients with a substrate-directed epilepsy may have a primary brain tumor, vascular anomaly or a malformation of cortical development (MCD) [10, 11, 14, 15, 18]. The common surgical pathologies encountered in patients with "lesional" or substrate-directed epilepsy include a low-grade glial neoplasm, cavernous hemangioma, and focal cortical dysplasia [10, 11]. Individuals with MTS and lesional pathology usually have an abnormal structural MRI study [2, 8, 10, 18–20].

MRI has a pivotal role in the selection and evaluation of patients for surgical treatment of intractable partial epilepsy [8, 10, 13, 16–18]. The MRI in these individuals may detect a specific intra-axial structural abnormality that may suggest the likely site of seizure onset and the surgical pathology [8, 20]. The rationale for the presurgical evaluation is to identify the site of ictal onset and initial seizure propagation, that is, epileptogenic zone, and determine the likely pathological findings underlying the epileptic brain tissue [12, 13]. In patients with an MRI-identified lesion or unilateral MTS the purpose of the electroclinical correlation is essentially to confirm the epileptogenicity of the structural abnormality [13, 15, 16, 18]. The demonstration of concordance between the pathological substrate and the ictal onset zone indicates a highly favorable operative outcome in selected individuals. Approximately 80% of patients with unilateral MTS, a low-grade glial neoplasm, or a cavernous hemangioma are rendered seizure-free following surgical treatment [2, 9, 11, 13–16, 18]. Over 90% of patients with these pathological findings will experience an excellent surgical outcome, that is, auras only or rare nondisabling seizures [9]. The operative outcome is distinctly less favorable in individuals with focal cortical dysplasia and other MCDs [19]. The most common operative strategy in patients with intractable partial epilepsy involves a focal cortical resection of the epileptogenic zone with an excision of the surgical pathology [10, 11]. The goals of surgical treatment are to render the individual seizure-free and allow the patient to become a participating and productive member of society [1, 2, 9].

5.2 Magnetic resonance imaging

MRI has been demonstrated to be the most sensitive and specific structural neuroimaging procedure in patients with partial or localization-related epilepsy [2, 8]. Importantly, MRI is a noninvasive technique that has no known biological toxicity and does not involve ionizing radiation [18]. The presence of an MRI-identified structural abnormality may suggest the localization of the site of seizure onset [4–8] (Figures 5.1–5.3). The high diagnostic yield of MRI to delineate foreign-tissue lesions, for example, tumor or vascular malformation, has been confirmed [11]. MRI findings have been used to select favorable candidates for epilepsy surgery, tailor the operative resection, and confirm the extent of corticectomy postoperatively [16].

The sensitivity and specificity of MRI in patients with partial epilepsy is directly related to the underlying pathology [8, 20]. The high diagnostic yield of MRI to

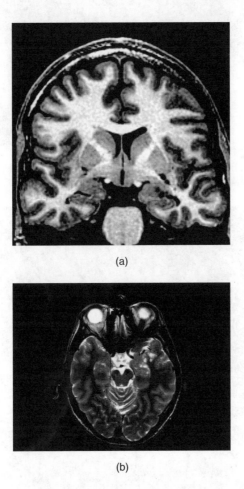

(a)

(b)

Figure 5.1 (a) MRI head: A T1-weighted pulse sequence in the coronal plane revealing an enhancing lesion in the region of the left amygdala and hippocampus. The pathological finding showed a dysembryoplastic neuroepithelioma (DNET). (Note: the left hemisphere is on the right side of the figure.) (b) MRI head: T2-weighted pulse sequence in the axial plane also demonstrates this lesion. (Note: the left hemisphere is on the right side of the figure.)

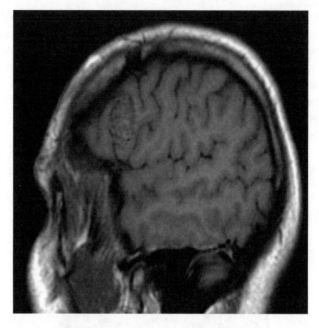

Figure 5.2 MRI head: A T1-weighted pulse sequence in the sagittal plane revealing frontal lobe cavernous hemangioma.

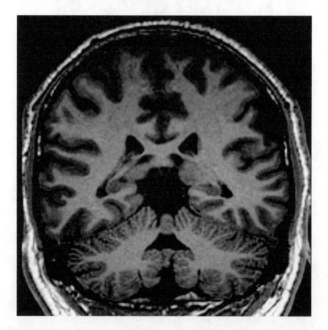

Figure 5.3 MRI head: A T1-weighted pulse sequence in the oblique-coronal plane a structural abnormality consistent with focal encephalomalacia related to remote head trauma in the left hemisphere. (Note: the left hemisphere is on the right side of the figure.)

"reveal" the common pathological alterations, for example, MTS, post-traumatic alterations, vascular malformation, tumor, MCD, has been demonstrated in patients undergoing epilepsy surgery. The optimal technique in adult patients with partial epilepsy must include coronal or oblique-coronal images using T1-weighted and T2-weighted sequences [15, 16]. Studies are performed on 1.5 or 3.0 T MRI scanners. The most common imaging alteration in the adult with intractable partial epilepsy is medial temporal lobe atrophy with a signal intensity change [15, 16]. Fluid attenuated inversion recovery (FLAIR) sequences have been shown to increase the sensitivity of MRI to indicate a signal change. An enhanced study will be performed if a probable structural lesion, for example, tumor, is detected in the unenhanced study.

Substrate-directed epilepsy

Low-grade, slowly growing tumors are most commonly associated with a chronic seizure disorder [21] (Figure 5.1). The histopathology includes the following tumors: oligodendroglioma, fibrillary astrocytoma, pilocytic astrocytoma, mixed glioma, ganglioglioma, and a dysembroblastic neuroepithelial tumor (DNET) [18, 20]. The DNET probably is more closely related to a disorder of cortical development that a primary brain neoplasm (Figure 5.1). Imaging features common to all these tumors include a typically small size, localization at or near a cortical surface, sharply defined borders, little or no surrounding edema and, with the exception of the pilocytic astrocytomas, little or no contrast enhancement. Most patients with primary central nervous system tumors and chronic epilepsy do not present with progressive neurological deficits, "changing" neurological examination or evidence for increased intracranial pressure.

There are four types of congenital cerebral vascular malformations: arteriovenous malformations (AVMs), cavernous hemangiomas, venous angiomas, and telangiectasias [11]. The epileptogenic potential of these pathological lesions is quite different. The common malformations resected for partial epilepsy are cavernous hemangiomas and AVMs (Figure 5.2). Seizures may in fact be the only clinical manifestation with these lesions. Venous angiomas and telangiectasias are often incidental findings in patients with seizure disorders. MRI is essential for the recognition and diagnosis of cavernous hemangiomas and occult AVMs. AVMs may be associated with a flow signal on MRI. Cavernous hemangiomas characteristically have a target appearance on T2-weighted images with a region of increased T2 signal intensity surrounded by an area of decreased signal produced by remote (often occult) hemorrhage with methemoglobin deposition [18]. Resection typically leads to complete or significant improvement in seizure control.

MCD is an important etiology for symptomatic partial epilepsy [19, 22] (Figures 5.4–5.6). The use of MRI has allowed recognition of these lesions and

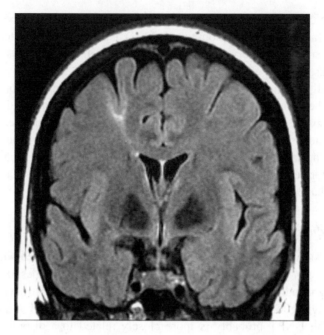

Figure 5.4   MRI head: Fluid attenuated inversion recovery sequence (FLAIR) in the oblique-coronal plane revealing an abnormality in the right frontal lobe consistent with a malformation of cortical development. The pathological finding showed focal cortical dysplasia. (Note: the right hemisphere is on the left side of the figure.)

demonstrated the frequency and importance of cortical developmental malformations in patients with intractable partial epilepsy. A variety of developmental abnormalities have been recognized that are commonly associated with medically refractory seizures and neurocognitive decline [22]. Cerebral developmental malformations could previously only be diagnosed by postmortem examination. MRI is essential for the diagnosis and proper classification of these pathological lesions. Central nervous system insults can produce a cerebral developmental malformation between the 5th and 10th weeks of gestation when the telencephalon is developed until the 25th week when cell migration is completed.

Medial temporal lobe epilepsy

Approximately 80% of patients with partial epilepsy have temporal lobe seizures [1, 2, 9]. The epileptogenic zone in the temporal lobe involves the amygdalohippocampal complex in nearly 90% of patients [16]. The pathological hallmark of medial temporal lobe epilepsy is MTS [17]. MRI findings in patients with MTS include hippocampal formation atrophy (HFA) and an increased mesial temporal signal intensity [8, 13–15] (Figure 5.7). Inspection of MRI will allow detection

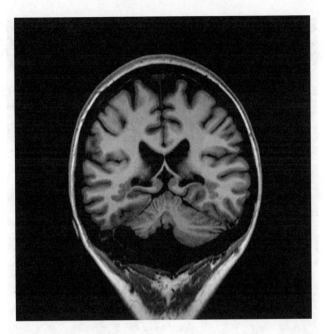

Figure 5.5 MRI head: A T1-weighted pulse sequence in the oblique-coronal plane bilateral periventricular gray matter heterotopia.

of 80–90% of the cases of MTS [8, 13–15]. The HFA is most obvious using the T1-weighted image in the oblique-coronal plane [13]. The signal intensity alteration can be identified using T2-weighted imaging or the FLAIR sequence in the oblique-coronal plane. The coronal or oblique-coronal planes are useful for MRI studies in patient MTS because of the capability to compare the two hippocampi for any side to side asymmetry [8, 13, 14]. Potential limitations of visual inspection of the MRI in patients with suspected MTS includes the following: head rotation, symmetrical bilateral HFA, subtle unilateral HFA or signal intensity alteration. Most importantly, visual inspection is a subjective determination that is strongly dependent on the inspector's expertise for appropriate interpretation. Three-dimensional images are helpful since they are reformatted into true anatomic coronal plane.

MRI-based hippocampal formation volumetric studies have been developed to objectively determine the degree of hippocampal volume loss in patients with MTS [13, 14, 16, 18]. Absolute hippocampal volume measurements are performed using a standardized protocol with the results being compared to age-matched normal controls to assign abnormal values [13]. A unilateral reduction in hippocampal volume has been shown to be a reliable indicator of the temporal lobe of seizure origin in patients with medically refractory partial epilepsy. Jackson *et al.* described T2 relaxometry to objectively determine the medial temporal lobe

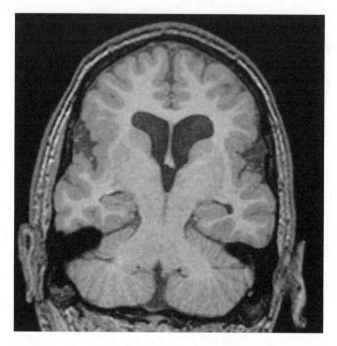

Figure 5.6 MRI head: A T1-weighted pulse sequence in the oblique-coronal plane showing changes consistent with bilateral perisylvian syndrome associated with polymicrogyria involving the sylvian fissure and opercular cortex.

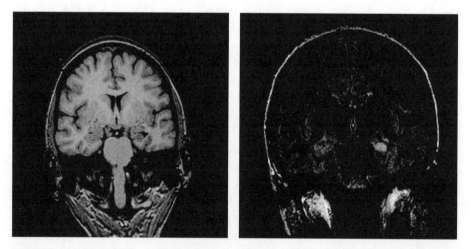

Figure 5.7 (a) MRI head: A T1-weighted pulse sequence in the oblique-coronal plane revealing left hippocampal atrophy. (Note: the left hemisphere is on the right side of the figure.) (b) MRI head: Fluid attenuated inversion recovery sequence (FLAIR) in the oblique-coronal plane revealing a left hippocampal signal intensity alteration. (Note: the left hemisphere is on the right side of the figure.)

signal intensity [17]. Quantitative MRI studies have limited clinical application because of the high diagnostic yield of visual inspection. The most important use of hippocampal formation volumetry and T2 relaxometry is for research studies. HFA correlates with an early age of seizure onset, a history of a febrile seizure of childhood, and the diagnosis of medial temporal lobe epilepsy [13, 14, 16–18]. A history of a neurologic illness in childhood, for example, febrile seizure, head trauma, or meningitis, appears to be an important risk factor for the development of MTS [16]. The duration of epilepsy and age at the time of surgery have not correlated with volumetric results in most studies [13, 14, 16].

The identification of MTS in the surgically excised temporal lobe has been a favorable prognostic indicator of seizure control following epilepsy surgery [9]. Nearly 90% of patients with unilateral hippocampal atrophy have been rendered seizure-free [16]. MRI is now recognized as being predictive of neurocognitive outcome in patients undergoing an anterior temporal lobectomy [18]. Patients with normal left hippocampal volumes are at greater risk for experiencing a significant decline in cognitive performance following a left medial temporal lobe resection than those with left HFA [16–18].

Potential limitations of visual inspection of the MRI in patients with suspected MTS includes the following: head rotation, symmetrical bilateral HFA, subtle unilateral HFA or signal intensity alteration. Most importantly, visual inspection is a subjective determination that is strongly dependent on the inspector's expertise for appropriate interpretation. Three-dimensional spoiled gradient echo images are helpful since they are reformatted into true anatomic coronal plane.

5.3 Functional neuroimaging

Patients with partial seizure disorders and a normal or indeterminate MRI study require additional neuroimaging procedures to assist in localizating the epileptic brain tissue [23]. The anatomical localization of the epileptogenic zone in these individuals commonly involves the neocortex, that is, extrahippocampal [15]. The most frequent site of seizure onset in patients with neocortical nonlesional partial epilepsy is the frontal lobe [15, 18]. The surgical pathology in these patients includes gliosis, focal cell loss, MCD, or no histopathological alteration [18]. The MRI may rarely be indeterminate in selected lesional pathology, for example, focal cortical dysplasia [18]. Only a minority of patients with neocortical, extratemporal seizures are rendered seizure-free following surgical treatment [15, 18]. An estimated 20–30% of these patients with extratemporal, mainly frontal lobe, seizures will enter a seizure remission following a focal cortical resection [18]. An important reason for the unfavorable operative outcome in patients with non-substrate-directed partial epilepsy is the inherent difficulty in identifying the epileptogenic zone [18]. The potential limitations of interictal and ictal extracranial and intracranial EEG monitoring in patients with partial seizures of extratemporal origin have been well defined [18]. The anatomical region of seizure onset may represent a continuum in these patients that lends itself to an incomplete focal resection of the epileptogenic zone. A large resection increases the likelihood of rendering the patient seizure-free, but it also increases the potential for operative morbidity [18, 20]. Advances in peri-ictal imaging (see below) have assisted the selection of operative candidates with MRI negative partial epilepsy, altered the preoperative evaluation, and tailored the surgical excision [23, 24].

Contemporary neuroimaging studies used to localize the epileptogenic zone in patients with MRI negative partial epilepsy being considered for surgical treatment include positron emission tomography (PET), magnetic resonance spectroscopy (MRS), and SPECT [23]. Selected epilepsy centers incorporate one or all of these techniques in the evaluation of potential surgical candidates. These imaging modalities may be of particular importance in the individuals with an indeterminate structural MRI and presumed extratemporal seizures.

Positron emission tomography

PET is a functional neuroimaging study that may be useful in identifying a localization-related abnormality that may assist the surgical planning in patients with intractable partial epilepsy [24–27]. PET also has been important for brain imaging research because regional glucose metabolism and cerebral blood flow can be quantified. The most common study used in the evaluation of intractable partial epilepsy is the ^{18}F-deoxyglucose (FDG)-PET [24, 25]. The disadvantages of PET include the difficulty in obtaining ictal studies, the cost of the procedure, and the limited number of scanners available [23–26]. A cyclotron is also required for the production of the short half-life radiopharmaceuticals. The high diagnostic yield of PET in patients with temporal lobe epilepsy has been confirmed [24–27]. PET is a reliable indicator of the temporal lobe of seizure origin in patients being evaluated for epilepsy surgery [27, 28]. The sensitivity of PET in these individuals approaches 90% [27, 28]. The false lateralization rate for PET in patients with unilateral temporal lobe epilepsy is approximately 1–2% [23–28]. The PET findings in patients with temporal lobe epilepsy are of prognostic importance. The most common interictal FDG-PET abnormality is a region of focal *hypometabolism* that corresponds to the localization of the epileptogenic zone [23–25] (Figure 5.8). The anatomical region associated with the interictal hypometabolism is characteristically larger than the pathological findings underlying the epileptogenic zone. The presence of the PET abnormality does not correlate with the focal cell loss in the hippocampus [24]. The focal hypometabolism may indicate a functional metabolic alteration related to the partial seizure activity. Unfortunately, PET has been shown to be less useful in patients with neocortical epilepsy [23]. In the absence of a structural intra-axial lesion the PET study is usually nondiagnostic or indeterminate in patients with extratemporal seizures. The inability to

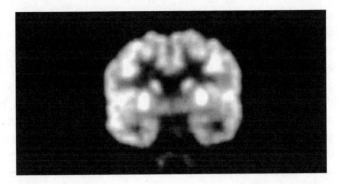

Figure 5.8 A FDG-PET scan shows left temporal hypometabolism in a patient with left temporal lobe epilepsy. MRI head was normal. (Note: the left hemisphere is on the right side of the figure.)

perform peri-ictal studies in patients with non-substrate-directed extratemporal seizures is a significant limitation of PET in the evaluation of potential operative candidates [20].

Evaluating neuronal receptors using PET may also be useful in patients with localization-related epilepsy. Central benzodiazepine receptors can be identified with (^{11}C) flumazenil PET [26]. Focal benzodiazepine receptor decreases may be present in patients with substrate-directed pathology [26]. Benzodiazepine receptor binding, reduced ipsilateral to both frontal and temporal epileptic foci, may be more restricted in extent than hypometabolism [29, 30].

(^{11}C) alpha methyl tryptophan (AMT) uptake is increased in epileptogenic tubers, and may help to identify lesions for resection in patients with tuberous sclerosis [31]. In children with neocortical malformations, increased AMT uptake appeared less sensitive but more specific than FDG-PET, showing more closely delineated abnormalities [32].

Magnetic resonance spectroscopy

Proton (^{1}H) MRS has been shown to be a reliable indicator of the temporal lobe of seizure origin in patients with medial temporal lobe epilepsy [33, 34]. ^{1}H MRS is highly sensitive in the lateralization of temporal lobe seizures by revealing a reduction in N-acetylated (NA) compound concentrations or abnormalities in the creatine (Cr)/NA or NA/choline ratios [33, 34]. The underlying pathogenesis for the metabolic changes are likely to be complex and may relate to focal neuronal loss, gliosis, or a functional alteration intimately associated with the frequency of seizure activity. The diagnostic yield of MRS is similar to structural MRI in patients with medial temporal lobe epilepsy related to MTS [33]. The detection of metabolic abnormalities by ^{1}H MRS also correlates with the outcome following temporal lobectomy for intractable partial epilepsy [33, 34]. Preoperative metabolic abnormalities in the contralateral temporal lobe were predictive of operative failure. ^{1}H MRS may be of particular benefit in patients with medial temporal lobe epilepsy and normal structural MRI studies [33, 34]. Proton spectroscopy may also lateralize the epileptic temporal lobe in patients with bilateral HFA. There is limited information regarding the diagnostic yield of ^{1}H MRS in patients with neocortical, extrahippocampal, seizures. The potential benefits of proton spectroscopy in patients with nonlesional extratemporal seizures remains to be determined. At present, ^{1}H MRS is an investigative diagnostic tool that is restricted to only selected epilepsy centers. Despite observations of focal metabolic abnormalities in selected patients with nonlesional extratemporal seizures, it is doubtful that this diagnostic innovation will have widespread use to demonstrate a localized abnormality in patients with non-substrate-directed partial epilepsy.

Single photon emission computed tomography

SPECT is most appropriate for peri-ictal imaging in patients with partial epileptic syndromes being considered for epilepsy surgery [23]. There is a broad consensus that ictal SPECT studies are superior to interictal images in localization-related epilepsy [35–45]. SPECT studies involve cerebral blood flow imaging using radiopharmaceuticals, principally either technetium-99m-hexamethylpropylene amine oxime (^{99m}Tc-HMPAO) or ^{99m}Tc-bicisate, that have a rapid first pass brain extraction with maximum uptake being achieved within 30–60 seconds of an intravenous injection [23, 35–45]. These studies may produce a "photograph" of the peri-ictal cerebral perfusion pattern that was present soon after the injection [37]. The SPECT images can be acquired up to four hours after the termination of the seizure so that the individual patient can recover from the ictus prior to being transported to the nuclear medicine laboratory. SPECT studies have an important clinical application in the potential identification of the epileptic brain tissue when the remainder of the noninvasive presurgical evaluation is unable to lateralize or localize the site of seizure onset [37].

The initial blood flow SPECT studies in patients with intractable partial epilepsy involved interictal imaging which variably detected a focal *hypoperfusion* in the region of the epileptogenic zone [37, 38]. Interictal SPECT images have proven to have a low sensitivity and a relatively high false positive rate in temporal lobe epilepsy [35–39]. Interictal SPECT has also been shown to have a low diagnostic yield in patients with extratemporal seizures [36]. Ictal SPECT studies have been confirmed to be useful in patients with temporal lobe epilepsy to identify a region of focal *hyperperfusion* [37]. The rationale for interictal SPECT imaging at present is to serve as a reference for a baseline study for the interpretation of ictal SPECT images. The diagnostic yield of ictal SPECT has been established to be superior to interictal SPECT in patients being considered for surgical ablation procedures. The recent development of stabilized radiotracers that do not require mixing immediately before injection, such as ^{99m}Tc-bicisate, has made ictal SPECT more practical in patients with extratemporal seizures that often are not associated with an aura and may have a shorter seizure duration [35–45]. A potential limitation of ictal SPECT is that the spatial resolution of these studies is inferior to that of PET [46].

Subtraction ictal SPECT co-registered to MRI (SISCOM)

The imaging paradigm using computer-aided subtraction ictal SPECT co-registered to MRI (SISCOM) has been introduced in patients with intractable partial epilepsy [37, 38]. SISCOM represents a recent innovation in neuroimaging that may be useful in the evaluation of patients with non-substrate-directed partial epilepsy. The localized blood flow alteration demonstrated using SISCOM may be intimately associated with the epileptogenic zone [35–39] (Figure 5.9). Subtracting normalized and co-registered ictal and interictal SPECT images, and then matching the resultant difference image to the high-resolution MRI for anatomical correlation has been shown to be a reliable indicator of the localization of the epileptogenic zone in patients with localization-related epilepsy [35–40]. The technique used at The Mayo Clinic that was introduced by O'Brien *et al.* has compared favorably to the traditional visual analysis of the interictal and ictal images [37]. SISCOM in a series of 51 patients had a higher rate of localization (88.2 versus 39.2%, p < 0.0001), better inter-observer agreement, and

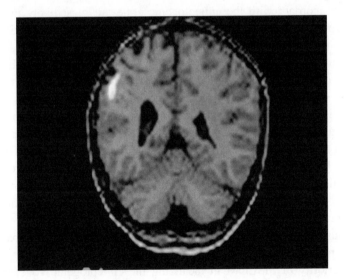

Figure 5.9 SISCOM: A region of cerebral hyperperfusion is identified in the right perirolandic region in a patient with extratemporal seizures. (Note: the right hemisphere is on the left side of the figure.)

was a better predictor of surgical outcome than visual inspection of the interictal and ictal images [37]. The study demonstrated the inherent problems with visual interpretation of either peri-ictal or interictal SPECT studies alone.

The methodology used for SISCOM at The Mayo Clinic involves co-registering of the interictal to the ictal SPECT study by matching the surface points on the cerebral binary images of the two procedures [35, 37–45]. The normalized interictal image is subtracted from the normalized ictal image to derive the difference (subtraction) in cerebral blood flow related to the partial seizure. Thresholding of the subtraction image to display only the pixels with intensities greater than two standard deviations above zero is performed. Finally, the images with intensities of more than two standard deviations are co-registered onto the structural MRI. Following implantation of subdural electrodes for chronic intracranial EEG monitoring the electrode positions can be segmented from a spiral CT scan and co-registered with the SISCOM image [38–40]. This allows the determination of the relationship between the localized peri-ictal blood flow alteration and the ictal onset zone.

The SISCOM region of blood flow alteration is a surrogate for the localization of the epileptogenic zone independent of the pathological finding [37]. The clinical parameters that are significant in determining the diagnostic yield of SISCOM include the duration of the seizure and the length of time of the injection from ictal onset [37]. The seizure should be at least 5–10 seconds in duration and the time from seizure onset should be less than 45 seconds [37]. The SISCOM findings also correlate with the operative outcome. Patients with a SISCOM alteration concordant with the epileptogenic zone are most likely to experience a significant reduction in seizure tendency if the focal cortical resection includes the region of peri-ictal blood flow change [31, 38, 40]. The disadvantages of a SISCOM study include the need for hospitalization and long-term EEG monitoring, the use of radioisotopes for two imaging procedures, and the required presence of habitual seizure activity. The indications for SISCOM in patients undergoing a presurgical evaluation include: non-substrate-directed partial epilepsy and conflicting findings in the noninvasive evaluation. SISCOM may be use to identify a "target" for placement on intracranial EEG electrodes [37, 40, 44]. The presence of a SISCOM alteration may obviate the need for intracranial EEG recordings in selected patients. For example, patients with non-substrate-directed partial epilepsy of temporal lobe origin may not require chronic intracranial EEG monitoring if the extracranial ictal EEG pattern and peri-ictal SPECT studies are concordant. SISCOM also improves the diagnostic yield of postictal studies in patients with intractable partial epilepsy [40].

The superiority of SISCOM in localizing the epileptogenic zone, particularly in extratemporal epilepsy, has been previously demonstrated [44]. The prognostic importance of the SISCOM *focus* in patients undergoing a focal cortical resection for partial epilepsy of extratemporal origin has been evaluated [44]. O'Brien and colleagues in a previous series evaluated the operative outcome in 36 patients with extratemporal epilepsy who had a SISCOM study prior to surgery [44]. The presence of a localizing SISCOM alteration concordant with the epileptogenic zone was a favorable predictor of an excellent surgical outcome ($p < 0.05$) [44]. Eleven of 19 patients (57.9%) with a concordant SISCOM *focus* and 3 of 17 patients (17.6%) with a nonlocalizing or discordant SISCOM, respectively, were rendered seizure-free or experienced only nondisabling seizures. Approximately three-quarters of the patients with a localized SISCOM abnormality had a normal structural MRI. In addition, this study demonstrated that the extent of resection of the SISCOM *focus* was also of prognostic importance ($p < 0.05$) [44]. Failure to resect the neocortical region intimately associated with the localized blood flow change concordant with the ictal onset zone was a predictor of an unfavorable operative outcome [44].

References

1. Dreifuss, F.E. (1987) Goals of surgery for epilepsy, in *Surgical Treatment of the Epilepsies*, 1st edn (ed. J. Engel Jr.), Raven Press, New York, pp. 31–49.
2. Cascino, G.D. (1996) Selection of candidates for surgical treatment of epilepsy, in *Neuroimaging in Epilepsy: Principles and Practice* (eds. G.D. Cascino and C.R. Jack Jr.), Butterworth-Heinemann, Boston, pp. 209–218.
3. Kwan, P. and Brodie, M.J. (2000) Early identification of refractory epilepsy. *N Engl J Med*, **342**, 314–319.
4. Mohanraj, R. and Brodie, M.J. (2005) Outcomes in newly diagnosed localization-related epilepsies. *Seizure*, **14**, 318–323.
5. Callaghan, B.C., Anand, K., Hesdorffer, D. *et al.* (2007) Likelihood of seizure remission in an adult population with refractory epilepsy. *Ann Neurol*, **62**, 382–389.
6. Luciano, A.L. and Shorvon, S. (2007) Results of treatment changes in patients with apparently drug-resistant chronic epilepsy. *Ann Neurol*, **62**, 375–381.
7. French, J.A., Kanner, A.M., Bautista, J. *et al.* (2004) Efficacy and tolerability of the new antiepileptic drugs II: treatment of refractory epilepsy: report of the Therapeutics and Technology Assessment Subcommittee and Quality Standards Subcommittee of the American Academy of Neurology and the American Epilepsy Society. *Neurology*, **62**, 1261–1273.
8. Duncan, J. (2009) The current status of neuroimaging for epilepsy. *Curr Opin Neurol*, **22**, 179–184.
9. Radhakrishnan, K., So, E.L., Silbert, P.L. *et al.* (1998) Predictors of outcome of anterior temporal lobectomy for intractable epilepsy: a multivariate study. *Neurology*, **51**, 465–471.
10. Cascino, G.D., Boon, P.A.J.M., and Fish, D.R. (1993) Surgically remediable lesional syndromes, in *Surgical Treatment of the Epilepsies*, 2nd edn (ed. J. Engel Jr.), Raven Press, New York, pp. 77–86.
11. Awad, I.A., Rosenfeld, J., Ahl, H. *et al.* (1991) Intractable epilepsy and structural lesions of the brain: mapping, resection strategies, and seizure outcome. *Epilepsia*, **32**, 179–186.
12. Engel, J. Jr. and Ojemann, G.A. (1993) The next step, in *Surgical Treatment of the Epilepsies*, 2nd edn (ed. J. Engel Jr.), Raven Press, New York, pp. 319–329.
13. Cascino, G.D., Trenerry, M.R., So, E. *et al.* (1996) Routine EEG and temporal lobe epilepsy: relation to long-term EEG monitoring, quantitative MRI, and operative outcome. *Epilepsia*, **37**, 651–656.

14. Cascino, G.D., Jack, C.R., Parisi, J. *et al.* (1993) Operative strategy in patients with MRI-identified dual pathology and temporal lobe epilepsy. *Epilepsy Res*, **14**, 175–182.

15. Mosewich, R.K., So, E.L., O'Brien, T.J. *et al.* (2000) Factors predictive of the outcome of frontal lobe epilepsy surgery. *Epilepsia*, **41**, 843–849.

16. Cambier, D.M., Cascino, G.D., So, E.L., and Marsh, W.R. (2001) Video-EEG monitoring in patients with hippocampal atrophy. *Acta Neurol Scan*, **103**, 1–7.

17. Jackson, G.D. (1996) Visual analysis in Mesial Temporal Sclerosis, in *Neuroimaging in Epilepsy: Principles and Practice* (eds. G.D. Cascino and C.R. Jack), Butterworth-Heinemann, Boston, pp. 73–110.

18. Cascino, G.D., Jack, C.R. Jr., Parisi, J.E. *et al.* (1992) MRI in the presurgical evaluation of patients with frontal lobe epilepsy and children with temporal lobe epilepsy: pathological correlation and prognostic importance. *Epilepsy Res*, **11**, 51–59.

19. Palmini, A., Andermann, F., Olivier, A. *et al.* (1991) Focal neuronal migrational disorders and intractable partial epilepsy: results of surgical treatment. *Ann Neurol*, **30**, 750–757.

20. Cascino, G.D. (2001) Advances in neuroimaging: surgical localization. *Epilepsia*, **42**, 3–12.

21. Britton, J.W., Cascino, G.D., Sharbrough, F.W., and Kelly, P.J. (1994) Low-grade glial neoplasms and intractable partial epilepsy: efficacy of surgical treatment. *Epilepsia*, **35**, 1130–1135.

22. Kuzniecky, R.I. (1996) Magnetic resonance imaging in cerebral developmental malformations and epilepsy, in *Neuroimaging in Epilepsy: Principles and Practice* (eds. G.D. Cascino and C.R. Jack Jr.), Butterworth-Heinemann, Boston, pp. 51–63.

23. Spencer, S. (1994) The relative contributions of MRI, SPECT, and PET imaging in epilepsy. *Epilepsia*, **35**, S72–S89.

24. Henry, T.R., Babb, T.L., Engel, J. Jr. *et al.* (1994) Hippocampal neuronal loss and regional hypometabolism in temporal lobe epilepsy. *Ann Neurol*, **36**, 925–927.

25. Swartz, B.E., Brown, C., Mandelkern, M.A. *et al.* (2002) The use of 2-deoxy-2-[18F]fluoro-D-glucose (FDG-PET) positron emission tomography in the routine diagnosis of epilepsy. *Mol Imaging Biol*, **4**, 245–252.

26. Henry, T.R. (1996) Functional neuroimaging with positron emission tomography. *Epilepsia*, **37**, 1141–1154.

27. Theodore, W.H., Sato, S., Kufta, C. *et al.* (1992a) Temporal lobectomy for uncontrolled seizures: the role of positron emission tomography. *Ann Neurol*, **32**, 789–794.

28. Carne, R.P., O'Brien, T.J., Kilpatrick, C.J. *et al.* (2004) MRI-negative PET-positive temporal lobe epilepsy: a distinct surgically remediable syndrome. *Brain*, **127**, 2276–2285.

29. Henry, T.R., Frey, K.A., Sackellares, J.C. *et al.* (1993) In vivo cerebral metabolism and central benzodiazepine-receptor binding in temporal lobe epilepsy. *Neurology*, **43**, 1998–2006.

30. Arnold, S., Berthele, A., Drzezga, A. *et al.* (2000) Reduction of benzodiazepine receptor binding is related to the seizure onset zone in extratemporal focal cortical dysplasia. *Epilepsia*, **41**, 818–824.

31. Chugani, D.C., Chugani, H.T., Muzik, O. *et al.* (1998) Imaging epileptogenic tubers in children with tuberous sclerosis complex using alpha-[11C]methyl-L-tryptophan positron emission tomography. *Ann Neurol*, **44**, 858–866.

32. Juhasz, C., Chugani, D.C., Muzik, O. *et al.* (2003) Alpha-methyl-L-tryptophan PET detects epileptogenic cortex in children with intractable epilepsy. *Neurology*, **60**, 960–968.

33. Cendes, F., Caramanos, Z., Andermann, F. *et al.* (1997) Proton magnetic resonance spectroscopy imaging and magnetic resonance imaging volumetry in the lateralization of temporal lobe epilepsy. *Ann Neurol*, **42**, 737–746.

34. Kuzniecky, R., Hugg, J.W., Hetherington, H. *et al.* (1998) Relative utility of ^{1}H spectroscopic imaging and hippocampal volumetry in the lateralization of mesial temporal lobe epilepsy. *Neurology*, **51**, 66–71.
35. O'Brien, T.J., So, E.L., Mullan, B.P. *et al.* (1996) Extent of resection of the ictal subtraction SPECT focus is an important determinant of epilepsy surgery outcome. *Epilepsia*, **37** (Suppl 5), S182.
36. Marks, D.A., Katz, A., Hoffer, P. *et al.* (1992) Localization of extratemporal epileptic foci during ictal single photon emission computed tomography. *Ann Neurol*, **31**, 250–255.
37. O'Brien, T.J., So, E.L., Mullan, B.P. *et al.* (1998) Subtraction ictal SPECT co-registered to MRI improves clinical usefulness of SPECT in localizing the surgical seizure focus. *Neurology*, **50**, 445–454.
38. O'Brien, T.J., O'Connor, M.K., Mullan, B.P. *et al.* (1998) Subtraction ictal SPECT co-registered to MRI in partial epilepsy: description and technical validation of the method with phantom and patients studies. *Nucl Med Commun*, **19**, 31–45.
39. So, E.L. (2000) Integration of EEG, MRI and SPECT in localizing the seizure focus for epilepsy surgery. *Epilepsia*, **41** (Suppl 3), S48–S54.
40. O'Brien, T.J., So, E.L., Mullan, B.P. *et al.* (1999) Subtraction SPECT co-registered to MRI improves postictal localization of seizure foci. *Neurology*, **52**, 137–146.
41. Brinkmann, B.H., O'Brien, T.J., Webster, D.B. *et al.* (2000) Voxel significance mapping using local image variances in subtraction ictal SPET. *Nucl Med Commun*, **21**, 545–551.
42. O'Brien, T.J., Brinkmann, B.H., Mullan, B.P. *et al.* (1999) Comparative study of 99mTc-ECD and 99mTc-HMPAO for SPECT: qualitative and quantitative analysis. *J Neurol Neurosurg Psychiatry*, **66**, 331–339.
43. So, E.L., O'Brien, T.J., Brinkmann, B.H. *et al.* (2000) The EEG evaluation of single photon emission computed tomography abnormalities in epilepsy. *J Clin Neurophysiol*, **17**, 10–28.
44. O'Brien, T.J., So, E.L., Mullan, B.P. *et al.* (2000) Subtraction peri-ictal SPECT is predictive of extratemporal epilepsy surgery outcome. *Neurology*, **55**, 1668–1677.
45. Fessler, J.A., Cascino, G.D., So, E.L. *et al.* (2000) Subtraction ictal SPECT co-registered to MRI (SISCOM) in the evaluation for repeat epilepsy surgery. *Neurology*, **54** (Suppl 3), A4.
46. Ho, S.S., Berkovic, S.F., Berlangieri, S.U. *et al.* (1995) Comparison of ictal SPECT and interictal PET in the presurgical evaluation of temporal lobe epilepsy. *Ann Neurol*, **37**, 738–745.

6 Video-EEG monitoring data

Elson L. So

Section of Electroencephalography, Mayo Clinic College of Medicine, Rochester, MN, USA

6.1 Introduction

The advent of digital video and EEG recordings has expanded the usefulness of the procedure beyond epilepsy monitoring, but it has also introduced complex issues relating to appropriate clinical indications, acceptable patient safety, and proper recording environment, equipment, and techniques. This chapter will address methods in optimizing recording techniques and skills in interpreting video-EEG data in adult patients. Most of these techniques are equally applicable to pediatric patients, especially in school-age children and in adolescents.

6.2 Pre-monitoring evaluation and preparation

The usefulness of the spell description in the neurological history has been doubted in a number of studies [1, 2]. Nonetheless, the neurological history gives clinicians the ability to determine whether or not there is an indication for video-EEG monitoring. Not all paroxysmal events require video-EEG monitoring. The basis for spells in some patients is obvious from their initial clinical evaluation. Considerable expense and inconvenience associated with video-EEG procedure can

Adult Epilepsy, First Edition. Edited by Gregory D. Cascino and Joseph I. Sirven.
© 2011 John Wiley & Sons, Ltd. Published 2011 by John Wiley & Sons, Ltd.

be avoided in these patients. In other patients, video-EEG monitoring may not be cost-effective because their spells are infrequent, unless the timing of spell occurrence is fairly predictable, or the spell occurrence can be enhanced by medication withdrawal or provocative tests. Factors that precipitate the patient's spells are identified during history taking, so that they may be duplicated during video-EEG monitoring to enhance the occurrence of spells. The following list serves as a guide during history taking so that paroxysmal events may be completely described and analyzed prior to considering video-EEG monitoring.

- Aura and prodrome
- Mode of progression
- Duration of each component of the spell
- Awareness and consciousness
- Distractibility
- Postictal state (behavior, confusion, weakness, dysphasia, amnesia)
- Time of occurrence
- Environment of occurrence
- Precipitants or triggers
- Aborting or relieving factors
- Frequency of spells
- Stereotypy of spells
- Injuries and disability
- Age of onset of spells
- Any medical disorders or psychosocial stressors when the disorder began.

6.3 Management during monitoring

Admission and medication management

It is appropriate to begin withdrawing AEDs before the day of admission when habitual spells are not intense and when they have not been affected beneficially by the AED. As a rule, we do not initiate AED withdrawal until the morning of admission. In general, AEDs are tapered daily at the rate of one-third of the original dose. Medications that are pharmacokinetically or pharmacodynamically long-acting may be discontinued (e.g., lamotrigine, zonisamide, phenobarbital, valproate). Occasionally, AED discontinuance or tapering may result in "withdrawal" symptoms such as restlessness, insomnia, and dysphoria. Barbiturates and benzodiazepine withdrawal are more commonly the basis, but such symptoms can also be encountered with carbamazepine withdrawal [3]. Diazepam or lorazepam are effective in sedating the patient, but may impede seizure recording if seizures have not been recorded sufficiently (25 mg of nortriptyline, or 25–50 mg of diphenhydramine, by mouth, is usually effective in controlling withdrawal symptoms, especially carbamazepine withdrawal symptoms). These two medications should not reduce the chance of recording seizures.

We attempt to duplicate factors that have been reported by patients to be potentially aggravating for their seizures. Although a recent study has cast doubts on the value of sleep deprivation in the monitoring setting [4], sleep deprivation is one of the most frequent reasons for seizure aggravation in the everyday living situation [5, 6]. We also implement exercise programs to prevent deep vein thrombosis and physical deconditioning from developing due to bedrest. When the risk of injury from seizures is high, we use a recumbent bike for the purpose.

Guidelines should be provided for the staff to treat prolonged or frequent seizures. A balance should be struck between the need for recording further spells and the need for initiating the "emergency" or "rescue" plan. Typical but not routine parameters for administering parenteral medications under the plan consist of: (i) two generalized convulsive seizures within two hours; or (ii) generalized convulsive activity lasting more than three minutes; or (iii) two partial seizures within one hour; or (iv) a partial seizure lasting five minutes or longer. Patient safety remains the primary concern in such considerations, and the parameters need to be modified according to the patient's health, seizure type, and epilepsy history [7]. The history in some patients may indicate the point at which their seizures are likely to become prolonged or clustered. Instead of intravenous administration of AED, oral treatment may be appropriate in less urgent instances. The sustained or continuous release form AEDs should not be used for this purpose of orally loading AED.

Spell evaluation

Analysis of video data and peri-ictal testing

Peri-ictal (ictal and postictal) examination of patients is important in bringing out semiologic features of their seizures that otherwise would not be apparent. Attempts should be made to test for the following functions:

- Response to communication
- Response to physical stimulation
- Memory, by presenting phrases or words for later recall
- Distractibility
- Weakness or lack of motor control
- Response to passive eye opening
- Plantar extensor response
- Speech (naming, reading).

Of the many possible types of spells in adults, epileptic seizures, psychogenic spells, and syncope are the most commonly encountered when conducting video-EEG studies. Three helpful semiologic clues to the epileptic nature of spells are: (i) localizing semiologic features; (ii) physiologic sequence of progression; (iii) peri-ictal signs of epileptic seizure mechanism.

Localizing semiologic features

Observable peri-ictal semiologic features can be grouped into the following: motor signs (positive and negative), automatisms, autonomic signs, and speech disturbance [8]. The following Table 6.1 lists specific peri-ictal signs and their diagnostic value. (The reader is referred to references [9, 10] for detailed discussion of the known or presumed mechanism underlying each sign.)

Temporal lobes and frontal lobes are two regions most frequently affected by partial epilepsy. Distinguishing between the two is important in evaluating medically intractable epilepsy patients for resective epilepsy surgery. Table 6.2 lists features that are more commonly associated with one type of seizure than with the other. Using the video-recorded features noted in Table 6.2, we found that seizures were localizable to the frontal lobe in about 83% of the frontal lobe patients, and to the temporal lobe in all temporal lobe epilepsy patients [11].

Physiologic sequence of progression

Physiologic sequence of progression of signs and symptoms is especially helpful in distinguishing between epileptic seizures and nonepileptic psychogenic spells (pseudoseizures). An example of epileptic seizures commonly seen in adults is partial seizures with secondary generalization [12]. With this type of seizure, the initial symptom or sign, such as aura or focal motor activity, indicates seizure onset at a cerebral focus. Ensuing loss of awareness with automatisms reflects limbic involvement, and subsequent contralateral extremity posturing is due to centripetal spread of epileptic discharge into the basal ganglia. Seizure generalization into tonic-clonic activity affects initially the contralateral face or extremities, followed by ipsilateral involvement. This physiologic sequence of spread of activity is lacking in psychogenic "seizures," in which motor or behavioral activities appear in a random sequence and distribution. Moreover, the motor or behavioral activity often occurs in bursts, rather than unfolding in a sequential manner as is seen in epileptic seizures. Features that are useful in distinguishing psychogenic spells from epileptic seizures are:

- Lingering prodrome
- Out-of-phase convulsive activity
- Nonphysiologic spread
- Pelvic thrusting.

Table 6.1 Peri-ictal signs and their diagnostic value

Positive motor signs

Sign	Hemisphere of seizure onset	Observed rate	Positive predictive value[a] (PPV)
Early nonforced head turn	Ipsilateral	30%	—
Late contraversive forced head turn	Contralateral	25–50% (52% in FLS patients)	(94%)
Late ipsiversive forced head turn	Ipsilateral	—	—
Eye deviation	Contralateral	Rarely solitary	High if occipital
Focal clonic	Contralateral	30% (52% in FLS patients)	>95% (81%)
Asymmetric clonic ending	Ipsilateral	70% of secondary generalized seizures (16% in FLS patients)	83% (80%)
Dystonic limb	Contralateral	67%	93%
Tonic limb	Contralateral	13% (32% in FLS patients)	85% (80%)
RINCH	Contralateral	—	—

Complex postures

M2E and fencing	Contralateral	3% of TLS patients 25% of FLS patients	90%
"Figure 4" sign	Contralateral to extended limb	70% of seizures generalizing from temporal lobe; 31% of extratemporal	89%
Truncal rotation	Contralateral if w/ forced head turn; ipsilateral if w/out	2% of TLS patients; 17% of FLS patients	? 100% (small n)

Negative motor signs

Sign	Hemisphere of seizure onset	Observed rate	Positive predictive value
Ictal paresis or immobile limb	Contralateral	5% of complex partial seizure patients	100%
Todd's paresis	Contralateral	13% of partial seizure patients	80–100%

Automatic behavior

Unilateral limb automatism	Ipsilateral to seizure focus; 90% PPV
Unilateral eye blinks	Ipsilateral to focus; 83% PPV
Postictal cough	40% of TLS patients, 0 of pseudoseizure or FLS patients
Postictal nose wiping	Ipsilateral; (seen in 36% of TLS vs. 3% of FLS)
Bipedal automatisms	30% of frontal and 10% of TLS patients
Ictal spitting, or drinking	Rare, but high association w/ right TLS

(Continued)

Table 6.1 (*Continued*)

Automatism w/ preserved responsiveness	Nondominant (usually right) temporal; or extratemporal on either side
Gelastic seizure	Hypothalamic; sometimes mesial temporal, or frontal cingulate origin
Ictal smile (in children)	11% of frontal, 3% of temporal, 26% of posterior cortical epilepsy; lateralizes seizure to the right
Autonomic signs	
Ictus emeticus	Rare, but usually right temporal
Ictal urinary urge	Rare (2%), but localizes to right temporal
Bilateral piloerection (goose bumps) unilateral piloerection	Mostly left temporal Ipsilateral
Peri-ictal speech	
Ictal speech arrest	Seen in 75% of TLS patients, but only 67% PPV for dominant hemisphere focus
Ictal speech preservation	Seen in only 15%, but PPV of 83% for nondominant hemisphere focus in TLS patients
Postictal dysphasia	90% dominant hemisphere involvement

[a]Positive predictive value (PPV) = number of true positives divided by the sum of true positives and false positives.

TLS: temporal lobe seizure; FLS: frontal lobe seizure; RINCH: rhythmic ictal nonclonic handmotions.

Table 6.2 Features more commonly associated with temporal lobe seizures versus frontal lobe seizures

Features	Temporal lobe seizures	Frontal lobe seizures
Somatosensory symptoms	Rare	More common
Onset	Slower	Abrupt, explosive
Progression	Slower	Rapid
Initial motionless stare	Common	Less common
Complex postures	Less frequent and prominent, occurring later as seizure starts to generalize	More frequent, prominent, and early
Hypermotor (hyperkinetic)	Rare	Common
Vocalization	Speech (nondominant temporal)	Loud nonspeech (grunting, screaming, moaning)
Automatisms	More common and longer	Less common
Bipedal automatism	Uncommon	Common and characteristic
Seizure duration	Longer	Brief
Postictal confusion	More prominent and longer	Absent, or less prominent or shorter
Postictal dysphasia	More frequent (dominant temporal)	Uncommon (unless spreads to dominant temporal lobe)
Seizure frequency	Less	Frequent, often multiple daily
Sleep activation	Less	Common and characteristic

- Side-to-side head or limb shaking
- Opisthotonus
- Eyes and mouth shut tight
- Geotrophic eye deviation
- Bursting "stop-go" ("reprisal phenomenon")
- Irregular progression
- Distractibility
- Abrupt cessation
- Disproportionate postictal mental status
- Feeble motor response or vocalization (whispering)
- Long duration of spells
- Tongue bitten at the tip
- Normal breathing or hyperventilation immediately after cessation of convulsion
- Lack of stereotypy between spells.

Note that the above list does not include "positive provocative test," which is the ability to induce a spell through suggestion. The reason is that as many as 15% of patients with epilepsy can be induced with IV saline into having *de novo* nonepileptic spells [13]. The suggestion used with the IV saline injection was even fairly mild, in that patients were told that the injection "occasionally precipitated seizures in patients with seizure tendencies." If stronger suggestions are made [14], the false positive rate for psychogenic spells is expected to be even higher. This situation can lead to disastrous consequences if the clinician fails to recognize the presence of epilepsy and withdraws the AED. Thus, it is very important that the clinician confirms that there is no other type of spells that needs to be evaluated. Provocative tests must be performed in the setting of video-EEG recording. The recorded event needs to be shown to the patient's family or friends to confirm that it is the same as habitual spells, and that no other type of spells is in question.

Other peri-ictal signs of epileptic seizure mechanism

The following are helpful in reinforcing a suspicion for epileptic seizures rather than psychogenic spells [15–21].

- Seizure arising out of sleep
- Tongue bitten
- Physical injury
- Postictal Babinski
- Postictal foaming at the mouth.

Analysis of EEG data

The EEG in epileptic seizures

Ictal discharge

Generalized ictal discharges include 3-Hz spike-and-wave paroxysms, bursts of atypical spike-and-waves or slow spike-and-waves; paroxysmal fast activity (generalized repetitive fast discharge); and electrodecrement [22]. Focal seizure discharges include focal or regional repetitive spike or sharp waves; rhythmic or sinusoidal theta, alpha, or beta frequency discharges; rhythmic or arrhythmic delta waves; periodic discharges, and electrodecrement [23]. The pattern of focal discharge at onset has some association with specific regions of the cerebral hemispheres (e.g., rhythmic theta discharge pattern in temporal lobe seizures versus the repetitive epileptiform pattern in frontal convexity seizures as reported by Foldvary and colleagues [24]; regular 5- to 9-Hz infero-temporal rhythm in hippocampal-onset seizures versus irregular polymorphic 2- to 5-Hz delta activity in temporal neocortical onset seizures as reported by Ebersole [25]). However, the association is not sufficiently reliable, and the primary basis for localizing seizures is still the location of seizure onset. One particular combination of scalp discharge pattern and location has high localization and prognostic value. A fast discharge in the beta frequency range at the onset of frontal seizures is highly indicative of the location of the epileptogenic zone [26]. Approximately 90% of patients with this frontal ictal beta discharge pattern at seizure onset became seizure-free following resection of the frontal lobe focus, even when the MRI is negative. In comparison, postsurgical seizure freedom occurred in only 16.7% of patients who did not have the focal ictal beta pattern.

The typical frequency and waveform evolution that we expect to see in EEG seizure discharges occur in 92% of seizures with clinical manifestations but in only 44% of subclinical seizures [27]. In fact, focal seizures may not even be accompanied by detectable EEG discharge. This is especially true of frontal lobe seizures and simple partial seizures [24, 28–30]. Minimally invasive EEG strategies for increasing the chance of recording ictal discharges include use of sphenoidal electrodes, anterior temporal scalp electrodes, subtemporal chain scalp electrodes, and closely spaced electrodes. Sphenoidal electrodes do not offer any advantage over anterior temporal electrodes in detecting interictal epileptiform discharges, especially when some discharges have already been detected by scalp electrodes [31–33]. However, fluoroscopically placed sphenoidal electrodes have been reported to be correctly localizing in more seizures than with anterior temporal electrodes (92% vs. 63%) [34] Studies comparing sphenoidal and scalp electrodes did not take advantage of modern digital review of records, in that paper EEG copies were used for the studies. Sphenoidal discharges do not necessarily indicate anterior or mesial temporal origin, as they can also arise from the inferior frontal region. It is also unclear whether sphenoidal recordings are superior in detecting midtemporal neocortical-onset seizures. At the least, the use of a subtemporal chain of electrodes should be considered, because they can be easily added to the standard EEG montage, and the chain includes the anterior temporal electrodes. The subtemporal chain is 10%, instead of 20%, inferior to the temporal chain of electrodes in the 10–20 system of electrode placement [35]. Routine application of closely spaced electrodes for recording frontal lobe epilepsy is not as useful. It does not yield information that is lacking in the regular 10–20 system scalp coverage [36]. Nonetheless, strategic placements of electrodes within an area predefined by semiology, neuroimaging, or interictal discharges may better localize seizures in selected patients, especially when the focus is at the perirolandic or occipital region.

Interictal, ictal, and postictal slowing

Interictal temporal delta slowing also suggests the location of the seizure focus. However, only temporal intermittent *rhythmic* delta activity (TIRDA) has a high association with an ipsilateral temporal lobe seizure focus, because temporal intermittent *polymorphic* delta activity (TIPDA) is present in 20% of extratemporal epilepsy patients [37].

Unequivocal onset of background slowing during or after a spell excludes a psychogenic explanation for the spell. The remaining major differential diagnosis is epileptic seizures, syncope, or migraine. Much less common possibilities are drug effects, acute metabolic disturbance, and strokes. These nonepileptic conditions usually have more prominent slowing during the spell, rather than following resolution of the clinical spell. Relatively more prominent EEG slowing following resolution of the clinical symptoms is more compatible with an epileptic seizure event.

The presence of lateralized postictal polymorphic delta activity (PPDA) in temporal lobe epilepsy is also highly suggestive of the side of seizure origin. Lateralized PPDA is concordant with the side of eventual temporal lobe epilepsy surgery in 96% of the EEGs [38].

EKG recording

Every effort should be made to ensure that the electrocardiogram (EKG) channel in the EEG recording montage is recording properly. The EKG is invaluable in recognizing cardiac-related artifacts, in determining seizure occurrence even when the EEG is indeterminate, and in diagnosing potentially fatal cardiac events. It is not uncommon for ictal tachycardia to be the only convincing objective evidence of an epileptic mechanism, because EEG discharge may not be observable, often because of muscle and movement artifacts from the clinical seizure activity. It has been difficult to say what degree of tachycardia suggests an epileptic mechanism, until Opherk and colleagues found that the change in heart rate in complex partial seizures is 120–218% of baseline heart rate, but only 84–126% during nonconvulsive psychogenic spells [39]. Heart rate during epileptic convulsive seizures is 136–236% of baseline heart rate, compared with 101–137% during convulsive psychogenic spells. These findings alone are not very useful clinically because of overlap in the values, but a derivation from the finding is that heart rate increase of at least 1.5 times over baseline has high sensitivity and specificity for epileptic seizure mechanism. Therefore, the multiple of 1.5 times baseline rate can be used as a minimum threshold for strongly indicating an epileptic explanation for the spell. Ictal tachycardia is also characteristically abrupt in onset [40], and often precedes the EEG seizure onset [41].

Ictal bradycardia syndrome is a serious disorder that can present as syncopal spells [42]. Epileptic seizures from either right or left temporal lobe induce hemodynamically significant bradycardia or arrest of the heart rhythm in patients with this syndrome. Video-EEG with EKG channel recording is needed for establishing the diagnosis. Many patients with the syndrome require demand cardiac pacing because their seizures are refractory to medical treatment and their degree of ictal cardiac inhibition is potentially fatal.

The EEG in psychogenic spells

The absence of EEG seizure discharges during a spell is often considered the hallmark of nonepileptic spells. However, the foregoing discussion shows that some epileptic seizures may not be accompanied by discernible EEG discharges. Four other EEG features that differentiate psychogenic spells from epileptic seizures are: (i) EEG showing sleep activity when the spell begins is very rare in psychogenic spells (<1% of psychogenic spell patients [20]). Although the patient with psychogenic spells may appear to be asleep when the spell occurs, the EEG shows a wake rhythm [16]; (ii) Ictal tachycardia favors epileptic mechanism (please see "The EEG in Epileptic Seizures" above); (iii) Normal wake rhythm in a mentally unresponsive patient is not physiologic and therefore favors psychogenic cause. (Note that EEG may appear normal in a *mentally confused* patient due to epileptic seizure occurrence, but EEG should not be normal when the patient is *unresponsive* and appears to be *comatose*.) Two other rare conditions where the EEG may be normal but the patient is unresponsive are locked-in syndrome and generalized motor paralysis such as pharmacologic neuromuscular blockade or Guillain-Barré syndrome; and (iv) Postictal slowing precludes psychogenic spells (please see "The EEG in Epileptic Seizures" above).

The EEG in syncopal attacks

Syncopal attacks can produce EEG changes that are similar to those seen in epileptic seizures. A full sequence of EEG changes can be seen in a typical syncopal attack but not necessarily in a near-faint [43]. The earliest EEG alteration in syncope is slowing of background rhythms. High-voltage delta slow waves follow, with the anterior head regions showing the highest amplitude. If cerebral perfusion is markedly compromised by hypotension, bradycardia or asystole, the EEG may become suppressed or "flattened." This EEG suppression often accompanies convulsive syncope or decorticate/decerebrate posturing. Seizure discharges are not present, even in patients who experienced convulsive syncope. As the patient is coming out of the syncopal attack, the sequence of the EEG changes reverses. Video-EEG monitoring is especially suitable in tracking the development of the clinical and EEG manifestations of syncope [44].

The EKG channel is necessary to detect cardiac arrhythmia as a cause of syncope. Of all types of syncope, syncope due to cardiac arrhythmia carries the most serious prognostic implications [45]. The EKG channel also helps in detecting bradycardia that can occur with noncardiac types of syncope, such as neurocardiogenic syncope and carotid hypersensitivity.

Integration of clinical and EEG data

EEG has sustained a reputation of being a standard test for evaluating spells. However, it has several limitations in the evaluation of many types of spells. Ictal EEG discharges are not always detectable on the scalp. Thus, the absence of EEG discharge cannot be taken alone as confirmatory of the nonepileptic nature of spells. When EEG discharges are present, they may be equivocal in their location or origin. In one study involving patients with unilateral mesial temporal lobe epilepsy [46], seizure onset could not be lateralized by EEG in about 25–30% of the seizures recorded. EEG localization of individual seizure episodes is often equivocal even in patients who had successful temporal lobectomy [47–49]. The limitation of ictal EEG is even greater in extratemporal epilepsy. Approximately 35–50% of extracranially recorded seizures in extratemporal epilepsy are nonlateralizing [47]. The nature and the anatomic origin of spells can be more confidently determined when EEG data are supplemented by other information [50, 51]. Also, the addition of video-recorded seizure semiology has been shown to improve the lateralization of seizures for temporal lobectomy [52]. With scalp EEG alone, only about 65% of temporal lobectomy candidates could be adequately lateralized. With the addition of video-recorded seizure semiology, the lateralization rate was improved to almost 95%.

Ideally, onset of electrographic seizure discharge should be earlier or coincident with the clinical seizure onset. If the EEG seizure onset is delayed, the possibility of false EEG localization should be entertained, because the EEG discharge detected could have been from a region of seizure propagation, rather than the region of seizure origination. Clinical seizures may not have developed until the EEG discharge has spread from the focus of onset to regions underlying the clinical semiology. On the other hand, when ictal EEG onset precedes the clinical onset, EEG localization is generally accepted as correctly localizing, so long as the two localizations are not discordant, and there is no other conflicting clinical or neuroimaging data.

6.4 Discharge management

It is imperative that recorded seizures be verified with patients and their relatives or friends to be certain that they are representative of habitual seizures. It is also important that enough seizure episodes are captured so that if there are previously unrecognized seizure foci, they will have a higher likelihood of being recorded.

It is best that serum concentrations be checked before discharge if phenytoin, phenobarbital or carbamazepine is resumed or initiated as the primary agent intended for seizure control. This is especially important if patients are at risk for convulsive seizures. Serum concentrations of other AEDs may not be as useful because of poor correlation between their dose and their therapeutic effect. Nonetheless, if any of those AEDs are intended as the main anticonvulsive agent, it may be necessary to defer discharge until an appropriate target dose and steady-state has been achieved.

One of the most difficult situations is in deciding whether AEDs should be stopped in patients whose recorded seizures are nonepileptic in nature. It is best to verify the following situations before considering AED discontinuance in such a case: (i) that there are no other type spells that have not been addressed; (ii) that the patient does not have risk factors for epilepsy (e.g., intracranial epileptogenic lesion, history of meningoencephalitis); (iii) that EEG shows no epileptiform discharges; (iv) that AED therapy had been ineffective; and (v) that the consequence of spell occurrence is not particularly grave. When these situations apply, patients may be counseled that the benefit of discontinuing AEDs outweighs the risk of exacerbating unrecognized epilepsy. Their decision to discontinue AEDs would have been based on the best medical evidence available from a complete evaluation of their spells. If suspicion remains regarding the possibility of concomitant epilepsy, one approach is to ask patients to continue at least one AED while they undergo the proper treatment for their nonepileptic spells. When they are free of spells for at least a year, considerations may be given to AED withdrawal at that time. This approach is based on the practice of permitting AED withdrawal in patients with factors that are favorable for seizure remission following AED withdrawal [53, 54].

Acknowledgments

This chapter was adapted with permission from "Nailing Down Spells in Adults: How to Analyze Video and EEG," in the American Academy of Neurology educational course syllabus titled "Video-EEG Monitoring in the Neurological Practice: Tools, Techniques, and Applications."

References

1. Rugg-Gunn, F.J., Harrison, N.A., and Duncan, J.S. (2001) Evaluation of the accuracy of seizure descriptions by the relatives of patients with epilepsy. *Epilepsy Res*, **43**, 193–199.
2. Deacon, C., Wiebe, S., Blume, W. *et al.* (2003) Seizure identification by clinical description in temporal lobe epilepsy. How accurate are we? *Neurology*, **61**, 1686–1689.
3. Duncan, J., Shorvon, S., and Trimble, M. (1988) Withdrawal symptoms from phenytoin, carbamazepine and sodium valproate. *J Neurol Neurosurg Psychiatr*, **51**, 924–928.
4. Malow, B., Passaro, E., Milling, C. *et al.* (2002) Sleep deprivation does not affect seizure frequency during inpatient video-EEG monitoring. *Neurology*, **59**, 1371–1374.
5. Neugebauer, R., Paik, M., Hauser, W. *et al.* (1994) Stressful life events and seizure frequency in patients with epilepsy. *Epilepsia*, **35**, 336–343.
6. Fucht, M., Quigg, M., Schwaner, C. *et al.* (2000) Distribution of seizure precipitants among epilepsy syndromes. *Epilepsia*, **41**, 1534–1539.
7. Noe, K. and Drazkowski, J. (2009) Safety of long-term video-electroencephalographic monitoring for evaluation of epilepsy. *Mayo Clin Proc*, **84**, 495–500.
8. So, E. (2006) Value and limitations of seizure semiology in localizing seizure onset. *J Clin Neurophysiol*, **23**, 353–357.
9. Loddenkemper, T. and Kotagal, P. (2005) Lateralizing signs during seizures in focal epilepsy. *Epilepsy Behav*, **7**, 1–17.
10. Lee, G., Arain, A., Lim, N. *et al.* (2006) Rhythmic ictal nonclonic hand (RINCH) motions: a distinct contralateral sign in temporal lobe epilepsy. *Epilepsia*, **47**, 2189–2192.
11. O'Brien, T., Mosewich, R., Britton, J. *et al.* (2008) History and seizure semiology in distinguishing frontal lobe seizures and temporal lobe seizures. *Epilepsy Res*, **82**, 177–182.
12. Jobst, B., Williamson, P., Neuschwander, T. *et al.* (2001) Secondarily generalized seizures in mesial temporal epilepsy: clinical characteristics, lateralizing signs, and association with sleep-wake cycle. *Epilepsia*, **42**, 1279–1287.
13. Walczak, T., Williams, D., and Berten, W. (1994) Utility and reliability of placebo infusion in the evaluation of patients with seizures. *Neurology*, **44**, 394–399.
14. Lancman, M., Asconape, J., Craven, W. *et al.* (1994) Predictive value of induction of psychogenic seizures by suggestion. *Ann Neurol*, **35**, 359–361.
15. Kanner, A., Morris, H., Luders, H. *et al.* (1990) Supplementary motor seizures mimicking pseudoseizures: some clinical differences. *Neurology*, **40**, 1404–1407.
16. Thacker, K., Devinsky, O., Perrine, K. *et al.* (1993) Nonepileptic seizures during apparent sleep. *Ann Neurol*, **33**, 414–418.
17. Walczak, T. and Rubinsky, M. (1994) Plantar responses after epileptic seizures. *Neurology*, **44**, 2191–2193.
18. De Toledo, J. and Ramsay, R. (1996) Patterns of involvement of facial muscles during epileptic and nonepileptic events: review of 654 events. *Neurology*, **47**, 621–625.
19. Benbadis, S.R., Lancman, M.E., King, L.M. *et al.* (1996) Preictal pseudosleep: a new finding in psychogenic seizures. *Neurology*, **47**, 63–67.
20. Orbach, D., Ritaccio, A., and Devinsky, O. (2003) Psychogenic, nonepileptic seizures associated with video-EEG-verified sleep. *Epilepsia*, **44**, 64–68.
21. Oliva, M., Pattison, C., Carino, J. *et al.* (2008) The diagnostic value of oral lacerations and incontinence during convulsive seizures. *Epilepsia*, **49**, 962–967.

22. Drury, I. and Henry, T. (1993) Ictal patterns in generalized epilepsy. *J Clin Neurophysiol*, **10**, 268–280.
23. Sharbrough, F. (1993) Scalp recorded ictal patterns in focal epilepsy. *J Clin Neurophysiol*, **10**, 281–297.
24. Foldvary, N., Klem, G., Hammel, M. *et al.* (2001) The localizing value of ictal EEG in focal epilepsy. *Neurology*, **57**, 2022–2028.
25. Ebersole, J.S. and Pacia, S.V. (1996) Localization of temporal lobe foci by ictal EEG patterns. *Epilepsia*, **37**, 386–399.
26. Worrell, G., So, E., Kazemi, J. *et al.* (2002) Focal ictal beta discharge on scalp EEG predicts excellent outcome of frontal lobe epilepsy surgery. *Epilepsia*, **43**, 277–282.
27. Blume, W., Young, G., and Lemieux, J. (1984) EEG morphology of partial seizures. *Electroencephalogr Clin Neurophysiol*, **57**, 295–302.
28. Bancaud, J. and Talairach, J. (1992) Clinical semiology of frontal lobe seizures. *Adv Neurol*, **57**, 3–58.
29. Quesney, L. (1992) Extratemporal epilepsy: clinical presentation, pre-operative EEG localization and surgical outcome. *Acta Neurol Scand Suppl*, **140**, 81–94.
30. Bautista, E., Spencer, D., and Spencer, S. (1998) EEG findings in frontal lobe epilepsies. *Neurology*, **50**, 1765–1771.
31. Sadler, R. and Goodwin, J. (1989) Multiple electrodes for detecting spikes in partial complex seizures. *Can J Neurol Sci*, **16**, 326–329.
32. Binnie, C., Marston, C., Polkey, C. *et al.* (1989) Distribution of temporal spikes in relation to the sphenoidal electrode. *Electroencephalogr Clin Neurophysiol*, **73**, 403–409.
33. So, E., Ruggles, K., Ahmann, P. *et al.* (1994) Yield of sphenoidal recordings in sleep-deprived outpatients. *J Clin Neurophysiol*, **11**, 226–230.
34. Kanner, A., Gil-Nagel, A., Soto, A. *et al.* (2002) The localizing yield of sphenoidal and anterior temporal electrodes in ictal recordings: a comparison study. *Epilepsia*, **43**, 189–196.
35. Sharbrough, F., Chatrian, G., Lesser, R. *et al.* (1991) American Electroencephalographic Society guidelines for standard electrode position nomenclature. *J Clin Neurophysiol*, **8**, 200–202.
36. Gross, D.W., Dubeau, F., Quesney, L.F. *et al.* (2000) EEG telemetry with closely spaced electrodes in frontal lobe epilepsy. *J Clin Neurophysiol*, **17**, 414–418.
37. Geyer, J., Bilir, E., Faught, R. *et al.* (1999) Significance of interictal temporal lobe delta activity for localization of the primary epileptogenic region. *Neurology*, **52**, 202–205.
38. Jan, M., Sadler, M., and Rahey, S. (2001) Lateralized postictal EEG delta predicts the side of seizure surgery in temporal lobe epilepsy. *Epilepsia*, **42**, 402–405.
39. Opherk, C. and Hirsch, L. (2002) Ictal heart rate differentiates epileptic from nonepileptic seizures. *Neurology*, **58**, 636–638.
40. Burgess, R., Pestana, E., and Shkurovich, P. (2004) Heart rate acceleration accompanying epileptic seizures. *Epilepsia*, **45** (Suppl 7), 361–362.
41. Luetmezer, F., Schernthaner, C., Lurger, S. *et al.* (2003) Electrocardiograhic change at the onset of epileptic seizures. *Epilepsia*, **44**, 348–354.
42. Reeves, A., Nollet, K., Klass, D. *et al.* (1996) The ictal bradycardia syndrome. *Epilepsia*, **37**, 983–987.
43. Brenner, R. (1997) Electroencephalography in syncope. *J Clin Neurophysiol*, **14**, 197–209.
44. Lempert, T., Bauer, H., and Schmidt, D. (1994) Syncope: a videometric analysis of 56 episodes of transient cerebral hypoxia. *Ann Neurol*, **36**, 233–237.
45. Martin, T.P., Hanusa, B.H., and Kappor, W.N. (1997) Risk stratification of patients with syncope. *Ann Emerg Med*, **29**, 540–542.
46. Pataraia, E., Lurger, S., Serles, W. *et al.* (1998) Ictal EEG in unilateral mesial temporal lobe epilepsy. *Epilepsia*, **39**, 608–614.

47. Walczak, T., Radtke, R., and Lewis, D. (1992) Accuracy and interobserver reliability of scalp ictal EEG. *Neurology*, **42**, 2279–2285.
48. Sirven, J., Liporace, J., French, J. *et al.* (1997) Seizures in temporal epilepsy: Reliability of scalp/sphenoidal ictal reading. *Neurology*, **48**, 1041–1046.
49. Blume, W., Ravindran, J., and Lowry, N. (1998) Late lateralizing and localizing features of scalp-recorded temporal lobe seizures. *J Clin Neurophysiol*, **15**, 514–520.
50. King, D., Gallagher, B., Murvin, A. *et al.* (1982) Pseudoseizure: diagnostic evaluation. *Neurology*, **32**, 18–23.
51. Sammaritano, M., de Lotbiniere, A., Andermann, F. *et al.* (1987) False lateralization by surface EEG of seizure onset in patients with temporal lobe epilepsy and gross focal cerebral lesions. *Ann Neurol*, **21**, 361–369.
52. Serles, W., Caramanos, Z., Lindinger, E. *et al.* (2000) Combining ictal surface-electroencephalography and seizure semiology improves lateralization in temporal lobe epilepsy. *Epilepsia*, **41**, 1567–1573.
53. Quality Standards Subcommittee of the American Academy of Neurology (1996) Practice parameter: a guideline for discontinuing antiepileptic drugs in seizure-free patients—Summary statement. *Neurology*, **47**, 600–602.
54. Berg, A. and Shinnar, S. (1994) Relapse following discontinuation of antiepileptic drugs: a meta-analysis. *Neurology*, **44**, 601–608.

7 Etiologies of seizures

Katherine H. Noe[1] and Korwyn Williams[2]

[1]*Department of Neurology, Division of Epilepsy, Mayo Clinic College of Medicine and Mayo Clinic Arizona, Phoenix, AZ, USA*
[2]*Department of Pediatrics, University of Arizona College of Medicine, Phoenix, AZ; Division of Neurology, Children's Neuroscience Institute, Phoenix Children's Hospital, Phoenix, AZ, USA*

7.1 Introduction

Seizures are common, and will occur in 10% of the population at some point in their lifetime [1]. Persons who have experienced a seizure will rightly question the cause and the likelihood of future seizures. For the clinician, the diagnostic evaluation should be informed by a knowledge of likely underlying etiologies of seizure activity in a given age group or population. Seizures can occur in response to an acute insult to the central nervous system (CNS), or can by symptomatic of chronic structural or functional disturbances in cerebral cortical function. Seizures can also arise from genetically mediated disorders altering neuronal excitation or inhibition, or may have no identifiable etiology. Establishing the underlying cause will help not only cement the diagnosis of seizure, but will contribute to determination of prognosis and decisions regarding the need for treatment.

7.2 Acute symptomatic seizures

Acute symptomatic seizures result from new and active insults to the CNS including toxic, metabolic, inflammatory, infectious, and structural disturbances

Adult Epilepsy, First Edition. Edited by Gregory D. Cascino and Joseph I. Sirven.

Table 7.1 Selected causes of acute symptomatic seizures

Metabolic
   Hypo- or hyperglycemia
   Hypo- or hypernatremia
   Hypocalcemia
   Uremia
Toxic
   Alcohol intoxication or withdrawal
   Carbon monoxide poisoning
   Illicit drugs (cocaine, amphetamines, PCP)
   Drug withdrawal (barbiturates, benzodiazepines)
   Prescription medications
Cerebral hypoxia
Trauma
   Traumatic brain injury/concussion
   Intracranial surgery (peri-operative)
Cerebrovascular
   Intracerebral hemorrhage
   Subdural hematoma
   Stroke
   Posterior reversible encephalopathy syndrome
   Cerebral venous thrombosis
CNS tumor (presenting symptom or peri-operative)
CNS infection

(Table 7.1). By definition, these seizures must occur in close temporal relationship to the provocative cause. For purposes of epidemiologic studies, proposed time-frame limits are seizures occurring within one week after acute stroke, traumatic, or anoxic brain injury; within 24 hours of acute toxic or metabolic disturbance; or during the course of active CNS infection [2]. Acute symptomatic seizures may also be referred to as provoked or reactive seizures.

Acute symptomatic seizures are not rare and constitute about 40% of all nonfebrile seizures [3]. In population-based studies the observed incidence is 29–39/100 000 person-years [3, 4]. While acute symptomatic seizures can occur at any age, the incidence is greatest in the first year of life and in the elderly [3]. Between 0.5 and 1% of children will have an acute symptomatic seizure, excluding febrile seizure [5].

The etiology of acute symptomatic seizures varies by age. In population-based epidemiologic studies from Rochester, Minnesota the leading causes for acute symptomatic seizures in the first year of life were CNS infection and metabolic derangements [3]. For older children infection and traumatic brain injury (TBI) were the most frequently identified etiology, while for adults 15–34 years of age TBI and alcohol/drug withdrawal were the most common [3]. In adults over 35 years cerebrovascular disease takes the lead and is the proximate cause of more than half of acute symptomatic seizures in the elderly [3]. Other important causes in adults age 35–64 are drug and alcohol withdrawal, TBI, and CNS tumor [3].

Acute symptomatic seizures are distinct from epilepsy and unprovoked seizures both for prognosis and treatment. The acute mortality for a first acute symptomatic seizure is almost nine times greater than that for a first unprovoked seizure [6]. Mortality in the first 30 days after an acute symptomatic seizure is about 20% [6, 7]. Mortality is greatest in elderly patients, and may be as high as 40% in this age group [7]. Not surprisingly, mortality is determined by the underlying etiology rather than seizures themselves. Acute symptomatic seizures are unlikely to recur, unless the provocative cause is recurrent (e.g., repeat episodes of profound hypoglycemia in a brittle diabetic). Compared to someone with a single unprovoked seizure, the patient with a single provoked seizure is 80% less likely to have recurrent events [6]. Because recurrence is unlikely, initiation of long-term anticonvulsant medication is not indicated. Rather, treatment of acute symptomatic seizures is aimed at reversing or removing the underlying cause.

Acute symptomatic seizures in traumatic brain injury

Seizures are a long-recognized complication of TBI. Acute symptomatic seizures from TBI, or postconcussive seizures, are typically defined as those occurring within a week of a head injury. The highest observed incidence is in penetrating head injuries in military combatants. In a cohort of veterans with penetrating head injury in the Vietnam War, over 20% had seizure in the first month (number with seizures in the first week not reported) [8]. For civilians hospitalized with nonpenetrating TBI the observed rates of early seizure range from 3–16.3% [9–12]. In a population-based study of civilian TBI in Rochester, MN from 1935 to 1984, 2.5% of 4541 children and adults had seizure within a month of head injury, all but 16 within the first week [13]. Risk factors for early seizures include increasing severity of head injury, skull fracture, brain contusion, and chronic alcoholism [9, 11]. Seizures may also be more common in children than adults with TBI [9, 10]. Early post-traumatic seizures are an important predictor for the subsequent development of epilepsy [10, 14, 15].

Acute symptomatic seizures in alcohol withdrawal

Alcohol withdrawal seizures are usually generalized tonic-clonic and develop within 48 hours from cessation of drinking. They may be the first or only symptom of alcohol withdrawal syndrome [16, 17]. They are a frequently encountered cause of seizures in the emergency department. In a study of emergency department visits for seizure in the United States based on national survey data, 6.4% were alcohol related [18]. These seizures are most commonly observed on Sunday and Monday after a weekend of heavy alcohol intake [16, 19]. Because alcohol can also provoke seizures in patients with epilepsy or underlying CNS structural abnormalities, it is important to distinguish these cases from seizures purely attributable to alcohol discontinuation alone. Investigation for additional contributing causes is warranted for patients with partial seizures or seizures developing later than 48 hours after cessation of alcohol intake [20].

Acute symptomatic seizures in infectious meningoencephalitis

Provoked seizures are reported in 15–23% of children and adults hospitalized with bacterial meningitis [21–23]. Seizures are more common in patients with alcoholism and with Streptococcus pneumoniae infection [21–23]. Patients with acute seizures have higher short-term mortality than those without seizures during the course of active infection [23]. In survivors of bacterial meningitis, a history of acute early seizures is an important predictor for the subsequent development of epilepsy [24].

For viral encephalitis the incidence of seizures is more difficult to estimate, as many cases have relatively mild symptoms that are unlikely to result in hospitalization and may remain undiagnosed. Among hospitalized patients with viral encephalitis, up to 40% have been observed to have acute symptomatic seizures [25, 26]. Seizures are most common in patients infected with herpes simplex virus or Japanese encephalitis virus, as compared to other forms of viral encephalitis [26]. For herpes simplex virus encephalitis seizures have been reported in 40–60% of hospitalized patients [27, 28]. This high rate likely reflects the preferential involvement of mesial temporal structures by this virus. In Japanese encephalitis seizures have been observed in 46–62% of children and adults in studies from India [28, 29, 78]. For viral encephalitis, as with bacterial meningitis, early seizures again predict the development of epilepsy in survivors [24].

7.3 Febrile seizures

Febrile seizures occur in children aged three months to five years with fever and no demonstrable CNS infection or other defined acute symptomatic cause and no history of unprovoked seizures. They are the most common seizure type in childhood, affecting 2–4% of children [5]. A simple febrile seizure lasts less than 15 minutes, is generalized at onset, and occurs only once in a 24-hour period; if any of these criteria are not met, it is considered a complex febrile seizure. Febrile seizures usually occur early in the course of febrile viral upper respiratory infections, gastroenteritis, urinary tract infection, or otitis media. Febrile seizures are generally benign and self-limited, but are also an important etiology of convulsive status epilepticus in children [30]. Simple febrile seizures indicate a slightly increased risk of later epilepsy (2–3%), while complex febrile seizures imply an even higher risk (5–20%) [30, 31].

Susceptibility to febrile seizures appears to predominantly genetic. Family history of febrile seizures is a strong risk factor, and a high concordance has been observed in twin studies [32–34]. Pre-existing neurologic deficits such as mental retardation or cerebral palsy also increase the risk of developing febrile seizures. For the majority of persons with febrile seizures, the inheritance pattern is polygenic and influenced by environmental factors. Complex segregation analysis of over 400 families in the population of Rochester, MN for probands presenting with febrile seizures between 1935 and 1964 with an affected parent or sibling suggested that a subset exhibit autosomal dominant inheritance with variable penetrance [35]. The single gene susceptibility model applied primarily to children presenting with multiple febrile convulsions [35]. In the subsequent 20 years, several genetic mutations linked to familial febrile seizures have been described. Generalized epilepsy with febrile seizures plus (GEFS+) is characterized by early febrile seizures, generalized and partial seizures with highly variable phenotypic expression and severity within affected families [36]. GEFS+ has been associated with mutations in sodium channel subunit genes SCN1A, SCN1B, SCN9A as well as GABA$_A$ receptor subunit genes GABARG2 and GABARD [37–42]. For other familial febrile seizure types, susceptibility loci without clear single gene mutations have been identified at chromosomes 8q13–q21 (FEB1), 19p13.3 (FEB2), and 2q23–q24 (FEB3) [43–45].

7.4 Unprovoked seizures

Seizures occurring without a clear acute symptomatic etiology are classified as unprovoked. There may be factors which contributed to seizure occurrence, such as sleep deprivation or illness, but by definition these should not be the sole precipitant as is the case with acute symptomatic seizures. The incidence of unprovoked seizures is 57–63/100 000 persons in the population [46–48]. When a person has experienced two or more unprovoked seizures this is classified as epilepsy. The incidence of epilepsy is 46–48/100 000 [46, 47].

Following a comprehensive evaluation, an underlying CNS lesion is identified for approximately 30–40% of unprovoked seizures (Table 7.2). Seizures resulting from a preexisting brain lesion or disorder are classified as remote symptomatic. The remaining seizures are categorized as cryptogenic when a structural cause is suspected but unproven with current technology, or as idiopathic when no cause is identified. Idiopathic seizures are of presumed genetic etiology. The proportion of symptomatic, idiopathic, and cryptogenic cases varies by age group. In young children, up to 80% of unprovoked seizures are idiopathic or cryptogenic [48–50]. The elderly (persons aged 65 years or more) are the only age group in which the majority of new onset unprovoked seizures are symptomatic [46, 48].

Etiologic classification is important in determining prognosis and treatment. Following first unprovoked seizure, many studies have shown recurrence risk is

Table 7.2 Etiologic classification of incident unprovoked seizures and epilepsy in children and adults

	Hauser et al. [46]	Zarelli et al. [51]	Loiseau et al. [52]	Lhatoo et al. [53]	Jallon et al. [54]	Olafsson et al. [48]
Study Location	Rochester, MN	Rochester, MN	Gironde, France	United Kingdom	France	Iceland
Design	Retrospective, population-based	Retrospective, population-based	Prospective, population-based	Prospective, population-based	Prospective, multicenter	Prospective, population-based
# of seizures at enrollment	≥1	≥2	≥1	≥1	≥1	≥1
Time frame	1935–1984	1980–1984	1984–1985	1984–1987	1995–1996	1995–1999
Sample size	880	157	281	481	1942	501
Idiopathic (%)	65	53	37	72	29	14
Cryptogenic	N/A	N/A	21%	N/A	53%	53%
Remote symptomatic (%)	35	47	42	28	18	33

increased for individuals with a clear remote symptomatic cause [1, 55, 56]. Based on a meta-analysis of 16 studies, following an unprovoked first seizure the recurrence risk at two years was 32% (95% CI 28–35%) if the seizure was idiopathic versus 57% (95% CI 51–63%) if remote symptomatic [1]. Persons with remote symptomatic seizures are less likely to enter long-term remission and successfully discontinue AEDs. In a cohort of children followed prospectively from first unprovoked seizure, the two-year remission rate was 35% for remote symptomatic etiology as compared to 67% for idiopathic and 69% for cryptogenic seizures [50]. Long-term mortality is also greater in persons with remote symptomatic seizures compared to idiopathic seizures [52, 53, 57]. The highest observed mortality is in persons with seizures secondary to cerebrovascular disease (Hazard Ratio 2.4), CNS tumor (HR 12.0), and congenital neurologic deficits (HR 10.9) [53].

There have been several large epidemiologic investigations into the causes of symptomatic epilepsies. In a study of epilepsy prevalence in the population of Rochester, MN in 1980 the leading symptomatic etiologies were cerebrovascular disease, TBI, and developmental abnormalities (e.g., congenital brain malformations, hypoxic-ischemic encephalopathy, mental retardation, cerebral palsy) (Figure 7.1) [58]. This study excluded persons with single unprovoked seizures. Since the Rochester study of 1980, the introduction of head imaging with CT and MRI, now in widespread use, could potentially increase the detection of underlying structural abnormalities. However, the reported percentages of symptomatic and idiopathic unprovoked seizures have been remarkably stable (Table 7.2). In a prospective population-based study of newly diagnosed unprovoked single seizures and epilepsy in France in the mid-1990s, Jallon *et al.* identified leading

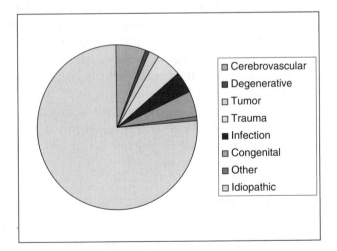

Figure 7.1 Prevalence of epilepsy by etiology in Rochester, MN, 1980. Source: Reproduced from Hauser, Annegers, and Kurland [58], with permission from John Wiley & Sons Ltd.

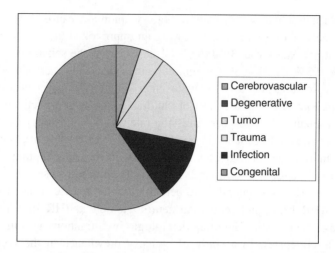

Figure 7.2 Etiology of newly diagnosed remote symptomatic seizures in children, aged 0–14 years; Rochester, MN, 1935–1984. Source: Reproduced from Hauser, Annegers, and Kurland [46], with permission from John Wiley & Sons Ltd.

symptomatic causes as developmental (4.4%), cerebrovascular disease (3.9%), and TBI (3.2%) [54]. The diagnostic evaluation included EEG in 99% and head imaging in 73% of subjects in the French study. In a population-based study from Iceland from the late 1990s, Olafsson *et al.* found 9% of unprovoked seizures were attributable to cerebrovascular disease, 6.6% to degenerative disorders, 5.8% to CNS neoplasm, and 4.6% to TBI [48]. EEG was performed in 89% of these subjects and head imaging in 85%. In developing countries it is likely that CNS infection is a leading cause of unprovoked seizures and epilepsy [59].

Remote symptomatic seizure etiologies also vary by age group. In epidemiologic studies of incidence of unprovoked seizures from Rochester, MN, and Iceland in young children (age 0–14 years) the leading symptomatic cause was developmental (Figure 7.2) [46, 48]. For adults the most commonly encountered causes were TBI, cerebrovascular disease, and CNS neoplasm (Figures 7.3 and 7.4) [46, 48]. In the elderly cerebrovascular disease accounts for two-thirds of all remote symptomatic seizures (Figure 7.5) [46]. Degenerative conditions such as Alzheimer's dementia are the second leading cause of symptomatic seizures in the population of persons aged 65 years or more [45, 48].

Unprovoked seizures after stroke

Many forms of cerebrovascular disease may lead to the development of epilepsy including ischemic and hemorrhagic stroke, subdural hematoma, subarachnoid hemorrhage, vascular malformations, and small vessel ischemic disease. For elderly patients in particular stroke is a major cause of new onset seizures.

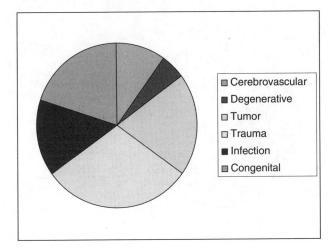

Figure 7.3 Etiology of newly diagnosed remote symptomatic seizures in young adults, aged 15–34 years; Rochester, MN, 1935–1984. Source: Hauser, Annegers, and Kurland [46], with permission from John Wiley & Sons Ltd.

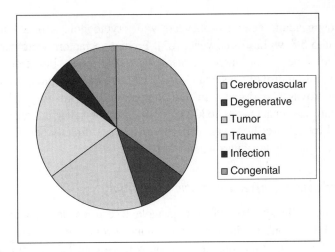

Figure 7.4 Etiology of newly diagnosed remote symptomatic seizures in adults, aged 35–64 years; Rochester, MN, 1935–1984. Source: Hauser, Annegers, and Kurland [46], with permission from John Wiley & Sons, Ltd.

A population-based study from Rochester MN of outcomes after ischemic stroke found 3% with epilepsy at 1 year, reaching 8.9% at 10 years [60]. Predictors of late seizures were early seizures and recurrent stroke [60]. In a more recent prospective multicenter study of acute stroke, seizures were noted 9% of the time, and 2.5% of the time lead to development of epilepsy [61]. In that series seizures were more common in hemorrhagic than ischemic stroke [61]. In a

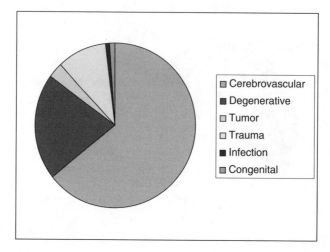

Figure 7.5 Etiology of newly diagnosed remote symptomatic seizures in the elderly, aged 65 years or greater; Rochester, MN, 1935–1984. Source: Hauser, Annegers, and Kurland [46], with permission from John Wiley & Sons, Ltd.

study of young adults aged 18–55 years with cryptogenic stroke, later seizures developed in 5.5% within three years [62]. Predictive factors were early seizure, cortical involvement, and large hemispheric stroke [62]. For elderly patients development of unprovoked seizures may be the first symptom of underlying chronic cerebrovascular disease. In this population head imaging will frequently reveal "silent" vascular lesions [63, 64]. Long-term mortality is greater for stroke complicated by seizure; however, the mortality is not directly seizure-related but reflects severity of underlying disease [61].

Unprovoked seizures after traumatic brain injury

Post-traumatic epilepsy, defined as unprovoked seizures developing a week or more after TBI, is one of the more commonly encountered etiologies of symptomatic seizures. With improved survival following severe TBI in both civilian and military populations, and with increasing numbers of veterans of recent military conflicts with TBI, it seems likely that the incidence of post-traumatic epilepsy will increase in the future. In military veterans with penetrating head trauma, the incidence of post-traumatic epilepsy is 30–50% [8, 15]. Most will manifest within the first year, but risk remains elevated even 15 years out from the initial injury [8]. For civilians with nonpenetrating TBI, late seizures develop in 2–25% [10, 12, 13]. In a recent large retrospective population-based study from Norway on TBI in children and young adults, as compared to general population the relative risk of epilepsy was 2.2 after mild TBI and 7.4 after severe TBI [65]. The risk of epilepsy is related to the severity of brain injury, and predicted by impaired consciousness at presentation, skull fracture, and early seizures [10, 13, 65].

Genetic basis of idiopathic epilepsies

Idiopathic epilepsies are presumed to have a genetic basis. For the majority of idiopathic epilepsies inheritance is complex, reflecting polygenetic, and environmental factors. Additional complexity arises in that multiple mutations may present with the same clinical phenotype, while a single gene mutation may have multiple phenotypic expressions. Despite these challenges, over the last decade there have been significant strides made in the understanding of genetic epilepsy syndromes. Study of select families with high penetrance, autosomal dominant epilepsies has allowed identification of a group of monogenetic disorders (Table 7.3). All are channelopathies with the exception of EF-hand domain containing 1 (EFHC1), which is proposed to effect the activity of voltage-gated calcium channels, and leucine-rich glioma inactivated gene 1 (LGI1), which influences seizure susceptibility in familial lateral temporal lobe epilepsy by an unknown mechanism [66, 67]. The

Table 7.3 Selected familial idiopathic epilepsy syndromes with monogenetic autosomal dominant inheritance

Syndrome	Gene	References
Benign familial neonatal seizures	KCNQ2	Singh et al. [68], Biervert et al. [69]
	KCNQ3	Charlier et al. [70]
Benign familial neonatal-infantile seizures	SCN2A	Heron et al. [71], Berkovic et al. [72]
GEFS+	SCN1A	Wallace et al. [37]
	SCN1B	Baulac et al. [38]
	SCN9A	Singh et al. [42]
	GABARG2	Baulac et al. [40]
	GABARD	Dibbens et al. [41]
Severe myoclonic epilepsy of infancy	SCN1A	Claes et al. [73]
Autosomal dominant lateral temporal lobe epilepsy	LGI1	Ottman et al. [66]
Autosomal dominant nocturnal frontal lobe epilepsy	CHRNA2	Aridon et al. [74]
	CHRNA4	Steinlein et al. [75]
	CHRNB2	DeFusco et al. [76]
Juvenile myoclonic epilepsy	GABAR1	Cossette et al. [77]
	EFHC1	Suzuki et al. [67]

KCNQ: potassium channel, KQT-like, subunit; SCN: sodium channel subunit; GABAR: GABA$_A$ receptor subunit; LGI: leucine-rich glioma inactivated gene; CHRN: nicotinic acetylcholine receptor subunit; EFHC: EF-hand domain containing.

identification of causative genes for epilepsy opens the door for genetic testing in highly selected patients. Such testing may facilitate improved prognosis as well having genetic implications for other family members. Increased understanding of epilepsy genetics in the future is likely to significantly impact how we diagnose, conceptualize, and treat both familial as well as sporadic idiopathic epilepsies.

References

1. Berg, A.T. and Shinnar, S. (1991) The risk of seizure recurrence following a first unprovoked seizure: a quantitative review. *Neurology*, **41**, 964–972.
2. Beghi, E., Carpio, A., Forsgren, L. *et al.* (2009) Recommendation for a definition of acute symptomatic seizure. *Epilepsia* Sep 3 [Epub ahead of print].
3. Annegers, J.F., Hauser, W.A., Lee, R.J., and Rocca, W.A. (1995) Incidence of acute symptomatic seizures in Rochester, Minnesota: 1935–1984. *Epilepsia*, **35**, 327–333.
4. Loiseau, J., Loiseau, P., Guyot, M. *et al.* (1990) Survey of seizure disorders in the French Southwest. I. Incidence of epileptic syndromes. *Epilepsia*, **31**, 391–396.
5. Hauser, W.A. (1994) The prevalence and incidence of convulsive disorders in children. *Epilepsia*, **35** (Suppl 2), S1–S6.
6. Hesdorffer, D.C., Benn, E.K., Cascino, G.D., and Hauser, W.A. (2009) Is a first acute symptomatic seizure epilepsy? Mortality and risk for recurrent seizure. *Epilepsia*, **50** (5), 1102–1108.
7. Hesdorffer, D.C. and D'Amelio, M. (2005) Mortality in the first 30 days following incident acute symptomatic seizures. *Epilepsia*, **46** (Suppl 1), 43–45.
8. Salazar, A.M., Jabbari, B., Vance, S.C. *et al.* (1985) Epilepsy after penetrating head injury. I. Clinical correlates: a report of the Vietnam Head Injury Study. *Neurology*, **35**, 1406–1414.
9. Desai, B.T., Whitman, S., Coonley-Hoganson, R. *et al.* (1983) Seizures and civilian head injury. *Epilepsia*, **24**, 289–296.
10. Asikainen, I., Kaste, M., and Sarna, S. (1999) Early and late posttraumatic seizures in traumatic brain injury rehabilitation patients: brain injury factors causing late seizures and influence of seizures on long-term outcome. *Epilepsia*, **40**, 584–589.
11. Wiedemayer, H., Triesch, K., Schafer, H., and Stolke, D. (2002) Early seizures following non-penetrating traumatic brain injury in adults: risk factors and clinical significance. *Brain Injury*, **16**, 323–330.
12. Englander, J., Bushnik, T., Duong, T.T. *et al.* (2003) Analyzing risk factors for late posttraumatic seizures: a prospective, multicenter investigation. *Arch Phys Med Rehabil*, **84**, 365–373.
13. Annegers, J.F., Hauser, W.A., Coan, S.P., and Rocca, W.A. (1998) A population-based study of seizures after traumatic brain injuries. *N Engl J Med*, **338**, 20–24.
14. Annegers, J., Grabow, J., Groover, R. *et al.* (1980) Seizures after head trauma: a population study. *Neurology*, **30**, 683–689.
15. Aarabi, B., Taghipour, M., Haghnegahdar, A. *et al.* (2000) Prognostic factors in the occurrence of posttraumatic epilepsy after penetrating head injury suffered during military service. *Neurosurg Focus*, **8**, e1.
16. Hillbom, M.E. (1990) Occurrence of cerebral seizures provoked by alcohol abuse. *Epilepsia*, **21**, 459–466.
17. Rathlev, N.K., Ulrich, A.S., Fish, S.S., and D'Onofrio, G. (2000) Clinical characteristics as predictors of recurrent alcohol-related seizures. *Acad Emerg Med*, **7**, 866–891.

18. Pallin, D.J., Goldstein, J.N., Moussally, J.S. *et al.* (2008) Seizure visits in U.S. emergency departments: epidemiology and potential disparities in care. *Int J Emerg Med*, **1**, 97–105.

19. Rathlev, N.K., Ulrich, A., Shieh, T. *et al.* (2002) Etiology and weekly occurrence of alcohol-related seizures. *Acad Emerg Med*, **9**, 824–828.

20. The ENFS Task Force on Diagnosis and Treatment of Alcohol-Related Seizures: Brathen, G., Ben-Menachem, E., Brodtkorb, E. *et al.* (2005) EFNS guidelines on the diagnosis and management of alcohol-related seizures: report on an EFNS task force. *Eur J Neurol*, **12**, 575–581.

21. Durand, M.L., Calderwood, S.B., Weber, D.J. *et al.* (1993) Acute bacterial meningitis in adults—a review of 493 episodes. *N Engl J Med*, **328**, 21–28.

22. Van de Beek, D., de Gans, J., Spanjaard, L. *et al.* (2004) Clinical features and prognostic factors in adults with bacterial meningitis. *N Engl J Med*, **351**, 1849–1859.

23. Zoons, E., Weisfelt, M., de Gans, J. *et al.* (2008) Seizures in adults with bacterial meningitis. *Neurology*, **70**, 2109–2115.

24. Annegers, J.F., Hauser, W.A., Beghi, E. *et al.* (1988) The risk of unprovoked seizures after encephalitis and meningitis. *Neurology*, **38**, 1407–1410.

25. Kim, M.A., Park, K.M., Kim, S.E., and Oh, M.K. (2008) Acute symptomatic seizures in CNS infection. *Eur J Neurol*, **15**, 38–41.

26. Misra, U.K. and Kalita, J. (2009) Seizures in encephalitis: predictors and outcome. *Seizure*, **18**, 583–587.

27. McGrath, N., Anderson, N.E., Croxson, M.C., and Powell, K.F. (1997) Herpes simplex virus encephalitis treated with acyclovir: diagnosis and long term outcome. *J Neurol Neurosurg Psychiatry*, **63**, 321–326.

28. Hsieh, W.B., Chiu, N.C., Hu, K.C. *et al.* (2007) Outcome of herpes simplex encephalitis in children. *J Microbiol Immunol Infect*, **40**, 34–38.

29. Kalita, J., Misra, U.K., Pandey, S., and Dhole, N. (2003) A comparison of clinical and radiological findings in adults and children with Japanese encephalitis. *Arch Neurol*, **60**, 1760–1764.

30. Shinnar, S. and Glauser, T.A. (2002) Febrile seizures. *J Child Neurol*, **17**, S44–S52.

31. Annegers, J.F., Hauser, W.A., Shirts, S.B., and Kurland, L.T. (1987) Factors prognostic of unprovoked seizures after febrile convulsions. *N Engl J Med*, **316**, 493–498.

32. Corey, L.A., Berg, K., Pellock, J.M. *et al.* (1991) The occurrence of epilepsy and febrile seizures in Virginian and Norwegian twins. *Neurology*, **41**, 1433–1436.

33. Bethune, P., Gordon, K.G., Dooley, J.M. *et al.* (1993) Which child will have a febrile seizure? *Am J Dis Child*, **147**, 35–39.

34. Berg, A.T., Shinnar, S., Shapiro, E.D. *et al.* (1995) Risk factors for a first febrile seizure—a matched case control study. *Epilepsia*, **36**, 334–341.

35. Rich, S.S., Annegers, J.F., Hauser, W.A., and Anderson, V.E. (1987) Complex segregation analysis of febrile convulsions. *Am J Hum Genet*, **41**, 249–257.

36. Scheffer, I.E. and Berkovic, S.F. (1997) Generalized epilepsy with febrile seizures plus. A genetic disorder with heterogeneous clinical phenotypes. *Brain*, **120**, 479–490.

37. Wallace, R.H., Wang, D.W., Singh, R. *et al.* (1998) Febrile seizures and generalized epilepsy associated with a mutation in the Na+ channel beta1 subunit gene SCN1B. *Nat Genet*, **19**, 366–370.

38. Baulac, S., Gourfinkel-An, I., Picard, F. *et al.* (1999) A second locus for familial generalized epilepsy with febrile seizures plus maps to chromosome 2q21-q33. *Am J Hum Genet*, **65**, 1078–1085.

39. Moulard, B., Guipponi, M., Chaigne, D. *et al.* (1999) Identification of a new locus for generalized epilepsy with febrile seizures plus on chromosome 2q24-q33. *Am J Hum Genet*, **65**, 1396–1400.

40. Baulac, S., Huberfeld, G., Gourfinkel-An, I. *et al.* (2001) First genetic evidence of GABA(A) receptor dysfunction in epilepsy: a mutation in the gamma2-subunit gene. *Nat Genet*, **28**, 46–68.

41. Dibbens, L.M., Feng, H.J., Richards, M.C. *et al.* (2004) GABRD encoding a protein for extra- or peri-synaptic GABAA receptors is a susceptibility locus for generalized epilepsies. *Hum Mol Genet*, **13**, 1315–1319.

42. Singh, N.A., Pappas, C., Dahle, E.J. *et al.* (2009) A role of SCN9A in human epilepsies, as a cause of febrile seizures and as a potential modifier of Dravet Syndrome. *PLoS Genet*, **5**, e10000649 [Epub].

43. Wallace, R.H., Berkovic, S.F., Howell, R.A. *et al.* (1996) Suggestion of a major gene for familial febrile convulsions mapping to 8q13-21. *J Med Genet*, **33**, 308–312.

44. Johnson, E.W., Dubovsky, J., Rich, S.S. *et al.* (1998) Evidence for a novel gene for familial febrile convulsions, FEB2, linked to chromosome 19p in an extended family from the Midwest. *Hum Mol Genet*, **7**, 63–67.

45. Peiffer, A., Thompson, J., Charlier, C. *et al.* (1999) A locus for febrile seizures (FEB3) maps to chromosome 2q23-24. *Ann Neurol*, **46**, 671–678.

46. Hauser, W.A., Annegers, J.F., and Kurland, L.T. (1993) Incidence of epilepsy and unprovoked seizures in Rochester, Minnesota: 1935–1984. *Epilepsia*, **34**, 453–468.

47. MacDonald, B.K., Cockerell, O.C., Sander, J.W., and Shorvon, S.D. (2000) The incidence and lifetime prevalence of neurologic disorders in a prospective community-based study in the UK. *Brain*, **123**, 665–676.

48. Olafsson, E., Ludvigsson, P., Gudmundsson, G. *et al.* (2005) Incidence of unprovoked seizures and epilepsy in Iceland and assessment of the epilepsy syndrome classification: a prospective study. *Lancet Neurol*, **4**, 6 27–634.

49. Sander, J.W., Hart, Y.M., Johson, A.L., and Shorvon, S.C. for the NGPSE (1990) National General Practice Study of Epilepsy: newly diagnosed epileptic seizures in a general population. *Lancet*, **336**, 1267–1271.

50. Shinnar, S., O'Dell, C., and Berg, A.T. (1999) Distribution of epilepsy syndromes in a cohort of children prospectively monitored from the time of their first unprovoked seizure. *Epilepsia*, **40**, 1378–1383.

51. Zarelli, M.M., Beghi, E., Rocca, W.A., and Hauser, W.A. (1999) Incidence of epileptic syndromes in Rochester, Minnesota: 1980–1984. *Epilepsia*, **40**, 1708–1714.

52. Loiseau, P., Loiseau, J., and Picot, M.C. (2005) One-year mortality in Bordeaux cohort: the value of syndrome classification. *Epilepsia*, **46** (Suppl 11), 11–14.

53. Lhatoo, S.D., Johnson, A.L., Goodridge, D.M. *et al.* (2001) Mortality in epilepsy in the first 11 to 14 years after diagnosis: multivariate analysis of a long-term, prospective, population-based cohort. *Ann Neurol*, **49**, 336–344.

54. Jallon, P., Loiseau, P., Loiseau, J., on behalf of Group CAROLE (2001) Newly diagnosed unprovoked epileptic seizures: presentation at diagnosis in CAROLE study. *Epilepsia*, **42**, 464–475.

55. Camfield, P., Camfield, C., Dooley, J. *et al.* (1989) A randomized study of carbamazepine versus no medication after a first unprovoked seizure in childhood. *Neurology*, **39**, 851–852.

56. Musicco, M., Beghi, E., Solari, A., and Viani, F. (1997) Treatment of first tonic-clonic seizure does not improve the prognosis of epilepsy. First Seizure Trial Group (FIRST Group). *Neurology*, **49**, 991–998.

57. Cockerell, O.C., Johnson, A.L., Sander, J.W., and Shorvon, S.D. (1997) Prognosis of epilepsy: a review and further analysis of the first nine years of the British National General Practice Study of Epilepsy, a prospective population-based study. *Epilepsia*, **38**, 31–46.

58. Hauser, W.A., Annegers, J.F., and Kurland, L.T. (1991) Prevalence of epilepsy in Rochester, Minnesota: 1940–1980. *Epilepsia*, **32**, 429–445.

59. Singh, G. and Prabhakar, S. (2008) The association between central nervous system (CNS) infections and epilepsy: epidemiological approaches and microbiological and epileptological perspectives. *Epilepsia*, **49** (Suppl 6), 2–7.

60. So, E.L., Annegers, J.F., Hauser, W.A. *et al.* (1996) Population-based study of seizure disorders after cerebral infarction. *Neurology*, **46**, 350–355.

61. Bladin, C.F., Alexandrov, A.V., Bellavance, A. *et al.* (2000) Seizure after stroke. A prospective multicenter study. *Arch Neurol*, **57**, 1617–1622.

62. Lamy, C., Domigo, V., Semah, F. *et al.* (2003) Early and late seizures after cryptogenic ischemic stroke in young adults. *Neurology*, **60**, 400–404.

63. Sung, C.Y. and Chu, N.S. (1990) Epileptic seizures in thrombotic stroke. *J Neurol*, **237**, 166–170.

64. Shorvon, S.D., Illiatt, R.W., Cox, T.C., and Yu, Y.L. (1984) Evidence of vascular disease from CT scanning in late onset epilepsy. *J Neurol Neurosurg Psychiatry*, **47**, 225–230.

65. Christensen, J., Pedersen, M.G., Pedersen, C.B. *et al.* (2009) Long-term risk of epilepsy after traumatic brain injury in children and young adults: a population-based cohort study. *Lancet*, **373**, 1105–1110.

66. Ottman, R., Winawer, M.R., Kalachikov, S. *et al.* (2004) LGI1 mutations in autosomal dominant partial epilepsy with auditory features. *Neurology*, **62**, 1120–1126.

67. Suzuki, T., Delgado-Escueta, A., Aguan, K. *et al.* (2004) Mutations in EFHC1 cause juvenile myoclonic epilepsy. *Nat Genet*, **36**, 842–849.

68. Singh, N.A., Charlier, C., Stauffer, D. *et al.* (1998) A novel potassium channel gene, KCNQ2, is mutated in an inherited epilepsy of newborns. *Nat Genet*, **18**, 25–29.

69. Biervert, C., Schroeder, B.C., Kubisch, D. *et al.* (1998) A potassium channel mutation in neonatal human epilepsy. *Science*, **279**, 403–406.

70. Charlier, C., Singh, N.A., Ryan, S.G. *et al.* (1998) A pore mutation in a novel KQT-like potassium channel gene in an idiopathic epilepsy family. *Nat Genet*, **18**, 53–55.

71. Heron, S.E., Crossland, K.M., Andermann, E. *et al.* (2002) Sodium-channel defects in benign familial neonatal-infantile seizures. *Lancet*, **360**, 851–852.

72. Berkovic, S.F., Heron, S.E., Giordano, L. *et al.* (2004) Benign familial neonatal-infantile seizures: characterization of a new sodium channelopathy. *Ann Neurol*, **55**, 550–557.

73. Claes, L., Del-Favero, J., Ceulemans, B. *et al.* (2001) De novo mutations in the sodium-channel gene SCN1A cause severe myoclonic epilepsy of infancy. *Am J Hum Genet*, **68**, 1327–1332.

74. Aridon, P., Marini, C., Di Resta, C. *et al.* (2006) Increased sensitivity of the neuronal nicotinic receptor alpha-2 subunit causes familial epilepsy with nocturnal wandering and ictal fear. *Am J Hum Genet*, **79**, 342–350.

75. Steinlein, O.K., Mulley, J.C., Propping, P. *et al.* (1995) A missense mutation in the neuronal nicotinic acetylcholine receptor alpha-4 subunit is associated with autosomal dominant nocturnal frontal lobe epilepsy. *Nat Genet*, **11**, 201–203.

76. De Fusco, M., Becchetti, A., Patrignani, A. *et al.* (2000) The nicotinic receptor beta-2 subunit is mutant in nocturnal frontal lobe epilepsy. *Nat Genet*, **26**, 275–276.

77. Cossette, P., Liu, L., Brisebois, K. *et al.* (2002) Mutation of GABRA1 in an autosomal dominant form of juvenile myoclonic epilepsy. *Nat Genet*, **31**, 184–189.

78. Misra, U.K. and Kalita, J. (2001) Seizures in Japanese encephalitis. *J Neurol Sci*, **190**, 57–60.

8 The evaluation of nonepileptic paroxysmal events

Joseph F. Drazkowski and Matthew Hoerth

Division of Epilepsy, Mayo Clinic Arizona, Phoenix, AZ, USA

8.1 Introduction

Making the correct diagnosis of the etiology of recurrent episodes of altered consciousness has important implications for the patient in question, the family members, and society. This chapter will cover adults who have episodic spells that could be considered to be possible seizures. Recurrent spells of altered consciousness are often a diagnostic challenge, especially if they are infrequent, occur on an irregular basis and are random/unpredictable, which describes most events of this type. The uncertainty that is associated with events of this type often does not allow for routine investigations to monitor or capture a typical event within a limited time frame dictated by the nature of such testing. The consequences that seizure-like events have on other spheres of life include difficulties with job performance (especially potentially hazardous jobs), social situations, recreational activities, and driving [1]. Social situations affected include difficulties with school performance, obtaining insurance benefits, and personal interaction with other family members, colleagues, and professors [2, 3]. The differential

Adult Epilepsy, First Edition. Edited by Gregory D. Cascino and Joseph I. Sirven.
© 2011 John Wiley & Sons, Ltd. Published 2011 by John Wiley & Sons, Ltd.

Table 8.1   Typical differential diagnosis of seizure-like events

Syncope
Transient ischemic attack
Transient global amnesia
Episodic vertigo
Sleep disorders
Seizure disorder
Psychiatric conditions
Nonepileptic seizures

diagnosis for transient neurologic events is outlined in Table 8.1, which includes the common etiologies of seizure-like events that could be mistaken for seizures or epilepsy.

A detailed history and physical examination remains crucial in arriving at a diagnosis for these conditions. The careful taking of a moment-by-moment history of the event by health care providers often leads to the ultimate diagnosis. However, the ability to obtain accurate histories from patients who have altered consciousness as part of their events is usually incomplete. Reliable witnesses to such events are also utilized in gathering data, but they are not usually medically trained observers. The events in question are generally dramatic, and often complex leading to a lack of details by witnesses. The person observing the spell or event is often scared and emotional that their colleague, friend, or loved-one has succumbed to what is often described as a dramatic event. The history and physical are supplemented by a directed evaluation of appropriate medical tests, generally depending on what clues may be ascertained during the initial evaluation. Depending on the nature of the specific complaints, this may allow for a more focused approach. Often, despite best efforts during an out-patient workup, as noted below, the patient with seizure-like events remains a mystery for extended periods of time.

When the diagnosis of episodic neurologic events is unclear, an Epilepsy Monitoring Unit (EMU) (continuous video-EEG monitoring unit) remains a critical tool in the ascertainment of the ultimate diagnosis. It is often argued that the events in question may not be numerous enough to justify the cost and social inconvenience of an admission to the EMU. However, as noted in a paper by Blum *et al.* [4], the number of events reported by the patient with the condition is often very misleading and typically under-reported. The under-reporting is largely due to the memory impairment that is often associated with these events, unnoticed events arising from sleep or the event being subtle. The under-reporting can be 50% or much higher as presented in this study, often depending on which hemisphere is involved for epilepsy. In our EMU, other conditions associated with similar impairment of consciousness are also poorly recalled by the patient. It is interesting to note also that when one evaluates a person with seizure-like events, admission to the EMU often helps make a diagnosis in a majority of patients, but also has an impact on the ultimate diagnosis. The diagnosis of seizure is made in the outpatient clinic, it is changed to another diagnosis such as nonepileptic seizures of physiologic seizure in approximately 25% of cases [5]. The reverse is also true when a person is thought to have pseudoseizures or psychogenic nonepileptic seizures (PNESs), they ultimately turn out to have an alternate diagnosis 25% of the time. Although patients admitted to the EMU represent a highly selected population that has been difficult to diagnose, including those who have not responded to treatment. Making the correct diagnosis or a change in diagnosis is meaningful for all concerned, especially if the spells are impacting the person's quality of life. In this chapter, we will explore the differential diagnosis for spells of uncertain etiology, looking at individual potential mimickers of seizures and epilepsy, and provide some clinical clues to assist the practitioner in making the ultimate correct diagnosis.

8.2 Syncope

The history does matter significantly with regard to diagnosing syncope. Syncope, like epilepsy, can be very dramatic, presenting with a sudden onset of altered consciousness usually followed by a loss of postural tone resulting in the subject hitting the floor or slumping over in a chair. A detailed history is often quite helpful in making the diagnosis and at times is sufficient to come to a correct conclusion [6]. Clues favoring the diagnosis of syncope are outlined in Table 8.2. There are many subtypes of syncope and a detailed examination of all of these is beyond the scope of this text; however, a cardiovascular etiology causing syncope has an extraordinarily high mortality of 30% at one year [7, 8]. Syncope remains a very common reason for admission to the Emergency Department, with about 3% of total admissions being seen in the Emergency Room due to a syncopal

Table 8.2 Features of the history favoring syncope events

Events provoked by pain

Prior history of acute myocardial infarction due to coronary artery disease or documented cardiac arrhythmia history

Position of the subject at the onset of the event (e.g., standing with all events)

Events triggered by a bodily function such as bowel movement or urination

Events triggered by specific situations such as after eating (postprandial) or haircutting

Triggering of events by exertion or exercise

Very brief duration (seconds versus minutes)

Rapid recovery with little altered consciousness postictally

History of palpitations prior to event

Either complaint of warmth, nausea, or sweats prior to the event

An observation of a flaccid fall to the ground by witnesses

---

event [9]. A patient's age may help in the determination of what type of syncope a person suffers from as syncope in younger people is more associated with a vaso-vagal etiology. A rapid drop in blood pressure due to an external stimulus would be an example of such an etiology. Older patients tend to have more of a cardiac arrhythmia associated syncope [7, 10]. It also should be kept in mind that the elderly may have only partial symptoms or atypical features that can be confusing and poorly described by the patient. An example of this would be a patient suffering from an arrhythmia, complaining of lightness or "butterflies" in the chest with a near syncope but not actual blacking out. Other symptoms such a sensation of feeling unsteady could be associated with presyncope [7, 10]. At times, these nonspecific symptoms can easily mimic other potential etiologies in the differential diagnosis including seizures.

Unfortunately, syncope can easily be mistaken for seizures as there is a fairly high percentage of syncope that is associated with abnormal movements. When the perfusion to the brain is reduced, convulsive, or twitching-type muscle activity can be observed and is referred to as "convulsive syncope" [11, 12]. Untrained witnesses will describe jerking or twitching of extremities and facial muscles during the event associated with loss of consciousness, potentially resulting in the diagnosis of convulsive epilepsy rather than syncope [13]. Even tongue biting and incontinence can be seen during syncopal events. Syncope has potentially important implications, especially when coexistent with preexisting medical conditions. Sudden falls due to syncope can cause head injury, fractures, or other traumatic injury, which can be quite disabling to the elderly. A careful moment-by-moment history and focused workup often leads to the diagnosis. During the event, it may be very helpful for bystanders to obtain blood pressure, heart rate, and blood sugar measurements if possible to help define the etiology of the events. The immediate measurement of vital signs during the event is unlikely even if equipment is readily available. Typically reliable evaluations are not made until the paramedics arrive minutes later at which time the patient physiology may normalize. Often syncopal events are fairly infrequent and typically brief in duration, making the chance of reliably recording physiologic data during an event rare.

Elements on the interictal physical exam that may be helpful in making the diagnosis of syncope could be a positive bedside orthostatic hypotension measurement. An irregular pulse on cardiac auscultation and pulse check for irregularity may also provide an insight into the diagnosis. A cardiac outflow murmur consistent with aortic stenosis or if an exam shows signs of congestive heart failure may also be important in the evaluation process. One item that may not often be considered is that of polypharmacy. Many of the elderly patients are on multiple medications that have potential to produce syncope; especially antihypertensives and medications that have a cardiovascular vascular effect. Carotid hypersensitivity is one of those issues that we suspect is mostly seen in the cardiac clinic, which occurs in the elderly due to atherosclerotic disease of the carotid sinus area. These events are triggered by carotid massage such as during shaving or other neck manipulation. This is defined as either a vasodepressor type where there is a drop of at least 50 mmHg in the systolic blood pressure or a cardioinhibitory response with associated asystole lasting more than three seconds. There are also patients that have a combination of both vasodepressor and cardioinhibitory syncope. Orthostasis due to an inadequate vasoconstriction response, whether this is due to medication, dehydration, or a blunted response due to an autonomic neuropathy, also can be part of the picture and should be looked for, especially in older patients [7].

The workup for syncope should include a 12-lead EKG, which is relatively cheap and if positive, an effective tool for evaluating these patients. Bradycardia, conduction blocks, and prolonged QT interval may be symptoms found during this simple bedside test. An echocardiogram is helpful for structural problems related to the heart that may produce transient altered consciousness. Valvular heart disease, particularly aortic stenosis, can easily be picked up on an echocardiogram. A cardiomyopathy or pericardial effusion would also be typically detected on this test, which can reduce cardiac outflow. A tilt table test should often be considered, especially if there is any hint that the spells themselves may have a positional component to them, that is, they only occur while sitting or standing. The tilt table is fairly sensitive for orthostatic changes. Bedside carotid massage has been used in the past and can be sensitive for diagnosing carotid hypersensitivity syndrome; it is generally left to our cardiology colleagues to perform this procedure. Long-term EKG monitoring is indicated for those patients who have prolonged intervals between spells or spells that occur at odd times [14]. The long-term monitoring can be basic as far as the initial evaluation is concerned with, perhaps, a 24-hour monitoring. But, often these events do not occur on a daily basis. An event monitor or implanted loop recorder may be more sensitive and specific for a rare event. Ambulatory blood pressure monitoring is available and may provide a clue if there is quite labile blood pressure during the monitoring period, which is typically 24 hours. If an arrhythmia is suspected of a malignant variety, it probably would be safer and wiser for inpatient monitoring to avoid any potential for sudden death, although this is basically a judgment call.

8.3 Transient ischemic events (TIAs)

The definition of what constitutes a TIA is changing from the old Definition of 24-hour reversible neurologic deficit due a vascular etiology, to a shorter duration definition where the event lasts minutes to hours. This change has been motivated in part by the advent of available thrombolytic agents that potentially minimize the devastating effects of strokes with early intervention. The change in duration to a shorter time period of these essentially reversible events crosses into the territory where seizures could be considered in the differential diagnosis. Seizures usually last minutes and not hours, and typically have positive symptoms versus negative symptoms associated with vascular events. A prolonged postictal deficit could easily be mistaken for an ischemic event lasting hours. Strokes themselves can generally be divided into anterior and posterior circulation for the means of this discussion. An anterior circulation stroke does not usually produce loss of awareness, but could potentially produce a brief aphasia, which to an untrained observer could be mistaken for a complex partial seizure. As a reminder, typically the stroke or TIA victim has a loss of function with the event, whereas a seizure produces a so-called positive phenomenon with increased function in the central nervous system such as automatisms, paresthesias, or visual changes [15]. This distinction between positive and negative symptomology can be helpful in distinguishing between seizure and TIA. Limb-shaking TIA is a condition that could certainly produce confusion between the two diagnoses. This event is considered to be a focal dysfunction due to a focal loss of blood supply near the motor strip, causing abnormal movements in the area of perfusion that is compromised [16]. Typically this abnormal movement is rhythmic postural in nature.

Vascular events occurring in the posterior circulation may produce altered consciousness, but when this occurs the events are associated with the signs or symptoms related to the brainstem dysfunction, such as vertigo, diplopia, facial weakness, dysarthria, dysphasia, or other similar symptoms which may provide clues to the diagnosis. The time course noted is generally longer for TIA compared to a partial seizure, but brief periods of loss of consciousness have been described with vertebral basilar insufficiency. It should be kept in mind that patients who have had a previous stroke have a higher likelihood of later developing epilepsy, with 9% of stroke victims developing seizures at nine months [17].

8.4 Transient global amnesia (TGA)

These events typically occur in middle-aged patients often those who are traveling or if they are undergoing stress. The hallmark of the disorder is retrograde amnesia without focal signs or symptoms. The patient remains awake but usually loses orientation to place and time, and without loss of identity. The transient global amnesia (TGA) begins suddenly in a person who is seemingly healthy moments just prior to the event. The typical TGA attack lasts less than 24 hours with the majority lasting between one and eight hours. Confusion and disorientation is reported by the patient during the spell, with the patient typically repeating the same question over and over, having just forgotten the answer even if this was just provided to them as a result of not being able to encode new information. Despite these ongoing cognitive deficits, the victim is still able to do typical activities of daily living. Once the attack resolves, there is no memory for events that occurred to them during the affected period. The etiology of these events has not been definitively understood, but reports of reversible involvement of hippocampus on MRI have been noted [18]. Usually, during these events the general physical exam and the vital signs remain normal. The neurological physical exam is otherwise normal without focal neurologic dysfunction; without weakness, sensory changes, or ataxia. An emergent EEG completed during these events is normal. The majority of TGA events are not recurrent, with less than 25% chance of recurrence [15, 19, 20]. Cases of TGA that do recur may be confused for partial epilepsy. There currently is no definitive preventive measure or therapy that has been reported for TGA. When workup is sufficiently negative for other potential causes, TGA patients should simply be counseled regarding the relative low risk of recurrence and reassured that this is not associated with other serious medical conditions.

8.5 Movement disorders

Common movement disorders such as Parkinson's disease, essential tremor, and chorea typically are more continuous in nature and as such usually do not present a significant diagnostic dilemma. The typical movement disorders that could be confused for seizures would be episodic in nature. The continuous nature of typical movement disorders makes them relatively easy to distinguish from seizures. One condition that may have the potential to mimic an epileptic attack would be hemifacial spasm. When active, the abnormal movements tend to be prolonged in duration and thus have the potential to be confused for a focal simple partial seizure. Hemifacial spasms often have somewhat variable intensity and may wax and wane for longer periods of time compared to a typical simple partial seizure lasting seconds to minutes, often evolving and resolving in a stereotypic manner. Depending on the location of the seizure focus, an EEG obtained during a simple partial seizure may or may not display an abnormality especially [21, 22] if the seizure focus is distant to the surface electrodes, as typically utilized during the routine EEG, and no EEG correlate is seen, an incorrect diagnosis could be made. Occasionally, myoclonus of a noncortical etiology can also potentially mimic seizures with its transient muscle activity also not having an EEG correlate on standard testing. Specialized movement disorder studies can help distinguish nonepileptic myoclonus from seizure [23].

8.6 Sleep disorders

Sleep disorders are generally easier to discern from seizure-like events after taking a proper history. However, sometimes with incomplete information or an atypical presentation, they could be mistaken for seizures. Excessive daytime sleepiness is a major complaint of most sleep disorders and screening the patient with Epworth Sleepiness Scale may be helpful in providing clues to the nature of transient events. It should be reminded that narcolepsy has characteristic features of excessive daytime sleepiness, but one of the features of narcolepsy could include cataplexy.

Cataplexy could potentially mimic seizures to the untrained eye in that the person typically falls to the ground due to lack of muscle control, which is precipitated by emotions, either good or bad. The connection between the trigger of emotionality is often felt to be functional, but is readily apparent once the association is made. Cataplexy would be extremely uncommon and is not considered in the differential. The diagnosis is made by running a sleep study and recording typical features of narcolepsy on polysomnography [24], including a multiple sleep latency test including at least two out of five naps that demonstrate REM sleep onset within 15 minutes.

Another form of sleep disorder, which could potentially be confused with seizures are the parasomnias, particularly REM behavior disorder. This is a condition where the patient is unable to inhibit motor movements that are typically suppressed during REM sleep. During an episode, the patient is said to act out their dreams and will do nonsensical motor activities while basically asleep, such as walking, running, or inappropriate behavior. Injuries do occur during these attacks and unless there is a witness, the patient may report not knowing how the injuries were sustained. The motor activity that occurs during the attack can be rather dramatic and appear violent [25]. A helpful feature in the history that may help differentiate this from seizures is that seizures are usually stereotypic, whereas REM enactment behavior may vary slightly in semiology and be potentially more complex. REM behavior disorder most commonly occurs in people over the age of 50 and has been associated with degenerative parkinsonian syndromes.

Other common parasomnias that have the potential to be mistaken for epilepsy include nightmares, somnambulism, night terrors, and confusional arousals. It can be very satisfying to make the diagnosis for these relatively rare conditions that make up approximately 15% of referrals to a typical sleep center [26]. Night terrors typically occur in children and arise out of slow-wave sleep. The person appears terrified and is generally not consolable during the event. The patient has no recall for the event, an event which consists of spontaneous crying, screaming, and lack of responsiveness. After the event, the patient typically falls back to sleep with the duration lasting a few minutes or so. Vocalizations during sleep are uncommon, but have been described typically in frontal lobe epilepsy. Nightmares usually are self-reported by patients and occur during REM sleep. The patient complains of the nightmare having recall of what occurs during them shortly after being awakened. In contrast to night terrors, the patient can typically be easily awakened during the event.

Nocturnal enuresis has sometimes been confused for nocturnal seizures with incontinence [27]. Enuresis occurs during non-REM sleep and is often considered normal until the age of approximately four years. Somnambulism or sleepwalking has the potential for being confused for seizures. These events typically arise out of slow-wave sleep and occur in as many as 15% of children and 0.7% of adults [28, 29]. They most often occur in adolescents aged 10–15 years. During the sleepwalking events when discovered by friends or family, the patients are often easily directed back to bed having no recall for the episode. It has been associated with Lewy body dementia.

8.7 Psychogenic nonepileptic seizures (PNESs)

PNES are common in the young and middle-aged patients. The events occur spontaneously, are unpredictable and typically associated with altered consciousness. Their appearance can be quite similar to epileptic seizures, often with similar duration. The health care provider should ask the patient about a history of being abused. Significant physical, emotional, or sexual abuse has been associated with the occurrence of PNES. PNES events may be reported by the patient to be triggered by acute stressful conditions [30]. Typical antiseizure medications are not usually effective in treating this condition and therefore, it can be confused with intractable epilepsy [31]. A careful description of each event is important to note. Events that are typically triggered by emotional reactions to confrontations at work or fights with a spouse, for example, would not be consistent with a typical epileptic seizure. The interictal EEG typically remains normal, even those that have been obtained under sleep deprivation conditions and with activation procedures. Unfortunately, many EEGs are over-interpreted leading to the erroneous diagnosis of epilepsy [32, 33]. The hallmark of making the diagnosis of PNES is a normal EEG during an event [34]. Events can typically be either recorded during an ambulatory EEG or more preferably a video-EEG monitoring session in the EMU [35].

In a person who has altered consciousness without physiologic changes on the EEG makes the diagnosis of PNES most likely. The duration of these events may be a clue as to their origin. Psychogenic seizures may fluctuate from minutes to even several hours without resolution, whereas typical epileptic seizures last a minute or two and then resolve. A rapid onset and rapid stop of the event with rapid reorientation postictally, also favors PNES. The diagnosis can be challenging at times as it is estimated that between 5 and 20% of patients admitted to the EMUs around the country have both epileptic seizures and PNES [36–38]. Many of the patients who are ultimately diagnosed with PNES also have concurrent personality or psychological disorders [39]. Over the years, many attempts have been made to associate clues on either the history or physical symptoms in PNES with the potential diagnosis. Both PNES and intractable ES do not respond to AED therapy [40]. Certain observations during the event such as pelvic thrusting, back arching (opisthotonic posturing), ictal stuttering, and pseudosleep have all been described as being associated with PNES [41–43]. Unfortunately, despite certain signs and symptoms having a higher association with PNES [44, 45], none of them is 100% reliable, and they typically require confirmation by observation or capturing an event during testing [46]. A comorbid history of chronic pain such as fibromyalgia, or having a seizure in an outpatient epilepsy clinic or waiting room has been associated with PNES [47]. Eye closure at the start of an event has also been associated with PNES [48]. Misdiagnosing PNES as epileptic seizures has consequences such as continuing therapy that is not necessary. In uncertain cases, the gold standard of making the diagnosis remains admission to the EMU. A recent article concerning the topic of EMU safety confirmed the evaluation process in epilepsy patients to be relatively safe [49]. The costs of misdiagnosis have been estimated to be substantial over a lifetime [50]. By the same token, if the diagnosis of PNES is made, the utilization of both inpatient and outpatient health services has been shown to be reduced [51, 52].

8.8 Summary

Patients with transient attacks associated with neurologic symptoms and signs can be sometimes perplexing. The evaluation process of these attacks should be inclusive, yet tailored to arrive at the diagnosis in an effective manner. While many of the conditions discussed in the differential diagnosis in this chapter typically do not have devastating consequences for the average person, there is a potential to impair quality of life and possibly of limb if the events persist. As society struggles with cost and quality issues in health care delivery, making and treating the correct diagnosis becomes paramount. The careful taking of a history remains the cornerstone of the evaluation process. Unfortunately, in cases such as these with intermittent symptoms and frequently less than optimal descriptions of the events, the health care provider is often challenged in arriving at the correct diagnosis. With this in mind, persistence is needed to work though the issue and when therapy is ineffective or the events change one should step back and consider the alternative diagnoses and reevaluate the situation.

References

1. Drazkowski, J.F. (2003) Management of the social consequences of seizures. *Mayo Clin Proc*, **78** (5), 641–649.
2. Fisher, R.S., Vickrey, B.G., Gibson, P. *et al.* (2000) The impact of epilepsy from the patient's perspective I. Descriptions and subjective perceptions. *Epilepsy Res*, **41** (1), 39–51.
3. Gilliam, F. (2003) The impact of epilepsy on subjective health status. *Curr Neurol Neurosci Rep*, **3** (4), 357–362.
4. Blum, D.E., Eskola, J., Bortz, J.J., and Fisher, R.S. (1996) Patient awareness of seizures. *Neurology*, **47** (1), 260–264.
5. Drazkowski, J.F. and Neiman, E.S. (2009) Electroencephalography and evoked potential studies, in *Clinical Adult Neurology*, 3rd edn (eds. J. Corey-Bloom and R.B. David), Demos Medical, New York, NY, pp. 15–33.

6. Strickberger, S.A., Benson, D.W., Biaggioni, I. *et al.* (2006) AHA/ACCF Scientific Statement on the evaluation of syncope: from the American Heart Association Councils on Clinical Cardiology, Cardiovascular Nursing, Cardiovascular Disease in the Young, and Stroke; the Quality of Care and Outcomes Research Interdisciplinary Working Group; and the American College of Cardiology Foundation: in collaboration with the Heart Rhythm Society: endorsed by the American Autonomic Society. *Circulation*, **113** (2), 316–327.

7. Kapoor, W.N., Karpf, M., Wieand, S. *et al.* (1983) A prospective evaluation and follow-up of patients with syncope. *N Engl J Med*, **309** (4), 197–204.

8. Soteriades, E.S., Evans, J.C., Larson, M.G. *et al.* (2002) Incidence and prognosis of syncope. *N Engl J Med*, **347** (12), 878–885.

9. Kapoor, W.N. (1990) Evaluation and outcome of patients with syncope. *Medicine*, **69** (3), 160–175.

10. Graf, D., Schlaepfer, J., Gollut, E. *et al.* (2008) Predictive models of syncope causes in an outpatient clinic. *Int J Cardiol*, **123** (3), 249–256.

11. Aminoff, M.J., Scheinman, M.M., Griffin, J.C., and Herre, J.M. (1988) Electrocerebral accompaniments of syncope associated with malignant ventricular arrhythmias. *Ann Int Med*, **108** (6), 791–796.

12. Zaidi, A., Clough, P., Cooper, P. *et al.* (2000) Misdiagnosis of epilepsy: many seizure-like attacks have a cardiovascular cause. *J Am Coll Cardiol*, **36** (1), 181–184.

13. Lin, J.T., Ziegler, D.K., Lai, C.W., and Bayer, W. (1982) Convulsive syncope in blood donors. *Ann Neurol*, **11** (5), 525–528.

14. Brignole, M., Menozzi, C., Maggi, R. *et al.* (2005) The usage and diagnostic yield of the implantable loop-recorder in detection of the mechanism of syncope and in guiding effective antiarrhythmic therapy in older people. *Europace*, **7** (3), 273–279.

15. Krumholz, A. (1994) Cerebrovascular imitators of epilepsy, in *Imitators of Epilepsy* (ed. R.S. Fisher), Demos Publications, New York, NY, pp. 109–123.

16. Tatemichi, T.K., Young, W.L., Prohovnik, I. *et al.* (1990) Perfusion insufficiency in limb-shaking transient ischemic attacks. *Stroke*, **21** (2), 341–347.

17. Bladin, C.F., Alexandrov, A.V., Bellavance, A. *et al.* (2000) Seizures after stroke: a prospective multicenter study. *Arch Neurol*, **57** (11), 1617–1622.

18. Bartsch, T., Alfke, K., Stingele, R. *et al.* (2006) Selective affection of hippocampal CA-1 neurons in patients with transient global amnesia without long-term sequelae. *Brain*, **129** (Pt 11), 2874–2884.

19. Miller, J.W., Petersen, R.C., Metter, E.J. *et al.* (1987) Transient global amnesia: clinical characteristics and prognosis. *Neurology*, **37** (5), 733–737.

20. Rowan, J.A. (2000) Diagnosis of non-epileptic seizures, in *Non-Epileptic Seizures*, 2nd edn (eds. J.R. Gates and A.J. Rowan), Butterworth-Heinemann, Boston, MA, pp. 15–29.

21. Devinsky, O., Sato, S., Kufta, C.V. *et al.* (1989) Electroencephalographic studies of simple partial seizures with subdural electrode recordings. *Neurology*, **39** (4), 527–533.

22. Drazkowski, J.F. (2009) Epileptiform activity, in *Clinical Neurophysiology* (eds. J.R. Daube and D.I. Rubin), Oxford University Press, New York, NY, pp. 137–150.

23. Evidente, V.G.H. and Caviness, J.N. (2009) Movement-related cortical potentials and event-related potentials, in *Clinical Neurophysiology* (eds. J.R. Daube and D.I. Rubin), Oxford University Press, New York, NY, pp. 229–234.

24. Coleman, R.M., Roffwarg, H.P., Kennedy, S.J. *et al.* (1982) Sleep-wake disorders based on a polysomnographic diagnosis. A national cooperative study. *J Am Med Assoc*, **247** (7), 997–1003.

25. Schenck, C.H. and Mahowald, M.W. (1991) Injurious sleep behavior disorders (parasomnias) affecting patients on intensive care units. *Intensive Care Med*, **17** (4), 219–224.
26. Schenck, C.H., Bundlie, S.R., Ettinger, M.G., and Mahowald, M.W. (1986) Chronic behavioral disorders of human REM sleep: a new category of parasomnia. *Sleep*, **9** (2), 293–308.
27. Oppel, W.C., Harper, P.A., and Rider, R.V. (1968) The age of attaining bladder control. *Pediatrics*, **42** (4), 614–626.
28. Kavey, N.B., Whyte, J., Resor, S.R. Jr., and Gidro-Frank, S. (1990) Somnambulism in adults. *Neurology*, **40** (5), 749–752.
29. Maselli, R.A., Rosenberg, R.S., and Spire, J.P. (1988) Episodic nocturnal wanderings in nonepileptic young patients. *Sleep*, **11** (2), 156–161.
30. Fargo, J.D., Schefft, B.K., Szaflarski, J.P. *et al.* (2004) Accuracy of self-reported neuropsychological functioning in individuals with epileptic or psychogenic nonepileptic seizures. *Epilepsy Behav*, **5** (2), 143–150.
31. Gates, J.R. (1998) Diagnosis and treatment of nonepileptic seizures, in *Psychiatric Comorbidity in Epilepsy: Basic Mechanisms, Diagnosis, and Treatment* (eds. P.S. Mc Connell and P.J. Snyder), Psychiatric Press, Washington, DC, pp. 187–204.
32. Benbadis, S.R. and Tatum, W.O. (2003) Overintepretation of EEGs and misdiagnosis of epilepsy. *J Clin Neurophysiol*, **20** (1), 42–44.
33. Cuthill, F.M. and Espie, C.A. (2005) Sensitivity and specificity of procedures for the differential diagnosis of epileptic and nonepileptic seizures: a systematic review. *Seizure*, **14** (5), 293–303.
34. Benbadis, S.R., Siegrist, K., Tatum, W.O. *et al.* (2004) Short-term outpatient EEG video with induction in the diagnosis of psychogenic seizures. *Neurology*, **63** (9), 1728–1730.
35. Buchhalter, J.R. (2009) Ambulatory electroencephalography, in *Clinical Neurophysiology*, 3rd edn (eds. J.R. Daube and D.I. Rubin), Oxford University Press, New York, NY, pp. 187–192.
36. Benbadis, S.R., Agrawal, V., and Tatum, W.O. (2001) How many patients with psychogenic nonepileptic seizures also have epilepsy? *Neurology*, **57** (5), 915–917.
37. Buchanan, N. and Snars, J. (1993) Pseudoseizures (nonepileptic attack disorder)—clinical management and outcome in 50 patients. *Seizure*, **2** (2), 141–146.
38. Martin, R., Burneo, J.G., Prasad, A. *et al.* (2003) Frequency of epilepsy in patients with psychogenic seizures monitored by video-EEG. *Neurology*, **61** (12), 1791–1792.
39. Cragar, D.E., Berry, D.T., Schmitt, F.A., and Fakhoury, T.A. (2005) Cluster analysis of normal personality traits in patients with psychogenic nonepileptic seizures. *Epilepsy Behav*, **6** (4), 593–600.
40. Davis, B.J. (2004) Predicting nonepileptic seizures utilizing seizure frequency, EEG, and response to medication. *European Neurol*, **51** (3), 153–156.
41. Benbadis, S.R., Lancman, M.E., King, L.M., and Swanson, S.J. (1996) Preictal pseudosleep: a new finding in psychogenic seizures. *Neurology*, **47** (1), 63–67.
42. Burneo, J.G., Martin, R., Powell, T. *et al.* (2003) Teddy bears: an observational finding in patients with nonepileptic events. *Neurology*, **61** (5), 714–715.
43. Vossler, D.G., Haltiner, A.M., Schepp, S.K. *et al.* (2004) Ictal stuttering: a sign suggestive of psychogenic nonepileptic seizures. *Neurology*, **63** (3), 516–519.
44. Gates, J.R., Ramani, V., Whalen, S., and Loewenson, R. (1985) Ictal characteristics of pseudoseizures. *Arch Neurol*, **42** (12), 1183–1187.
45. Geyer, J.D., Payne, T.A., and Drury, I. (2000) The value of pelvic thrusting in the diagnosis of seizures and pseudoseizures. *Neurology*, **54** (1), 227–229.
46. Hoerth, M.T., Wellik, K.E., Demaerschalk, B.M. *et al.* (2008) Clinical predictors of psychogenic nonepileptic seizures: a critically appraised topic. *Neurologist*, **14** (4), 266–270.

47. Benbadis, S.R. (2005) A spell in the epilepsy clinic and a history of "chronic pain" or "fibromyalgia" independently predict a diagnosis of psychogenic seizures. *Epilepsy Behav*, **6** (2), 264–265.

48. Chung, S.S., Gerber, P., and Kirlin, K.A. (2006) Ictal eye closure is a reliable indicator for psychogenic nonepileptic seizures. *Neurology*, **66** (11), 1730–1731.

49. Noe, K.H. and Drazkowski, J.F. (2009) Safety of long-term video-electroencephalographic monitoring for evaluation of epilepsy. *Mayo Clin Proc*, **84** (6), 495–500.

50. Martin, R., Bell, B., Hermann, B., and Mennemeyer, S. (2003) Nonepileptic seizures and their costs: the role of neuropsychology, in *Clinical Neuropsychology and Cost Outcome Research: A Beginning* (ed. G.P. Prigatano), Psychology Press, New York, NY, pp. 235–258.

51. Lesser, R.P. (2003) Treatment and outcome of psychogenic nonepileptic seizures. *Epilepsy Curr/Am Epilepsy Soc*, **3** (6), 198–200.

52. Walczak, T.S., Papacostas, S., Williams, D.T. *et al.* (1995) Outcome after diagnosis of psychogenic nonepileptic seizures. *Epilepsia*, **36** (11), 1131–1137.

Section 3

Principles of medical management

9 Mechanisms of action of antiepileptic drugs

Jeffrey W. Britton[1], Tarek M. Zakaria[2], and Eduardo Benarroch[3]

[1]*Department of Neurology, Divisions of Clinical Neurophysiology-EEG and Epilepsy, Mayo Clinic, Rochester, MN, USA*
[2]*Epilepsy Monitoring Unit; Epilepsy surgery program, Norton Neuroscience Institute, Louisville, KY*
[3]*Department of Neurology, Division of Autonomic Disorders, Mayo Clinic, Rochester, MN, USA*

9.1 Introduction

Historically, treatments for epilepsy were selected without a firm understanding of the pathophysiology of ictogenesis or pharmaceutical mechanism of action. The antiepileptic pharmacotherapy era began in 1850 with the introduction of bromides, the use of which was based on the theory that epilepsy was caused by an excessive sex drive [1]. In 1910, phenobarbital, which was initially used as a soporific agent, was selected for treatment of seizures based on its sedative properties. This became the drug of choice for many years, and a number of barbiturates were subsequently developed, including primidone which is still in limited use. In 1940, phenytoin was developed as a compound with structural properties similar to barbiturates but which lacked the latter's sedative effects. Despite the fact that these drugs were developed prior to development and understanding of the mechanisms of ictogenesis or their mechanism of action, these drugs have

Adult Epilepsy, First Edition. Edited by Gregory D. Cascino and Joseph I. Sirven.
© 2011 John Wiley & Sons, Ltd. Published 2011 by John Wiley & Sons, Ltd.

remained valid antiepileptic drug (AED) options in the treatment of epilepsy and seizures [2, 3].

The mechanisms of action of subsequently developed early generation AEDs in many cases became understood only well after their clinical use was established, and in the case of some remain unknown [4]. For example, ethosuximide has been used since 1958 for the treatment of absence seizures; however, its currently understood mechanism of action was identified 30 years later and is still being clarified. In 1962, carbamazepine was approved first for the treatment of trigeminal neuralgia. Approval for the treatment of partial seizures occurred much later in 1974. Valproate was serendipitously found to have antiepileptic properties without an a priori understanding of its mechanism. It was approved for use in Europe in 1960 and the United States in 1978. These first generation anticonvulsants were the mainstays of epilepsy treatment until the 1990s when the second generation AEDs became available.

In contrast with early generation treatments, the development of the second generation AEDs was more consistently based on a firmer foundation of the underlying mechanisms of seizure initiation and inhibition [5, 6]. In many cases, the mechanisms targeted in the drug design process held true, but in other cases (such as with gabapentin, which was originally developed as a gamma aminobutyric acid (GABA) analog then subsequently found not to have GABAergic properties) they were found to act via mechanisms other than that for which they were designed. In this chapter, the mechanisms of action of the AEDs as currently understood are reviewed with respect to known mechanisms of neuronal excitation and inhibition.

9.2 Treatment of epilepsy

Understanding the mechanisms of action of AEDs is important in clinical practice, especially when considering multidrug regimens. Second generation AEDs were selected for development based in part on findings of favorable properties referable to their influence on neuronal inhibition and excitation [5]. However, the mechanisms of action of currently marketed AEDs are not fully understood in all cases. The common link among the various proposed mechanisms for many of the AEDs involves the ability of a drug to modulate excitatory and inhibitory neurotransmission through effects on ion channels, neurotransmitter receptors, and neurotransmitter metabolism, with an end result favoring inhibition or decreased excitation [7]. The mechanisms of action of the most common AEDs and their primary mechanisms of action are summarized in Figure 9.1 and Table 9.1.

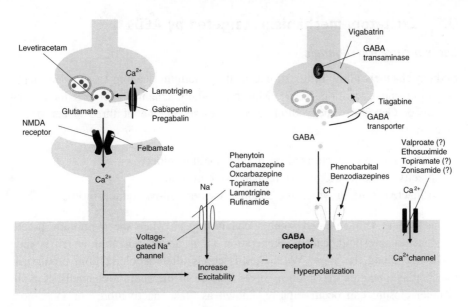

Figure 9.1 Mechanisms of action of AEDs. From Benarroch, E.E. (2006) *Basic Neuroscience with Clinical Applications*, Butterworth-Heinemann/Elsevier, Copyrighted and used with permission of Mayo Foundation for Medical Education and Research, all rights reserved.

Table 9.1 Main mechanisms of action of the AEDs

Drug	Na channel blockade	T-type Ca channel blockade	Non-T-type Ca channel blockade	Increase GABAergic transmission	Inhibit glutamate transmission	Carbonic anhydrase inhibition
Phenytoin	+++	—	—	—	—	—
Carbamazepine	+++	—	—	—	—	—
Oxcarbazepine	+++	—	—	—	—	—
Lamotrigine	+++	—	+	—	+	—
Valproic acid	++	+	—	++	+	—
Topiramate	++	—	+	++	++	+
Zonisamide	++	+	—	++	++	+
Phenobarbital	—	—	—	++	—	—
Benzodiazepines	—	—	—	+++	—	—
Vigabatrin	—	—	—	+++	—	—
Tiagabine	—	—	—	+++	—	—
Gabapentin	—	—	++	+	—	—
Pregabalin	—	—	—	—	—	—
Levetiracetam	—	—	+	—	+	—
Felbamate	+	—	+	+	++	—
Ethosuximide	+	+++	—	—	—	—
Rufinamide	++	—	—	—	—	—
Lacosamide	++	—	—	—	—	—

9.3   Excitatory mechanisms targeted by AEDs

Sodium currents/channels

Sodium channels allow influx of extracellular sodium, leading to neuronal depolarization and excitation [8, 9]. Multiple sodium channel subtypes have been identified. Generally, the sodium channel exists in one of three states at any given time:

- A resting state characterized by limited sodium influx.
- An active state marked by significant sodium influx.
- An inactive state in which the channel does not allow sodium influx.

The typical voltage-gated sodium channel opens when the membrane potential reaches threshold, causing generation of an action potential which is then conducted along the axon. Within milliseconds after depolarization, repolarization begins, one step of which involves closure of the sodium channels. Sodium channel closure can occur rapidly, known as "fast inactivation," or in a more gradual, sustained manner known as "slow inactivation" [10]. Slow inactivation is an important mechanism in regulation and modulation of burst discharges in neurons and axons [10, 11]. Many AEDs, like carbamazepine or lamotrigine, enhance fast inactivation, reducing the ability of neurons to fire repetitive action potentials. As fast inactivation only occurs in neurons firing action potentials, these drugs preferentially inhibit axons in active cells, such as those involved in seizure activity [12]. However, some AEDs primarily affect "slow inactivation." Lacosamide promotes slow inactivation at thresholds lower than is present in the normal state, thereby preferentially affecting neurons which are partially depolarized for relative long periods, such as those hypothetically present in the epileptogenic zone region [13].

Calcium channels

Voltage-gated calcium channels are classified as high- and low-voltage subtypes based on depolarization threshold [14, 15]. The high-voltage calcium channels are further classified as L, N, P/Q, and the R types; the T-channel is the primary low-voltage calcium channel type.

L-type calcium channels

The L-type calcium channels (Ca_V 1.2) are expressed in the neuronal dendrites and cell bodies. Their main function is to allow a large influx of calcium, which in turn activates a cascade of protein kinase pathways that promote gene transcription required for long-term synaptic plasticity in the hippocampus and cerebral cortex.

N-, P/Q-, and R-type calcium channels

N-, P/Q-, and R-type calcium channels are present in presynaptic terminals, where they are involved with triggering neurotransmitter release. N-channels promote release from GABAergic, sympathetic noradrenergic, and dorsal root ganglion terminals. The P/Q calcium channels are associated with glutamate release in the central nervous system (CNS). The R-type calcium channels contribute to exocytosis in many regions, including the hippocampus, where they play a major role in presynaptic long-term potentiation.

T-type channels

T-type calcium channels have a widespread distribution in the CNS including the neocortex, hippocampus, thalamus, cerebellum, and inferior olivary nucleus. T-type calcium channels are responsible for rhythmic burst firing pattern in thalamic neurons and thalamocortical circuits, as occurs both during non-rapid eye movement (REM) sleep and in pathological conditions such as absence seizures [15].

There is some evidence, based mainly on genetic animal models involving mutations of voltage-gated calcium channels, that they play a role in the pathophysiology of generalized spike-and-wave discharges underlying generalized absence seizures [16, 17]. Most of these mutations have been found to result in a gain of T channel activity or loss of P/Q channel activity [18, 19].

Several AEDs affect voltage-gated calcium channels in vitro. Gabapentin and pregabilin reduce calcium channel subunit expression in the presynaptic terminal. Lamotrigine inhibits N- and P/Q-type channels; levetiracetam predominantly affects N-type channels; and topiramate inhibits R-type channels. Ethosuximide, zonisamide, and valproate probably have an affect on thalamocortical circuits by blocking T-type calcium channels, which might explain their efficacy against absence seizures [18, 20].

Glutamate receptors

Glutamate receptors are classified as ionotropic and metabotropic types. The ionotropic glutamate receptors are nonselective cation channels that trigger fast depolarization [21]. The ionotropic glutamate receptors are further classified based on their relative affinity for certain ligands, namely N-methyl-D-aspartate (NMDA), alpha-amino-3-hydroxy-5-methylisoxazole-4-propionic acid (AMPA), and kainic acid. The NMDA receptor is a voltage-dependent channel that is highly permeable to calcium. It has two distinct subunits NR1 and NR2. NMDA receptor channel activation requires binding of glutamate to the NR2 subunit; binding of glycine to an allosteric site on the NR1 subunit; and membrane depolarization, which removes voltage-dependent magnesium blockade of the channel pore.

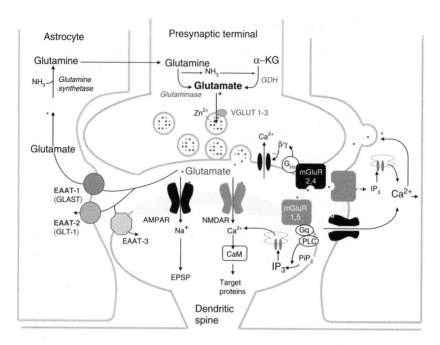

Figure 9.2 A glutamatergic synapse with different glutamate receptors and related neuro-transmitters. Glutamate, the main excitatory neurotransmitter in the CNS, binds to multiple receptor sites that differ in activation and inactivation time courses, desensitization kinetics, conductance, and ion permeability. The three main glutamate receptor subtypes are N-methyl-D-aspartate (NMDA), metabotropic, and non-NMDA (alpha-amino-3-hydroxy-5-methylisoxazole-4-propionic acid (AMPA) and kainate receptors). From Benarroch, E.E. (2006) *Basic Neuroscience with Clinical Applications*, Butterworth-Heinemann/Elsevier, Copyrighted and used with permission of Mayo Foundation for Medical Education and Research, all rights reserved.

Both the NMDA ionotropic and metabotropic glutamate receptors have been found to be important modulators of seizure activity in animal models. Many different glutamate receptor types may coexist in an individual synaptic cleft, resulting in a differential response to glutamate in different synapses. A gluta-matergic synapse is shown on Figure 9.2. AEDs that are currently thought to confer antiepileptic activity through antiglutamatergic mechanisms include: fel-bamate through inhibition of the glycine site [22], topiramate [23], levetiracetam [24], and lamotrigine indirectly via reduced presynaptic glutamate release [25].

9.4   Inhibitory mechanisms targeted by AEDs

GABA_A receptors/channels

GABA is produced through activity of the enzyme glutamic acid decarboxy-lase (GAD), which requires pyridoxal phosphate and is stored via the vesicular

GABA transporter (VGAT). After release into the synaptic cleft, GABA undergoes degradation by GABA-transaminase (GABA-T) to succinic semialdehyde (SSA), which is metabolized in the mitochondria to α-ketoglutarate (α-KG), the main substrate for Lglutamate synthesis.

The fast inhibitory effects of GABA are mediated by $GABA_A$ receptors, which are ligand-gated chloride channels that are allosterically activated by benzodiazepines and some neurosteroids. Neuronal $GABA_A$ receptors are pentameric proteins consisting of five subunits (classified as α, β, γ, and δ subtypes) arranged around a central pore. There are several $GABA_A$ receptor subtypes, the functions of which vary based on the combination of α-, β-, γ-, and δ- subunits in a given receptor.

There are two forms of $GABA_A$ receptor-mediated inhibition, phasic and tonic. Phasic inhibition is mediated by $GABA_A$ receptors that contain γ subunits, which are clustered at the postsynaptic terminals and are allosterically activated by benzodiazepines. Tonic inhibition is mediated by $GABA_A$ receptors which express δ subunits and are distributed at extrasynaptic sites; these receptors are not modulated by benzodiazepines but are targets of general anesthetics, alcohol, and neurosteroids. Steroids may act as positive (progesterone and allopregnanolone) or negative (estrogens, glucocorticoids) modulators. Allosteric antagonists of the $GABA_A$ receptor chloride channel include picrotoxin, pentylenetetrazol, and penicillin.

Impaired $GABA_A$ receptor-mediated inhibition is an important pathophysiologic mechanism of increased neuronal excitability which can lead to epilepsy. Dysfunction of $GABA_A$ receptors, either genetic or acquired, has been recently described in patients with idiopathic generalized epilepsy, catamenial epilepsy, and status epilepticus [26].

AEDs modulate GABAergic activity through a number of mechanisms (Figure 9.3). Tiagabine produces a nonselective increase in GABA levels through inhibition of GABA reuptake. Vigabatrin inhibits GABA degradation by inhibition of GABA-T [5]. Valproate increases regional neuronal concentrations of GABA by inhibiting GABA degradation and increasing GABA synthesis [27]. Benzodiazepines increase the probability of chloride channel opening by GABA [28]; this effect is blocked by flumazenil. Barbiturates are also positive modulators of the $GABA_A$ receptor by increasing the average channel opening duration [29].

The $GABA_B$ receptor is a G protein-coupled receptor that increases conductance of G-protein activated inward rectifying potassium (GIRK) channels and decreases conductance of presynaptic N- and P/Q calcium channels.

Carbonic anhydrase inhibition

Inhibition of the enzyme carbonic anhydrase increases the concentration of intracellular hydrogen ions. This leads to a shift of potassium ions to the extracellular

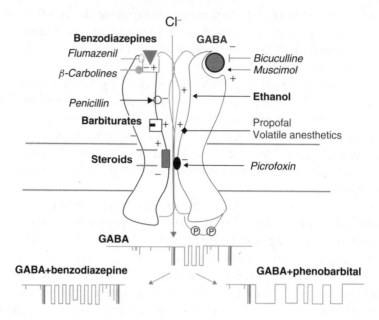

Figure 9.3   The GABA receptor and AED mechanisms of action. From Benarroch, E.E. (2006) *Basic Neuroscience with Clinical Applications*, Butterworth-Heinemann/Elsevier, Copyrighted and used with permission of Mayo Foundation for Medical Education and Research, all rights reserved.

compartment resulting in hyperpolarization. Acetazolamide has been used as an adjunctive therapy in refractory seizures. Topiramate and zonisamide also are weak inhibitors of this enzyme, which may contribute to their anticonvulsant effect.

9.5   Mechanism of action-specific drugs

Phenytoin and carbamazepine

Several studies have shown that therapeutic concentrations of phenytoin and carbamazepine prevent sustained repetitive neuronal firing through blockade of voltage-dependent sodium channels [30, 31].

Ethosuximide

The mechanism of action of ethosuximide was not elucidated until 1989, when it was shown to reduce low-threshold T-type calcium currents in thalamic neurons. Voltage-dependent reduction in T-type current was observed at clinically relevant ethosuximide concentrations, suggesting that this mechanism may be the basis for its efficacy in absence seizures [30]. By preventing calcium-dependent depolarization of thalamocortical neurons, ethosuximide is believed to inhibit the synchronized rhythmic activation thought to underlie the rhythmic spike-wave discharges characteristic of absence seizures [32]. However, recent evidence suggests that the antiepileptic effects of this drug may not be fully explained by this mechanism and may also involve blockade of sodium channels.

Valproic acid

The main antiepileptic mechanisms underlying valproate are still incompletely defined. Three different mechanisms of action have been proposed. First, in vitro studies support an inhibitory effect on voltage-sensitive sodium channels [33]. Second, it has been shown to reduce T-type calcium currents in primary afferent neurons [34]. This may contribute to its efficacy in absence seizures. Finally, valproic acid has been associated with an increase in whole-brain GABA levels and found to potentiate GABAergic activity at high drug concentrations [27, 35]. This effect, coupled with its effect on the voltage-sensitive sodium channel, may contribute to its efficacy against kindled seizures in rats and against partial seizures [36].

Benzodiazepines and barbiturates

Benzodiazepines bind to an allosteric site in γ-subunit-containing GABA receptors; this interaction increases the chloride channel opening frequency without affecting channel-opening duration [37]. Barbiturates bind to a different allosteric site and increase the mean duration of chloride channel-opening without affecting opening frequency. Barbiturates can potentiate chloride currents directly in the absence of GABA, whereas benzodiazepine activity is dependent on the presence of GABA. This difference is believed to explain why benzodiazepines attenuate spike-wave seizures in both rodents and humans, whereas barbiturates may exacerbate spike-wave discharges in some cases [38]. Benzodiazepines and barbiturates limit high-frequency repetitive action potential generation, but this is only at high drug concentrations.

Felbamate

Similar to valproate, felbamate has a broad preclinical profile and clinical spectrum. It possesses several neuropharmacological properties involving more than one potential anticonvulsant mechanism of action. Felbamate reduces sustained repetitive firing through inhibition of voltage-dependent sodium channels. Felbamate at low concentrations also appears to inhibit dihydropyridine-sensitive, high-threshold voltage-sensitive calcium currents. Furthermore, at higher concentrations, felbamate has been reported to enhance GABA-evoked chloride currents and to inhibit NMDA-glutamatergic activity [39, 40]. Felbamate appears to inhibit the function of the NMDA receptor complex through an interaction with the strychnine-insensitive glycine recognition site, as demonstrated in studies of rat and human postmortem brain tissue. This may lead to anticonvulsant and neuroprotective effects by inhibiting NMDA receptor function through allosteric modulation of the glycine site [22].

Gabapentin and pregabalin

Gabapentin and pregabalin bind to the alpha (22)-delta subunit of voltage-gated L-, P/Q-, and N-type calcium channels. These drugs decrease expression and activity of this subunit and reduces N- and P/Q channel-dependent release of several neurotransmitters [23, 41, 42].

Lamotrigine

Lamotrigine is a sodium channel blocker that leads to inhibition of presynaptic glutamate release [25, 43–46]. This observation might explain its additional efficacy against some generalized seizure types [47].

Oxcarbazepine

Oxcarbazepine is structurally related to carbamazepine. Oxcarbazepine is rapidly and completely reduced to its active metabolite (10,11-dihydro-10-hydroxy-carbamazepine, known as the monohydroxy-derivative or MHD), which is believed to confer its anticonvulsant effect. Similar to carbamazepine, in vitro studies indicate that MHD induces blockade of voltage-sensitive sodium channels, resulting in neuronal membrane stabilization, inhibition of repetitive neuronal discharges, and diminution of propagation of synaptic impulses [48].

Topiramate

Topiramate has several pharmacologic effects which likely contribute to its anticonvulsant activity. It inhibits sustained repetitive firing in a use- and concentration-dependent manner by reducing voltage-activated sodium currents in cultured neocortical neurons [49]. Topiramate also enhances GABA-mediated chloride influx and potentiates GABA-evoked whole-cell currents in vitro [50, 51]. Topiramate has also been shown to reduce kainate-evoked depolarization; this contributes to decreased neuronal excitability. In other preclinical studies, topiramate was also shown to inhibit certain carbonic anhydrase isoforms, a property that may contribute to its anticonvulsant effect.

Tiagabine

Tiagabine is a potent inhibitor of neuronal and glial GABA re-uptake. Tiagabine binds selectively and reversibly to the GABA reuptake carrier (GAT-1) [50]. This increases synaptic concentrations of GABA, which is the likely basis of its anticonvulsant activity in partial seizures. However, this effect may also lead to aggravation of spike-wave seizures and nonconvulsive status epilepticus. This may result from potentiation of GABA-induced hyperpolarization of thalamic neurons leading to T-channel triggered rhythmic burst firing in thalamocortical circuits [52, 53].

Vigabatrin

Vigabatrin irreversibly binds to and inactivates GABA-T, the enzyme responsible for GABA degradation. This results in increased GABA levels and GABA-mediated neuronal inhibition; which likely explains the clinical efficacy of vigabatrin against partial seizures [54, 55].

Zonisamide

Zonisamide blocks sustained repetitive firing of neurons in vitro through a variety of mechanisms [56]. These include blockade of voltage-sensitive sodium channels, inhibition of T-type calcium channels, changes in expression of glutamate and GABA transporters, and weak carbonic anhydrase inhibition [56, 57].

Levetiracetam

The mechanism for the anticonvulsant effect of levetiracetam is not known with certainty. This drug binds to SV2A, a protein that is present in synaptic vesicles and is expressed throughout the brain [58]. The function of SV2A is poorly understood, although it may be important in calcium-dependent neurotransmitter release [59]. SV2A knock-out mice have seizures, which supports a potential role of this protein in epilepsy [60]. More recently, Lee et al. reported that levetiracetam might modulate the presynaptic P/Q-type voltage-dependent calcium channel leading to a reduction in glutamate release [61].

Lacosamide

Lacosamide is a modified amino acid that acts as an antagonist of the glycine allsoteric site of the NMDA receptor, leading to decreased glutamate-mediated neuronal hyperexcitability. Lacosamide also selectively enhances sodium channel slow inactivation [62].

Rufinamide

The exact mechanism of action is unknown. In vitro studies suggest that rufinamide prolongs the inactive state of the sodium channel.

9.6   Conclusions

In recent years, there have been significant advances in the understanding of the mechanisms associated with seizures and the anticonvulsant activity of AEDs. Newer AEDs have been found to act through a number of mechanisms that reduce neuronal excitability, burst firing, or abnormal synchronization in various combinations. A thorough understanding of the mechanisms of action of currently available drugs should increase knowledge regarding the pathophysiology of seizures, and should allow development of novel therapies in the future.

References

1. Friedlander, W.J. (2000) The rise and fall of bromide therapy in epilepsy. *Arch Neurol*, **57**, 1782–1785.
2. Krall, R.L., Penry, J.K., Kupferberg, H.J., and Swinyard, E.A. (1978) Antiepileptic drug development: I. History and a program for progress. *Epilepsia*, **19**, 393–408.
3. Shorvon, S.D. (2009) Drug treatment of epilepsy in the century of the ILAE: the first 50 years, 1909–1958. *Epilepsia*, **50** (Suppl 3), 69–92.
4. Ziporyn, T. (1985) Antietileptics: age-old search for effective therapy continues. *J Am Med Assoc*, **254**, 329–333.
5. Macdonald, R.L. and Kelly, K.M. (1994) Mechanisms of action of currently prescribed and newly developed antiepileptic drugs. *Epilepsia*, **35** (Suppl 4), S41–S50.
6. Shorvon, S.D. (2009) Drug treatment of epilepsy in the century of the ILAE: the second 50 years, 1959–2009. *Epilepsia*, **50** (Suppl 3), 93–130.
7. Macdonald, R.L. and Kelly, K.M. (1995) Antiepileptic drug mechanisms of action. *Epilepsia*, **36** (Suppl 2), S2–S12.
8. Catterall, W.A., Nunoki, K., Lai, Y. *et al.* (1990) Structure and modulation of voltage-sensitive sodium and calcium channels. *Adv Second Messenger Phosphoprotein Res*, **24**, 30–35.
9. Catterall, W.A., Goldin, A.L., and Waxman, S.G. (2005) International Union of Pharmacology. XLVII. Nomenclature and structure-function relationships of voltage-gated sodium channels. *Pharmacol Rev*, **57**, 397–409.
10. Benarroch, E.E. (2007) Sodium channels and pain. *Neurology*, **68**, 233–236.
11. Ulbricht, W. (2005) Sodium channel inactivation: molecular determinants and modulation. *Physiol Rev*, **85**, 1271–1301.
12. Kuo, C.C. (1998) A common anticonvulsant binding site for phenytoin, carbamazepine, and lamotrigine in neuronal Na+ channels. *Mol Pharmacol*, **54**, 712–721.
13. Errington, A.C., Stohr, T., Heers, C., and Lees, G. (2008) The investigational anticonvulsant lacosamide selectively enhances slow inactivation of voltage-gated sodium channels. *Mol Pharmacol*, **73**, 157–169.

14. Catterall, W.A., Perez-Reyes, E., Snutch, T.P., and Striessnig, J. (2005) International Union of Pharmacology. XLVIII. Nomenclature and structure-function relationships of voltage-gated calcium channels. *Pharmacol Rev*, **57**, 411–425.

15. Catterall, W.A. and Few, A.P. (2008) Calcium channel regulation and presynaptic plasticity. *Neuron*, **59**, 882–901.

16. Iftinca, M., Hamid, J., Chen, L. *et al.* (2007) Regulation of T-type calcium channels by Rho-associated kinase. *Nat Neurosci*, **10**, 854–860.

17. Qin, N., Yagel, S., Momplaisir, M.L. *et al.* (2002) Molecular cloning and characterization of the human voltage-gated calcium channel alpha(2)delta-4 subunit. *Mol Pharmacol*, **62**, 485–496.

18. Khosravani, H. and Zamponi, G.W. (2006) Voltage-gated calcium channels and idiopathic generalized epilepsies. *Physiol Rev*, **86**, 941–966.

19. Imbrici, P., Jaffe, S.L., Eunson, L.H. *et al.* (2004) Dysfunction of the brain calcium channel CaV2.1 in absence epilepsy and episodic ataxia. *Brain*, **127**, 2682–2692.

20. Perez-Reyes, E. (2003) Molecular physiology of low-voltage-activated T-type calcium channels. *Physiol Rev*, **83**, 117–161.

21. Tang, F.R., Bradford, H.F., and Ling, E.A. (2009) Metabotropic glutamate receptors in the control of neuronal activity and as targets for development of anti-epileptogenic drugs. *Curr Med Chem*, **16**, 2189–2204.

22. McCabe, R.T., Sofia, R.D., Layer, R.T. *et al.* (1998) Felbamate increases [3H]glycine binding in rat brain and sections of human postmortem brain. *J Pharmacol Exp Ther*, **286**, 991–999.

23. Bialer, M., Johannessen, S.I., Kupferberg, H.J. *et al.* (1999) Progress report on new antiepileptic drugs: a summary of the fourth Eilat conference (EILAT IV). *Epilepsy Res*, **34**, 1–41.

24. Ueda, Y., Doi, T., Nagatomo, K. *et al.* (2007) Effect of levetiracetam on molecular regulation of hippocampal glutamate and GABA transporters in rats with chronic seizures induced by amygdalar FeCl3 injection. *Brain Res*, **1151**, 55–61.

25. O'Donnell, R.A. and Miller, A.A. (1991) The effect of lamotrigine upon development of cortical kindled seizures in the rat. *Neuropharmacology*, **30**, 253–258.

26. Benarroch, E.E. (2007) GABAA receptor heterogeneity, function, and implications for epilepsy. *Neurology*, **68**, 612–614.

27. Whitlow, R.D., Sacher, A., Loo, D.D. *et al.* (2003) The anticonvulsant valproate increases the turnover rate of gamma-aminobutyric acid transporters. *J Biol Chem*, **278**, 17716–17726.

28. Doble, A. and Martin, I.L. (1992) Multiple benzodiazepine receptors: no reason for anxiety. *Trends Pharmacol Sci*, **13**, 76–81.

29. DeLorey, T.M. and Olsen, R.W. (1992) Gamma-aminobutyric acidA receptor structure and function. *J Biol Chem*, **267**, 16747–16750.

30. Czapinski, P., Blaszczyk, B., and Czuczwar, S.J. (2005) Mechanisms of action of antiepileptic drugs. *Curr Top Med Chem*, **5**, 3–14.

31. Mantegazza, M., Curia, G., Biagini, G. *et al.* (2010) Voltage-gated sodium channels as therapeutic targets in epilepsy and other neurological disorders. *Lancet Neurol*, **9**, 413–424.

32. Coulter, D.A., Huguenard, J.R., and Prince, D.A. (1989) Characterization of ethosuximide reduction of low-threshold calcium current in thalamic neurons. *Ann Neurol*, **25**, 582–593.

33. Taverna, S., Mantegazza, M., Franceschetti, S., and Avanzini, G. (1998) Valproate selectively reduces the persistent fraction of Na+ current in neocortical neurons. *Epilepsy Res*, **32**, 304–308.

34. Kryzhanovskii, G.N., Karpova, M.N., Abrosimov, I. *et al.* (1993) Anticonvulsant activity of sodium valproate and various calcium antagonists during their combined use in mice. *Biull Eksp Biol Med*, **115**, 231–233.

35. Lee, W.S., Limmroth, V., Ayata, C. *et al.* (1995) Peripheral GABAA receptor-mediated effects of sodium valproate on dural plasma protein extravasation to substance P and trigeminal stimulation. *Br J Pharmacol*, **116**, 1661–1667.

36. Kelly, K.M., Gross, R.A., and Macdonald, R.L. (1990) Valproic acid selectively reduces the low-threshold (T) calcium current in rat nodose neurons. *Neurosci Lett*, **116**, 233–238.

37. Concas, A., Pepitoni, S., Atsoggiu, T. *et al.* (1988) Aging reduces the GABA-dependent 36Cl- flux in rat brain membrane vesicles. *Life Sci*, **43**, 1761–1771.

38. Twyman, R.E., Rogers, C.J., and Macdonald, R.L. (1989) Differential regulation of gamma-aminobutyric acid receptor channels by diazepam and phenobarbital. *Ann Neurol*, **25**, 213–220.

39. Rho, J.M., Donevan, S.D., and Rogawski, M.A. (1994) Mechanism of action of the anticonvulsant felbamate: opposing effects on N-methyl-D-aspartate and gamma-aminobutyric acidA receptors. *Ann Neurol*, **35**, 229–234.

40. Steinhoff, B.J. (1994) The pharmacologic and clinical profile of the new anticonvulsant felbamate: an overview. *Fortschr Neurol Psychiatr*, **62**, 379–388.

41. Taylor, C.P., Angelotti, T., and Fauman, E. (2007) Pharmacology and mechanism of action of pregabalin: the calcium channel alpha2-delta (alpha2-delta) subunit as a target for antiepileptic drug discovery. *Epilepsy Res*, **73**, 137–150.

42. Tremont-Lukats, I.W., Megeff, C., and Backonja, M.M. (2000) Anticonvulsants for neuropathic pain syndromes: mechanisms of action and place in therapy. *Drugs*, **60**, 10 29–1052.

43. Cheung, H., Kamp, D., and Harris, E. (1992) An in vitro investigation of the action of lamotrigine on neuronal voltage-activated sodium channels. *Epilepsy Res*, **13**, 107–112.

44. Leach, M.J., Marden, C.M., and Miller, A.A. (1986) Pharmacological studies on lamotrigine, a novel potential antiepileptic drug: II. Neurochemical studies on the mechanism of action. *Epilepsia*, **27**, 490–497.

45. Lees, G. and Leach, M.J. (1993) Studies on the mechanism of action of the novel anticonvulsant lamotrigine (Lamictal) using primary neurological cultures from rat cortex. *Brain Res*, **612**, 190–199.

46. Miller, A.A., Wheatley, P., Sawyer, D.A. *et al.* (1986) Pharmacological studies on lamotrigine, a novel potential antiepileptic drug: I. Anticonvulsant profile in mice and rats. *Epilepsia*, **27**, 483–489.

47. Coulter, D.A. (1997) Antiepileptic drug cellular mechanisms of action: where does lamotrigine fit in? *J Child Neurol*, **12** (Suppl 1), S2–S9.

48. McLean, M.J. and Macdonald, R.L. (1986) Carbamazepine and 10,11-epoxycarbamazepine produce use- and voltage-dependent limitation of rapidly firing action potentials of mouse central neurons in cell culture. *J Pharmacol Exp Ther*, **238**, 727–738.

49. Zona, C., Ciotti, M.T., and Avoli, M. (1997) Topiramate attenuates voltage-gated sodium currents in rat cerebellar granule cells. *Neurosci Lett*, **231**, 123–126.

50. Perucca, E. and Bialer, M. (1996) The clinical pharmacokinetics of the newer antiepileptic drugs. Focus on topiramate, zonisamide and tiagabine. *Clin Pharmacokinet*, **31**, 29–46.

51. White, H.S., Brown, S.D., Woodhead, J.H. *et al.* (1997) Topiramate enhances GABA-mediated chloride flux and GABA-evoked chloride currents in murine brain neurons and increases seizure threshold. *Epilepsy Res*, **28**, 167–179.

52. Schachter, S.C. (1999) Tiagabine. *Epilepsia*, **40** (Suppl 5), S17–S22.

53. Meldrum, B.S. and Chapman, A.G. (1999) Basic mechanisms of gabitril (tiagabine) and future potential developments. *Epilepsia*, **40** (Suppl 9), S2–S6.

54. Willmore, L.J., Abelson, M.B., Ben-Menachem, E. *et al.* (2009) Vigabatrin: 2008 update. *Epilepsia*, **50**, 163–173.

55. Tolman, J.A. and Faulkner, M.A. (2009) Vigabatrin: a comprehensive review of drug properties including clinical updates following recent FDA approval. *Expert Opin Pharmacother*, **10**, 3077–3089.

56. Leppik, I.E. (2004) Zonisamide: chemistry, mechanism of action, and pharmacokinetics. *Seizure*, **13** (Suppl 1), S5–S9; discussion S10.

57. Leppik, I.E. (2002) Three new drugs for epilepsy: levetiracetam, oxcarbazepine, and zonisamide. *J Child Neurol*, **17** (Suppl 1), S53–S57.

58. Noyer, M., Gillard, M., Matagne, A. *et al.* (1995) The novel antiepileptic drug levetiracetam (ucb L059) appears to act via a specific binding site in CNS membranes. *Eur J Pharmacol*, **286**, 137–146.

59. Crowder, K.M., Gunther, J.M., Jones, T.A. *et al.* (1999) Abnormal neurotransmission in mice lacking synaptic vesicle protein 2A (SV2A). *Proc Natl Acad Sci USA*, **96**, 15268–15273.

60. Stahl, S.M. (2004) Psychopharmacology of anticonvulsants: levetiracetam as a synaptic vesicle protein modulator. *J Clin Psychiatry*, **65**, 1162–1163.

61. Lee, C.Y., Chen, C.C., and Liou, H.H. (2009) Levetiracetam inhibits glutamate transmission through presynaptic P/Q-type calcium channels on the granule cells of the dentate gyrus. *Br J Pharmacol*, **158**, 1753–1762.

62. Doty, P., Rudd, G.D., Stoehr, T., and Thomas, D. (2007) Lacosamide. *Neurotherapeutics*, **4**, 145–148.

10 Antiepileptic drugs: pharmacology, epilepsy indications, and selection

Jeffrey W. Britton[1] and Julie Cunningham[2]

[1]*Department of Neurology, Divisions of Clinical Neurophysiology-EEG and Epilepsy, Mayo Clinic, Rochester, MN, USA*
[2]*Department of Pharmacy, Mayo Clinic, Rochester, MN, USA*

10.1 Introduction

Several antiepileptic drugs (AEDs) now exist for the treatment of epilepsy. Prior to the 1990s, there were few options available, and many of these had suboptimal pharmacokinetic and side effect properties. However, these medications, often referred to as "traditional" or "first generation" AEDs, have been proven effective over the test of time and remain in clinical use today. Ten medications have been approved in the US for use in the treatment of epilepsy since 1993 [1]. These are often referred to as "second generation" AEDs. A few of these are used only in special clinical situations due to potential toxicity or to their particular efficacy in a niche of epilepsy care. These have been referred to as "subspecialty" AEDs. The existence of multiple options is welcome given the diversity of the epilepsies and the differences between the individuals affected by it. However, the task of selecting a particular medication from the many available and developing

Adult Epilepsy, First Edition. Edited by Gregory D. Cascino and Joseph I. Sirven.
© 2011 John Wiley & Sons, Ltd. Published 2011 by John Wiley & Sons, Ltd.

a working knowledge of each can be daunting. In this chapter, the selection, pharmacologic properties, indications, clinical considerations, and use of the AEDs are reviewed.

10.2 AED selection

Selecting a particular AED for a given patient requires consideration of several factors. These include seizure type, medical comorbidities, side-effect profile, concurrent medical therapies, and drug–drug interaction potential, gender, age, ease of use, clinical urgency, and cost. First generation therapies remain appropriate for use in the treatment of epilepsy. A study evaluating the efficacy of AED medications in newly diagnosed epilepsy showed little difference between first and second generation therapies in terms of seizure control [2]. However, second generation AEDs offer improvements in pharmacological properties and different side-effect profiles which may make them more appropriate in certain clinical scenarios.

Epilepsy syndrome and seizure type

Accurate seizure classification is an important first step in the AED selection process (see Table 10.1). A few points are worth emphasizing in this regard. First, complex partial and generalized absence seizures can be mistaken on clinical grounds, yet some of the AEDs appropriate for complex partial seizures (e.g., carbamazepine, oxcarbazepine, phenytoin) are ineffective in generalized absence seizures. Second, generalized tonic-clonic seizures can occur as a manifestation of idiopathic primary generalized epilepsy, or by secondary generalization of partial seizures. Distinguishing primary generalized from secondary generalized seizures is important as certain AEDs effective in partial seizures, such as carbamazepine, phenytoin, phenobarbital, tiagabine, lamotrigine, and vigabatrin may lead to exacerbation of certain seizure types that may accompany generalized tonic-clonic seizures in patients with idiopathic generalized epilepsy [3]. Third, certain AEDs, including valproate, topiramate, felbamate, zonisamide, and levetiracetam, are considered to have a "broad spectrum" of activity, that is, are effective in most generalized and partial seizure types, therefore may have a role in cases where the epilepsy diagnosis is unknown [4]. And finally, although second generation AEDs have been found to have efficacy against a broad spectrum of seizure types, in one large series, valproate was shown to have the greatest efficacy compared to the rest [5]. Given the potential side effects and risks of valproate, however, it is clear that factors other than efficacy alone as discussed below, need to be considered when selecting an AED.

Table 10.1 Seizure classification and AED selection. AEDs are organized by their position as first or second generation therapies (those approved from the 1990s or later), and those used primarily in epilepsy subspecialty care

AED	Partial	Absence	Myoclonic, tonic, atonic, astatic	GTC
First generation				
Carbamazepine	+	0[a]	0[a]	±
Clonazepam	0	0	+	0
Divalproex sodium/valproate	+	+	+	+
Ethosuximide	0	+	0	0
Phenobarbital	+	0[a]	0[a]	+
Phenytoin	+	0[a]	0[a]	±
Primidone	+	0	0	+
Second generation				
Gabapentin	+	0	0	0
Lacosamide	+	0	0	0
Lamotrigine	+	+	+[a]	+
Levetiracetam	+	±	+	+
Oxcarbazepine	+	0	0	±
Pregabalin	+	0	0	0
Tiagabine	+	0[a]	0	0
Topiramate	+	±	+	+
Zonisamide	+	±	±	+
Subspecialty				
Felbamate	+	+	+	+
Rufinamide	0	0	+	0
Vigabatrin	+	0[a]	0[a]	+

[a] Has been associated with exacerbation of listed seizure type.
+: use established; ±: occasionally appropriate; 0: use not generally appropriate.

Medical comorbidities and side-effect profile

Certain medical conditions may influence AED selection. The presence of significant renal insufficiency may favor AEDs degraded through hepatic pathways, and conversely the presence of hepatic disease may warrant treatment with AEDs eliminated via renal mechanisms. The influences of hepatic and renal insufficiency on AED dosing are summarized in Tables 10.2 and 10.3. Table 10.4 lists medical conditions which may influence AED selection given the potential for adverse effects of that particular AED for the listed condition. Similarly, certain common side effects characteristic of a particular AED may affect selection in a given patient who may already struggle with similar symptoms. Common side effects associated with the AEDs are listed in Table 10.5. The potential major

Table 10.2 AEDs: first generation drugs—pharmacologic properties, interaction potential, and dosing in hepatic and renal insufficiency states. Protein-binding and half-life data derived from Levy et al. [6]. Therapeutic ranges from Mayo Medical Labs effective December 2009. Recommendations for hepatic and renal dosing Lacerda et al. [7, 8].

AED	Protein binding	Serum half-life	Therapeutic range total and (unbound)	Interaction potential: AED on other meds	Interaction potential: other meds on AED	Dosage in hepatic disease	Dosage in renal disease
First generation							
Carbamazepine	70–80%	8–20 h	2–10 µg/ml	+++	+++	+ Reduction	No change
Clonazepam	86%	20–60 h	10–50 µg/ml	+	+	+ Reduction	No change
Divalproex Na+/valproic acid	90%	11–20 h (mono) 5–9 h w/EIAED	40–100 µg/ml (4–15 µg/ml)	++	++	+ Reduction	+ Reduction (protein binding)
Ethosuximide	Minimal	40–60 h	40–75 µg/ml	+	+	+ Reduction	+ Reduction, dialyzable
Phenobarbital	55%	50–160 h	15–40 µg/ml	+++	+++	+ Reduction	No change, dialyzable
Phenytoin	90%	~24 h (longer @ high conc)	10–20 µg/ml (1–2 µg/ml)	+++	+++	+ Reduction	+ Reduction (protein binding)
Primidone	9–20%	3–22 h 10–25 (PEMA)	PB 15–40 µg/ml PEMA 4–12.5	+++	+++	+ Reduction	No change, dialyzable

w/EIAED: with enzyme-inducing antiepileptic drug; PB: phenobarbital; PEMA: phenylethylmalonamide—active metabolites of primidone; +++: high; ++: moderate; +: low; ±: marginal propensity; dialyzable: removable through hemodialysis.

Table 10.3 AEDs: second generation and "subspecialty" drugs—pharmacologic properties, interaction potential, and dosing in hepatic and renal insufficiency states. Protein-binding and half-life data derived from Levy et al. [6]. Therapeutic ranges from Mayo Medical Labs effective December 2009. Recommendations for hepatic and renal dosing Lacerda et al. [7, 8]

AED	Protein binding	Serum half-life	Therapeutic range	Interaction potential: AED on other meds	Interaction potential: other meds on AED	Dosage in hepatic disease	Dosage in renal disease
Second generation							
Gabapentin	Minimal	5–7 h	>2 µg/ml	None	None	No change	+++ Reduction, dialyzable
Lacosamide	<1%	~12 h	N/A	None	None	+ Reduction	+++ Reduction, dialyzable
Lamotrigine	55%	25 h (mono) 11–15 h w/EIAED 54–94 h w/VPA	2.5–15 µg/ml	None	++	+ Reduction	± Reduction
Levetiracetam	Minimal	6–8 h	Peak 10–63 µg/ml (trough 3–34)	None	None	No change	+++ Reduction, dialyzable
Oxcarbazepine	40% (MHD)	8–15 h (MHD)	Peak < 40 µg/ml (trough 6–10)	+	++	± Reduction	+ Reduction

(Continued)

Table 10.3 (*Continued*)

AED	Protein binding	Serum half-life	Therapeutic range	Interaction potential: AED on other meds	Interaction potential: other meds on AED	Dosage in hepatic disease	Dosage in renal disease
Pregabalin	Minimal	5–7 h	N/A	None	None	No change	++ Reduction
Tiagabine	96%	7–9 h	5–520 µg/ml	None	++	+ Reduction	None
Topiramate	9–17%	20–30 h	Peak 9–12 µg/ml (trough 2–4)	+	+	+ Reduction	++ Reduction, dialyzable
Zonisamide	40–60%	50–70 h 25–35 w/EIAED	10–40 µg/ml	None	+	Unknown	Dialyzable
Subspecialty							
Felbamate	22–25%	12–22 h (mono) 11–20 w/EIAED VPA > 24 h	25–100 µg/ml	+++	++	Avoid	++ Reduction
Rufinamide	~25%	6–10 h	N/A	+	None	Unknown	None
Vigabatrin	Minimal	5–7 h	N/A	None	None	No change	+++ Reduction, dialyzable

w/EIAED: with enzyme-inducing AED; VPA: valproic acid; N/A: not available; MHD: the monohydroxy-derivative (active metabolite) of oxcarbazepine; +++: high; ++: moderate; +: low; ±: marginal propensity; dialyzable: removable through hemodialysis.

Table 10.4 Medical co-morbidities and effect on AED selection

AED	Chronic anticoagulant therapy	Urolithiasis	Cardiac conduction abnormalities	Hyponatremia	Sulfonamide allergy	Glaucoma	Liver disease	Visual impairment	Blood dyscrasias	Hepatic porphyria	Cognitive impairment
First generation											
Carbamazepine	++	—	+	++	—	—	+	—	++	+++	+
Clonazepam	—	—	—	—	—	++	—	—	—	—	+
Divalproex Na+/valproic acid	++	—	—	—	—	—	++	—	+	+++	+
Ethosuximide	—	—	—	—	—	—	—	—	—	—	—
Phenobarbital	+++	—	—	—	—	—	—	—	+	+++	+
Phenytoin	++	—	—	—	—	—	+	—	—	+++	+
Primidone	+++	—	—	—	—	—	—	—	—	+++	+
Second generation											
Gabapentin	—	—	—	—	—	±	—	—	—	—	—
Lacosamide	—	—	++	—	—	—	—	—	—	—	—
Lamotrigine	—	—	—	—	—	—	—	—	—	—	—
Levetiracetam	—	—	—	—	—	—	—	—	—	—	+
Oxcarbazepine	—	—	—	++	—	—	—	—	++	—	—
Pregabalin	—	—	—	—	—	—	—	—	—	—	—
Tiagabine	—	—	—	—	—	—	—	—	—	—	—
Topiramate	—	++	—	—	—	++	—	—	—	++	±
Zonisamide	—	++	—	—	+++	+	—	—	—	—	+
Subspecialty											
Felbamate	++	—	—	—	—	—	+++	—	+++	++	—
Rufinamide	—	—	—	—	—	—	—	—	—	—	—
Vigabatrin	—	—	—	—	—	—	—	+++	—	—	—

+++: significant or listed as contraindication; ++: moderate; +: low; ±: marginal potential difficulties with specific condition; blank: no adverse effect for the given comorbidity known with the listed AED.

Table 10.5   AEDs: Characteristic side effects

AED	Most common side effects affecting tolerability
First generation	
Carbamazepine	Ataxia, diplopia, blurred vision, cognitive, hyponatremia, leukopenia
Clonazepam	Sedation, cognitive
Divalproex Na+/ valproic acid	Weight gain, tremor, hair loss, cognitive, polycystic ovary syndrome, nausea, thrombocytopenia
Ethosuximide	Nausea, anorexia, psychiatric
Phenobarbital	Cognitive, sedation, frozen shoulder, Dupuytren's, depression, macrocytic anemia
Phenytoin	Cognitive, gum hypertrophy, peripheral neuropathy, dyskinesia, neuropathy, ataxia, macrocytic anemia
Primidone	Cognitive, vertigo, nausea, sedation, frozen shoulder, Dupuytren's
Second generation	
Gabapentin	Ataxia, weight gain, somnolence
Lacosamide	Dizziness, nausea, blurred vision, P-R interval prolongation
Lamotrigine	Insomnia, ataxia, blurred vision
Levetiracetam	Irritability, aggression, somnolence, dizziness
Oxcarbazepine	Ataxia, diplopia, blurred vision, cognitive, hyponatremia, leukopenia
Pregabalin	Unsteadiness, weight gain, edema, somnolence, dizziness
Tiagabine	Confusion, dizziness, fatigue
Topiramate	Cognitive, word finding, paresthesias, weight loss, nausea, glaucoma
Zonisamide	Nausea, cognitive, glaucoma, psychiatric
Subspecialty	
Felbamate	Weight loss, insomnia, nausea
Rufinamide	Somnolence, dizziness, diplopia, nausea
Vigabatrin	Somnolence, weight gain, ataxia, psychiatric, anemia, neuropathy

toxicities associated with the different AEDs are summarized in Table 10.6, which also may affect AED selection in the presence of certain medical comorbidities.

Drug–drug interactions: concurrent medical therapies

Concurrent medical therapies may influence AED selection, or at least the target dose. Many first and some second generation AEDs are metabolized by or affect the activity of hepatic enzyme pathways, which may lead to drug–drug interactions when taken concurrently with other medications undergoing degradation by the same processes.

The hepatic enzyme systems of relevance to AED drug–drug interactions are the cytochrome P450 system, the uridine glucuronyl transferase (UGT) system, and epoxide hydrolase [9, 10]. AEDs that influence or undergo extensive metabolic degradation through the cytochrome p450 system include carbamazepine, phenytoin, phenobarbital, primidone, ethosuximide, oxcarbazepine,

Table 10.6   Major toxicities associated with the AEDs

AED	Major potential drug-related toxicities
First generation	
Carbamazepine	Stevens-Johnson/toxic epidermal necrolysis (TEN), hepatotoxicity, aplastic anemia, multiorgan hypersensitivity
Clonazepam	Nonconvulsive status epilepticus
Divalproex Na+/valproic acid	Pancreatitis, hepatotoxicity, hyperammonemic encephalopathy, multiorgan hypersensitivity, hypothermia
Ethosuximide	Aplastic anemia, drug-associated lupus
Phenobarbital	Multiorgan hypersensitivity
Phenytoin	Stevens-Johnson/TEN, blood dyscrasia, hepatotoxicity, multiorgan hypersensitivity
Primidone	Blood dyscrasias
Second generation	
Gabapentin	None reported
Lacosamide	PR interval prolongation, multiorgan hypersensitivity
Lamotrigine	Stevens-Johnson/TEN, multiorgan hypersensitivity
Levetiracetam	None reported
Oxcarbazepine	Stevens-Johnson/TEN, angioedema, multiorgan hypersensivity
Pregabalin	Angioedema
Tiagabine	Nonconvulsive status epilepticus, encephalopathy
Topiramate	Urolithiasis, metabolic acidosis, oligohidrosis, hyperthermia, acute angle-closure glaucoma, hyperammonemic encephalopathy
Zonisamide	Stevens-Johnson/TEN, urolithiasis, oligohidrosis, hyperthermia, acute angle-closure glaucoma, aplastic anemia
Subspecialty	
Felbamate	Aplastic anemia, hepatotoxicity
Rufinamide	QT interval shortening, multiorgan hypersensitivity
Vigabatrin	Progressive visual field loss

tiagabine, zonisamide, felbamate, and valproate [11]. Of these, carbamazepine, phenytoin, phenobarbital, and primidone induce cytochrome p450 enzyme activity; valproate inhibits; and felbamate has both inducing and inhibiting effects. AEDs in which glucuronidation by the UGT system plays a significant role include lamotrigine, the oxcarbazepine monohydroxy derivative (MHD), and valproate [11]. The latter also undergoes extensive beta-oxidation. Epoxide hydrolase is an enzyme involved with the elimination of the active carbamazepine metabolite, carbamazepine-9,10-epoxide, which has both antiepileptic and side effect-related properties. Valproate and felbamate inhibit epoxide hydrolase, leading to accumulation of carbamazepine-9,10-epoxide, which may lead to drug toxicity.

Another pharmacological property of some AEDs that can contribute to drug–drug interactions is protein binding. Interactions involving displacement of

AEDs from protein-binding sites may escape detection unless serum-free levels are measured. The AEDs most commonly affected by protein-binding interactions are phenytoin and valproate. Finally, shared pharmacologic effects of one drug may be additive to another without affecting the other's pharmacokinetics. Such interactions are known as "pharmacodynamic" interactions. Examples of the latter include excess sedation that may occur with concurrent use of barbiturates and benzodiazepines, or in the concurrent use of sedating AEDs with medications of other classes in which CNS depression can occur such as opiates and tricyclic medications.

Common drug–drug interactions associated with the AEDs are summarized in Table 10.7. This table is not a definitive summary. Drug–drug interactions are not consistently reported to regulatory bodies or in the medical literature, so there are limitations in the references available when these issues arise. The reader is advised to consult with a pharmacist when new medications are being added to a patient on other existing therapies. Review of the approved medication labeling for the AED using online resources, or doing a drug–drug interaction check using one of the numerous public and proprietary online drug information resources available is strongly recommended before prescribing AED therapy in patients on other medication treatments.

Gender

Certain AEDs have properties which are suboptimal for use in women [13]. For example, some AEDs lead to reduced serum concentration of the active ingredients in oral contraceptive drugs which may render them less effective. A list of first and second generation AEDs which affect oral contraceptive therapies are summarized in Table 10.8. The teratogenic potential of AEDs is an additional concern. Certain AEDs, specifically phenytoin, carbamazepine, and particularly valproate, are considered to have relatively high teratogenic risk compared to other AEDs [14]. In certain clinical situations, a second generation AED may be more appropriate when teratogenicity is a particular concern or when polypharmacy is deemed clinically necessary [15]. Breast-feeding risk is another common concern in women taking AED therapy. While many AEDs are only present in trace quantities in breast milk due to their high serum protein binding, other medications with low protein binding such as primidone and levetiracetam may be transferred into breast milk in amounts that could be clinically significant [16].

Age

Several factors associated with aging may affect AED selection. Age-associated medical comorbidities, concomitant medication therapy and age-related changes in factors which influence AED elimination such as renal insufficiency, may

Table 10.7 Pharmacokinetic drug–drug interactions involving the AEDs

AED	Interactions with other AEDs	Interactions with nonAEDs
Carbamazepine	*Decreases*: LTG, TGB, ZNS, TPM *Decreased by*: PHT, PB, PRM *CBZ-epoxide increased by*: VPA, FBM	*Decreases*: certain chemotherapeutics, warfarin, OCPs, amlodipine, cyclosporine, voriconazole, aripiprazole, quetiapine, olanzapine, methadone *Increased by*: erythromycin, clarithromycin, fluoxetine, isoniazid, cimetidine, azoles, protease inhibitors, propoxyphene, quetiapine, risperidone, verapamil *Decreased by*: rifampin
Clonazepam		
Ethosuximide	*Decreased by*: PHT, CBZ, PB, PRM *Increases*: PHT *Increases or decreased by*: VPA	— *Increased by*: isoniazid
Felbamate	*Decreased by*: PHT, CBZ, PB, PRM *Increases*: PHT, CBZ epoxide, VPA, PB	*Decreases*: OCPs *Increases*: warfarin
Gabapentin	*Increases*: FBM	*Decreases*: hydrocodone *Increased by*: morphine
Lacosamide	None	None[a]
Lamotrigine	*Decreased by*: PHT, CBZ, PB, PRM, OXC *Increased by*: VPA	*Decreased by*: OCPs
Levetiracetam	None[a]	None
Oxcarbazepine	*Increases*: PHT *Decreased by*: CBZ, PHT, PB, PRM, VPA	*Decreases*: OCPs, amlodipine, simvastatin, cyclosporine, clopidogrel *Decreased by*: verapamil
Phenobarbital/primidone	*Decreases*: CBZ, TGB *Increases*: CBZ-epoxide *Increased by*: VPA, FBM, PHT	*Decreases*: certain chemotherapeutics, warfarin, OCPs, quetiapine *Decreased by*: rifampin *Increased by*: amiodarone, isoniazid, fluconazole, fluoxetine, chloramphenicol, propoxyphene

(Continued)

Table 10.7 (*Continued*)

AED	Interactions with other AEDs	Interactions with nonAEDs
Phenytoin	*Decreases:* CBZ, TGB, TPM, LTG *Increases:* CBZ-epoxide *Increased by:* FBM, VPA (free PHT), OXC	*Decreases:* chemotherapeutics, warfarin, OCPs, darunavir, aripiprazole, quetiapine *Decreased by:* rifampin, antacids *Increased by:* amiodarone, isoniazid, fluconazole, fluoxetine, chloramphenicol, omeprazole, diltiazem *Increased or decreased by:* phenobarbital, primidone
Pregabalin	None	None
Rufinamide	*Increases:* PHT, PB *Increased by:* VPA *Decreased by:* PHT, PB, PRM, CBZ *Decreases:* CBZ, LTG	*Decreases:* OCPs
Tiagabine	*Decreased by:* PHT, CBZ, PB, PRM	—
Topiramate	*Decreased by:* PHT, CBZ, PB, PRM	*Decreases:* OCPs, risperidone, pioglitazone *Increases:* metformin *Increased by:* meformin, thiazides, posaconazole
Valproate	*Increases:* free PHT, CBZ-epoxide, LTG, PB, PRM *Increased by:* FBM *Decreases:* PHT	*Increases:* warfarin (free level), tricyclic antidepressants *Increased by:* sertraline, isoniazid, cimetidine *Decreased by:* carbapenem antibiotics
Vigabatrin	*Increases or decreases:* CBZ	—
Zonisamide	*Decreased by:* PHT, CBZ, PB, PRM	—

PHT: phenytoin; CBZ: carbamazepine; CBZ-epoxide: carbamazepine-9,10-epoxide metabolite; VPA: valproic acid; FBM: felbamate; PB: phenobarbital; PRM: primidone; LTG: lamotrigine; OXC: oxcarbazepine; TPM: topiramate; TGB: tiagabine; ZNS: zonisamide.

aNotable pharmacodynamic interaction present (see text).

Sources: approved medication labeling and Micromedex *DRUG-REAX*® online software, Thomson-Reuters, Inc. [12]; reviewed January 11, 2010.

Table 10.8 Effect of AEDs on efficacy of oral contraceptive pill (OCP) therapy

Impairment of OCP efficacy	No identified effect on OCP efficacy
Carbamazepine	Gabapentin
Felbamate	Lacosamide
Oxcarbazepine	Lamotrigine
Phenobarbital	Levetiracetam
Phenytoin	Pregabalin
Primidone	Tiagabine
Rufinamide	Valproate
Topiramate	Vigabatrin
	Zonisamide

Source: Data from Red Book 2009: Pharmacy's Fundamental Reference [20].

influence choice of therapy [13]. The drug–drug interaction potential and renal dosing for each of the AEDs are summarized in Tables 10.2 and 10.3. Typical doses used in younger patients may not be tolerated, and escalation of therapy should generally proceed at a slower rate in the elderly in order to help mitigate side effects. Selection of AEDs with a more favorable cognitive profile such as lamotrigine or levetiracetam may be preferred over AEDs with a greater incidence of cognitive side effects (e.g., carbamazepine, valproate, topiramate, phenobarbital, and primidone) in this age group.

Ease of use

A therapy's ease of use is correlated with compliance. It is estimated that patients take 75% of medications prescribed for their epilepsy [17]. Factors impacting ease of use in AED treatment include dose frequency and complexity of the treatment regimen. Treatment plans consisting of greater than one dosage per day or involving more than one AED may be difficult for patients, but can be facilitated by the use of a pill box. Using an alarm clock as a reminder may be helpful as well. Single daily dose regimens may also improve compliance. Examples of AEDs that can be taken as single daily dose therapy include phenobarbital and extended-release formulations of lamotrigine, levetiracetam, valproate, and phenytoin.

Clinical urgency

Sometimes clinical urgency guides AED selection. Certain AEDs can be initiated at maintenance doses at treatment initiation, while others require a relatively protracted titration period due to the potential for toxicity associated with rapid escalation. The initiation rates of the AEDs are summarized in Table 10.9.

Table 10.9   AEDs: treatment initiation rates

May initiate at target maintenance dose	
Phenytoin	
Phenobarbital	
Valproate	
Titrate to target dose over two to three weeks	
Carbamazepine	Oxcarbazepine
Ethosuximide	Rufinamide
Felbamate	Vigabatrin
Gabapentin	Zonisamide
Levetiracetam	
Titrate to target dose over several weeks	
Lacosamide	Primidone
Lamotrigine	Tiagabine
Topiramate	Pregabalin

Cost

Cost is of significant importance when selecting an AED. The least expensive AED is phenobarbital which costs a few US dollars per month, followed by phenytoin which is significantly less expensive than second generation AEDs. However, these medications may be less optimal than their more expensive counterparts in certain situations where more desirable pharmacokinetic or other indication attributes are particularly crucial. It is important to note that factors other than efficacy, pharmacokinetics, and tolerability contribute significantly to drug pricing. For example, gabapentin is one of the more expensive AED options available yet it has the lowest published responder rate of all the second generation AEDs when compared in a meta-analysis of AED clinical trials [18]. This largely stems from its widespread use in the treatment of pain, and has little to do with its favorable drug–drug interaction profile. Basic economic factors also influence drug-pricing sometimes to a greater extent than the value of the drug related to efficacy and pharmacological factors. For example, vigabatrin, which has a unique niche in epilepsy care and is distributed through a single pharmacy secondary to its potential for causing progressive visual field impairment, is the most expensive AED approved for use in the US at the present, in part due to the lack of source competition.

Cost is an increasingly important aspect in treatment selection. Multiple factors affect drug pricing, and counseling patients as to the costs they may be facing for a particular treatment plan can be challenging [19]. While pharmacy benefit plans significantly offset medication costs, many are not fortunate enough to be enrolled in one. Pharmacy benefit plan formulary rules also may restrict the treatment options and may require prior authorizations which complicate the efficiency of patient care. Generic AEDs offer a lower cost alternative for the treatment of epilepsy. However, while the expiration of patents for branded AED products allowed the licensing of cheaper generic equivalent products, the loss of patent protection had the unfortunate consequence of removing the incentive for pharmaceutical companies to make these drugs available as samples for dispensing to the economically disadvantaged. It is also important to realize that the cost of generic second generation AEDs is still substantial and in many cases remains more expensive than the cost of branded first generation AEDs (see Table 10.10) [20].

10.3 Generic AED therapy

Generic AED therapy is assuming a larger role in epilepsy management. The FDA (US Food and Drug Administration) has approved generic bioequivalents for several second generation AEDs, and many pharmacy benefit plans have stringent rules favoring their use over branded alternatives. While generic AEDs provide an opportunity for cost savings, the prospect of switching a stable patient from a branded AED to a generic alternative can be a source of anxiety for physicians and patients.

The "Drug Price Competition and Patent Term Restoration Act of 1984," (aka Hatch-Waxman Act) provided authority to the FDA to utilize an expedited process for approval of generic medications. This allowed utilization of the standard of "bioequivalence" to form the basis of approval, as opposed to requiring verification of clinical equivalence. Manufacturers seeking FDA approval for a generic medication are currently required to complete an Abbreviated New Drug Application (ANDA) process, which is less arduous than the New Drug Application (NDA) process required for approval of a new drug [21].

The ANDA process requires submission of data supporting bioequivalence between the generic product and its branded equivalent, and does not require evidence of clinical equivalence vis à vis seizure control. The standards for determining "bioequivalence" are outlined in a publication called Approved Drug Products with Therapeutic Equivalence Evaluations (aka "the Orange Book"), published by the Department of Health and Human Services and available for free download on the FDA.gov web site [21]. The premise of the standard of bioequivalence is that pharmacokinetic equivalence between an approved drug and a generic version should result in clinical equivalence. According to the Orange Book, bioequivalence may be established by performance of a crossover study involving "usually 24–36" healthy adult volunteers [21]. Single doses of the generic drug and reference product are administered to healthy volunteers and the resulting area under the curve (AUC) of the graph plotting plasma concentration over time, and peak serum concentrations (CMax) are compared. The standard is considered satisfied when the 90% confidence interval of the ratios of the AUC and Cmax of the branded and generic products using log-transformed data falls between the range of 0.8–1.25.

Table 10.10 Cost comparison: branded AEDs and generic bioequivalents based on average wholesale price (AWP) for dosage shown

Drug	Formulation	Daily dosage	Cost of 30-day supply (AWP cost[a])
Carbamazepine (Tegretol®)	200 mg tablets	200 mg four times daily	$107
Carbamazepine (generic)	*200 mg tablets*	*200 mg four times daily*	*$36*
Carbamazepine (Tegretol XR®)	400 mg XR tablets	400 mg twice daily	$120
Carbamazepine SR (generic)	*400 mg SR tablets*	*400 mg twice daily*	*$112*
Divalproex acid (Depakote®)	500 mg tablets	500 mg three times a day	$347
Divalproex acid (generic)	*500 mg tablets*	*500 mg three times a day*	*$287*
Divalproex acid ER (Depakote®)	500 mg ER tablets	1500 mg once daily	$301
Divalproex acid ER (generic)	*500 mg ER tablets*	*1500 mg once daily*	*$266*
Gabapentin (Neurontin®)	600 mg tablets	600 mg three times a day	$328
Gabapentin (generic)	*600 mg tablets*	*600 mg three times a day*	*$215*
Lamotrigine (Lamictal®)	200 mg tablets	200 mg twice daily	$417
Lamotrigine (generic)	*200 mg tablets*	*200 mg twice daily*	*$339*
Levetiracetam (Keppra ®)	1000 mg tablets	1000 mg twice daily	$532
Levetiracetam (generic)	*1000 mg tablets*	*1000 mg twice daily*	*$405*
Phenytoin (Dilantin®)	100 mg capseals®	300 mg daily	$35
Phenytoin (generic)	*100 mg capsules*	*300 mg daily*	*$30*
Topiramate (Topamax®)	200 mg tablets	200 mg twice daily	$543
Topiramate (generic)	*200 mg tablets*	*200 mg twice daily*	*$424*
Zonisamide (Zonegran®)	100 mg capsules	100 mg twice daily	$189
Zonisamide (generic)	*100 mg capsules*	*100 mg twice daily*	*$124*

[a]Where multiple generic products are available, the lowest pricing was used (December 2009).
Source: Data from *Red Book 2009: Pharmacy's Fundamental Reference* [20]

Despite the assurance of pharmacokinetic bioequivalence, patients and physicians often harbor concerns whether a generic AED will work as well as a branded product. A limited number of controlled trials comparing the clinical efficacy of first generation AEDs and generic bioequivalents have been performed. These studies have not shown differences in efficacy of branded AEDs over generic [22, 23]. Nonetheless, some observational studies have raised questions regarding the clinical equivalency of generic AEDs, finding increased switchback rates and greater rates of emergency services and hospitalization associated with mandated generic substitution policies [24].

In response to these concerns, the American Academy of Neurology has issued a position paper recommending that physicians be allowed to approve or disapprove generic AED substitutions for the treatment of epilepsy [25]. Some states require physician notification when generic substitution has occurred, but most do not. It is also not well known that there may be several different generic manufacturers for a given branded product. No laws currently prevent dispensing pharmacies from switching between generic manufacturers, which can potentially lead to treatment variability and patient confusion.

Generic AED therapy will clearly remain a part of epilepsy care into the future. In the majority of cases, the transition between branded and generic therapy is uneventful. The savings are often welcomed by patients, and affordability may lead to improved compliance in some cases. When switching, it may be prudent to check serum levels following the transition to help assure stability in some cases. It should also be recognized that switching from generic to branded AED therapy may be associated with toxicity as well, particularly in treatment with AEDs associated with a narrow therapeutic window such as phenytoin.

10.4 The AEDs: summary of clinical use, pharmacokinetics, and efficacy

In this section, general information regarding indications, pharmacokinetics, and efficacy of the first generation, second generation, and subspecialty AEDs are provided. The AEDs are discussed in alphabetical order. Tables 10.2, 10.3, 10.5, and 10.6 summarize AED pharmacokinetics and side effects. Table 10.7 summarizes AED drug–drug interactions that are frequently encountered in practice. The drug interactions listed are those identified in the individual drug's approved medication labeling, and in the proprietary online drug interaction software tool DRUG REAX® provided by Micromedex through Thomson Reuters (Healthcare) Inc. [12].

For more detailed information about AEDs, the reader is referred to the approved medication labeling for each drug which can be found online on the National Library of Medicine's web site "Daily Med": http://dailymed .nlm.nih.gov/dailymed/about.cfm. Additional medication information can be found on www.epilepsy.com. For a detailed textbook on the AEDs, the reader is referred to the comprehensive reference titled *Antiepileptic Drugs*, R.H. Levy *et al.* (eds.) [6].

First generation medications

Carbamazepine

Indications, usage, and potential side effects

Carbamazepine is approved for use in the treatment of partial and generalized tonic-clonic seizures. Carbamazepine may be associated with exacerbation of absence and myoclonic seizures, so should not be used to treat these seizure types [3].

Advantages of carbamazepine are its relative low cost and lack of cosmetic side effects compared to phenytoin. It occasionally may have beneficial effects on mood as well. Disadvantages include the potential for side effects such as dizziness, fatigue, blurred vision, and propensity towards drug–drug interactions. Similar to phenytoin, carbamazepine can be associated with peripheral neuropathy, ataxia, and osteopenia with chronic use. Hypersensitivity drug rash and hepatotoxicity can occur. In addition, leukopenia can be seen in up to 10% of patients. This is usually minor and does not require drug discontinuation, but may necessitate periodic monitoring. Carbamazepine can also be associated with hyponatremia secondary to a SIADH mechanism.

Dosage, pharmacokinetics, and potential interactions

Carbamazepine is available in a standard release tablet formulation, which is recommended to be taken on a t.i.d. schedule. An extended release formulation is also available which allows b.i.d. dosing. An oral suspension and chewable tablets are available, but a parenteral form is not. It should be noted that auto-induction of carbamazepine metabolism can occur during the first month of treatment. Because of auto-induction, the initial steady-state serum concentration may decrease in the first month or two of therapy despite maintaining compliance.

Carbamazepine is prone to pharmacokinetic interactions (see Table 10.7) [10]. Carbamazepine induces the hepatic cytochrome P450 and UDP-glucuronyl transferase enzyme systems, which increases degradation of medications metabolized through these pathways. Likewise, carbamazepine elimination may be increased by enzyme-inducing drugs such as phenytoin and rifampin. Conversely, carbamazepine or its metabolites including carbamazepine-9,10-epoxide may accumulate when taken with drugs that inhibit hepatic enzyme systems such as erythromycin, clarithromycin, propoxyphene, isoniazid, fluoxetine, and valproate.

Clonazepam (Klonopin)

Indications, usage, and potential side effects

Clonazepam is used as adjunctive therapy in the treatment of Lennox-Gastaut syndrome, myoclonic seizures, and occasionally in the treatment of absence seizures. The main side effects associated with clonazepam are sedation and cognitive dysfunction. Clonazepam has been implicated as a trigger of nonconvulsive status epilepticus in some cases, particularly when taken in combination with valproate. Caretakers should be cautioned to look for evidence of decreased responsiveness in patients with severe symptomatic or cryptogenic generalized epilepsy on treatment with clonazepam given this risk.

Dosage, pharmacokinetics, and potential interactions

Clonazepam should be initiated at low doses and titrated gradually. While it is metabolized through hepatic enzyme pathways, it is not a significant inducer of hepatic enzyme activity. Even though there are minimal pharmacokinetic interactions between clonazepam and other medications, pharmacodynamic interactions may occur, particularly if used in combination with other GABAergic drugs, such as tiagabine, vigabatrin, phenobarbital, primidone, valproate, and benzodiazepine receptor agonists. Psychotropic medications with sedating properties and opiates should also be used with caution if combined with clonazepam.

Ethosuximide

Indications, usage, and potential side effects

Ethosuximide is indicated exclusively for the treatment of generalized absence seizures. It is not approved for the treatment of generalized tonic-clonic, myoclonic or partial seizures. In patients with seizure types other than absence seizures, additional AEDs are usually required, or a broad spectrum AED should be considered instead. Ethosuximide is associated with side effects in a significant proportion of cases, including gastrointestinal symptoms such as nausea and abdominal discomfort; and CNS side effects including drowsiness, dizziness, behavior changes, and headaches. Hypersensitivity cutaneous reactions, a lupus-like syndrome, and blood dyscrasia can occur as well.

Dosage, pharmacokinetics, and potential interactions

Ethosuximide is available in capsule and syrup dosage forms. A parenteral form is not available. In adults, ethosuximide is typically started at 250 mg per day. The dosage is then adjusted higher as needed to desired clinical effect. The potential for drug–drug interactions with ethosuximide is low.

Phenytoin

Indications, usage, and potential side effects

Phenytoin is approved for use in generalized tonic-clonic and partial seizures. The advantages of phenytoin are its low cost and the potential for once a day dosing. Disadvantages include potential morphological side effects include hirsuitism, coarsening of facial features, and gum hypertrophy. Gum hypertrophy can be prevented to some extent by periodic dental visits. Other common side effects include cognitive symptoms, ataxia, and fatigue. Phenytoin also has a relatively high potential for drug–drug interactions. Peripheral neuropathy and osteopenia may occur which should be monitored when used long term. Other possible side effects include hypersensitivity drug rash, blood dyscrasias and hepatotoxicity.

Dosage, pharmacokinetics, and potential interactions

Phenytoin is available in capsular, tablet, and suspension form. While phenytoin is available in a parenteral formulation, a derivative, fosphenytoin, is preferred for parenteral use as it is much more soluble at physiologic pH, less irritative during IV infusion, and not prone to development of the purple glove syndrome. Unlike parenteral phenytoin, fosphenytoin can be mixed in dextrose-containing solutions and may be administered intramuscularly. The typical IV loading dose for IV fosphenytoin in status epilepticus is 18–20 mg/kg phenytoin equivalents (PEs) administered at a rate of 100–150 mg PE/min. IV fosphenytoin loading doses should only be administered in a setting where hemodynamic and ECG monitoring can be provided [26].

In less urgent situations, an oral loading dose of phenytoin can be administered in three divided doses over a 12–24 hour period. In cases where a loading dose is not needed, the predicted maintenance dose (usually 300 mg/day in adults) can be started on day 1, without the need for gradual titration. The absorption of oral phenytoin is poor in neonates, decreased if taken with antacids, and may be erratic when administered via enteral feeding tubes. Some patients are rapid metabolizers of phenytoin, requiring maintenance dosages significantly higher than 300 mg per day. Given the narrow therapeutic window associated with phenytoin and the variation seen in the serum concentration-dose relationship between individuals, follow-up serum concentration measurements should be performed two to four weeks after initiation.

Phenytoin's pharmacokinetic properties follow nonlinear zero-order kinetics, attributed to the capacity for saturation of serum protein binding and hepatocellular enzyme sites. This property leads to disproportionate increases or decreases in serum concentrations resulting from even small dose changes when baseline levels are in the higher end of the therapeutic range. When a dose increase is contemplated in a patient with high baseline serum concentrations, small adjustments should be used. The 30 mg capsules and 50 mg tablets are useful in this setting.

Phenobarbital

Indications, usage, and potential side effects

Phenobarbital is indicated for treatment of primary and secondary generalized tonic-clonic and partial seizures, but not absence or myoclonic seizures. Advantages of phenobarbital include its low cost and once-daily dosing. The disadvantages of phenobarbital are its cognitive and sedative effects, and potential for drug–drug interactions. Chronic use may be associated with osteopenia, Dupuytren's contracture, and frozen shoulder.

Dosage, pharmacokinetics, and potential interactions

Phenobarbital is available in tablet, suspension, and parenteral form. It has fallen out of favor in epilepsy care given the availability of other treatments with fewer side effects, shorter half-lives, and less potential for drug–drug interactions. Phenobarbital can be administered intravenously in a loading dose in urgent epilepsy-related clinical situations. However, rapid intravenous infusion may be associated with hypotension and respiratory suppression, and therefore should only be administered in a setting capable of providing hemodynamic monitoring and the immediate availability of ventilatory support.

Phenobarbital has a long half-life spanning a few days' duration which allows once a day dosing. As a result, the effects of dose adjustments may take several days to be reflected by a change in drug levels. Phenobarbital is metabolized extensively by hepatic enzyme pathways and can induce metabolism of other medications metabolized through the same pathways including oral contraceptives (OCPs), warfarin, and phenytoin. Drugs that inhibit hepatic enzymes, such as valproate and isoniazid, may decrease phenobarbital elimination leading to toxicity.

Primidone

Indications, usage, and potential side effects

Primidone is indicated for the treatment of partial and secondary generalized seizures. It is not as well tolerated as other AEDs which significantly limits its use [27]. Initiation of primidone may be complicated by dizziness and nausea. This can be offset by starting therapy at low doses. The more common long-term side effects associated with primidone include sedation and cognitive dysfunction. Side effects with chronic use include osteopenia and Dupuyten's contractures.

Dosage, pharmacokinetics, and potential interactions

Primidone is available in tablet form. Given the need to titrate the dose slowly, primidone is not appropriate for the acute treatment of seizures. Dosing should start at low doses and be gradually increased over four to eight weeks in order to prevent drug discontinuation due to intolerance. It induces hepatic enzyme activity and may be associated with drug–drug interactions. Primidone is metabolized into two active metabolites, phenobarbital and phenylethylmalonamide (PEMA), both of which contribute to its antiepileptic activity. Drugs which induce hepatic enzyme activity, such as phenytoin and carbamazepine, promote conversion of primidone to its metabolites.

Valproate (divalproex sodium, valproic acid)

Indications, usage, and potential side effects

Divalproex sodium and valproic acid, collectively referred to as "valproate," are considered "broad spectrum" AEDs due to their efficacy against several seizure types including absence, myoclonic, partial, and primary and secondary generalized tonic-clonic seizures. Valproate may be less effective than carbamazepine in the treatment of complex partial seizures [28]. Common side effects include weight gain, hair loss, and tremor. Valproate is also associated with polycystic ovary syndrome, hirsuitism, and is associated with the highest teratogenic risk amongst the AEDs [29]. Mild thrombocytopenia is common, but this rarely becomes clinically significant. Potential major side effects associated with valproate therapy are pancreatitis and a Reye's-like form of hepatotoxicity.

Dosage, pharmacokinetics, and potential interactions

Divalproex sodium is available in unscored standard and extended release tablets. It also is available in a 125 mg "sprinkles" formulation which can be sprinkled on food for patients with an aversion to taking tablets or capsules. Valproic acid is available in capsular and syrup dosage forms. A parenteral formulation of divalproex sodium is available, which is officially approved for use in providing maintenance therapy when oral administration is not possible. However, it has been used off-label in the acute treatment of seizures. There is no need for gradual titration of valproate upon initiation of therapy.

Valproate's high protein-binding and inhibitory effect on hepatic enzyme activity can lead to clinically significant drug–drug interactions [9]. Drug–drug interactions involving valproate secondary to enzyme inhibition have been described with lamotrigine, phenobarbital, and carbamazepine. Competition for protein-binding sites with other protein-bound medications such as phenytoin may lead to toxicity. In such cases, total phenytoin levels may be normal making the diagnosis difficult unless serum-free levels are obtained.

Second generation medications

Gabapentin

Indications, usage, and potential side effects

Gabapentin is approved for use as adjuvant therapy for partial seizures with or without secondary generalization. It is not approved for the treatment of primary generalized tonic-clonic, absence, or myoclonic seizures in idiopathic generalized epilepsy. Gabapentin has not been approved as a monotherapy agent. The main side effects are ataxia, dizziness, and lethargy [30].

Dosage, pharmacokinetics, and potential interactions

Gabapentin is available in multiple strengths in tablet, capsular, and suspension form. Neither parenteral nor extended release formulations are available. Because of its short half-life, it is typically administered on a t.i.d. or q.i.d schedule [31]. The usual starting dose is 300 mg daily with daily 300 mg dose increments until an optimal dose is reached. The minimally effective dose for epilepsy in clinical trials is 300 mg t.i.d. Significantly higher dosages are generally used. However, it is important to note that the bioavailability of gabapentin decreases substantially at higher dosages, presumably secondary to saturation of transport mechanisms in the lining of the GI tract. In patients requiring higher dosages, the prescriber may want to consider pregablin instead which has a similar mechanism of action and a more reliable absorption potential at higher dosages.

Gabapentin is excreted unchanged in the urine and does not undergo hepatic metabolism. Therefore, the risk of pharmacokinetic interactions with gabapentin would be predicted to be low. However, gabapentin has been associated with a reduction in the bioavailability of hydrocodone, and morphine has been associated with increased levels of gabapentin [12]. Given the lack of dependency on hepatic elimination, gabapentin is a consideration in patients with coexisting liver disease. Due to its dependency on renal elimination, the gabapentin dosage must be significantly reduced in patients with moderate to severe renal insufficiency [7]. It's also important to remember that while the potential for pharmacokinetic interactions is minimal with gabapentin, pharmacodynamic interactions with other CNS medications may occur, particularly in the elderly [32].

Efficacy

Gabapentin is indicated for the treatment of partial epilepsy. The efficacy in partial epilepsy was evaluated in five placebo-controlled add-on trials [33]. In these trials, roughly 20% of patients receiving gabapentin experienced a 50% or greater reduction in seizure frequency. A modest dose–response relationship has been observed: in one trial, the responder rate at 600 mg per day was 18%, it increased slightly to 26% at 1800 mg per day [34]. Significantly higher doses can be safely prescribed as the therapeutic window associated with gabapentin is quite wide and GI absorption limited; however, there is no evidence that higher dosages are any more effective than those used in clinical trials.

Lacosamide

Indications, usage, and potential side effects

Lacosamide, formerly known as harkoseride, is approved as adjunctive therapy for partial seizures. It has minimal potential for drug–drug interactions so is useful in patients who are on other medication therapies. Side effects that occurred in greater than 10% of subjects in clinical trials included arthralgias, ataxia, blurred vision, diplopia, dizziness, fatigue, headache, nausea, tremor, and vomiting [35]. Cardiac conduction abnormalities were noted in preclinical trials. The FDA-approved labeling advises caution when used in patients with preexisting PR interval prolongation, other known cardiac conduction abnormalities (e.g., first- and second-degree AV block), in those taking drugs known to induce PR interval prolongation, and in those with severe cardiac disease such as myocardial ischemia or heart failure. Lacosamide is classified in the US as a controlled substance, which somewhat complicates prescribing.

Dosage, pharmacokinetics, and potential interactions

Lacosamide is available in tablet form in several dosage strengths and in parenteral form, which is approved for use as temporizing therapy for situations in which oral dosing is not feasible. The initial recommended dose in adults is 50 mg twice daily, followed by weekly dose increases of 50 mg twice daily to a target of 200 mg twice daily. Pharmacokinetic studies show that it is renally excreted, minimally bound to plasma proteins and has no known clinically relevant drug–drug interactions [12, 36]. Lacosamide does not appear to interfere with oral contraceptive pharmacokinetics [37]. The potential for pharmacodynamic interactions referable to the PR interval should be kept in mind when prescribing lacosamide in patients taking other medications that affect atrioventricular conduction.

Efficacy

Open-label studies showed a 14–47% reduction in seizure frequency with lacosamide, and placebo-controlled trials demonstrated a 26–40% reduction. The 50% responder rates ranged from 32.7 to 41.2% [35]. Doses below 400 mg per day did not reach statistical significance over the seizure reduction seen in placebo groups. The parenteral form has not been studied in the setting of acute epilepsy emergencies or status epilepticus.

Lamotrigine

Indications, usage, and potential side effects

Lamotrigine is approved as adjuvant treatment and for conversion to monotherapy in partial seizures. It is also approved for use in generalized tonic-clonic seizures in generalized epilepsy and Lennox-Gastaut syndrome, and has shown efficacy in absence seizures [38]. Lamotrigine may cause worsening of myoclonic seizures in some patients [39]. The risk of greatest concern is the potential for systemic hypersensitivity reactions, such as Stevens-Johnson syndrome and toxic epidermal necrolysis (TEN). Cutaneous hypersensitivity reactions occur in up to 13% of patients treated with lamotrigine, most of which are minor and resolve with discontinuation [40]. According to the package insert dated October 2009, the incidence of Stevens-Johnson syndrome has been calculated in children and adults to be 0.8 and 0.3% respectively. Early reports suggested a higher prevalence of hypersensitivity reactions when used in combination with valproic acid. Subsequent research shows the risk associated with valproate combination therapy can be mitigated by using lower lamotrigine dosages during initiation [40]. Other side effects include insomnia, dizziness, and ataxia.

Dosage, pharmacokinetics, and potential interactions

Lamotrigine is available in standard release, chewable, oral disintegrating, and extended release tablets. Parenteral and suspension forms are not currently available. Lamotrigine is usually prescribed on a b.i.d. schedule, but once-daily dosage is possible using the extended release formulation. Due to the risk of hypersensitivity, lamotrigine should be gradually introduced over a six to eight week period of time beginning at a low dose. It therefore is disadvantageous for use in urgent treatment scenarios.

Lamotrigine is conjugated with glucuronic acid in the liver by the UGT system, and the conjugated metabolite is excreted in the urine. Lamotrigine elimination and serum concentrations are significantly affected by medications which induce or inhibit the UGT enzyme pathway [41]. A higher target dose is typically needed when used in combination with drugs that induce UGT, including OCPs and certain enzyme-inducing AEDs such as phenytoin, phenobarbital, primidone, and carbamazepine. It is also important to reduce the dose when used in combination with drugs that inhibit this pathway, such as valproate, which doubles lamotrigine's elimination half-life.

Efficacy

In a meta-analysis of placebo-controlled trials involving the second generation AEDs, lamotrigine was found to be associated with a 50% reduction in seizures in 26% of patients [18]. Lamotrigine, phenytoin, and carbamazepine appear to be equally effective in partial seizures. In a comparative trial of lamotrigine and carbamazepine, 26% of patients in the lamotrigine arm were seizure-free during the last 40 weeks of the trial compared to 29% in the carbamazepine arm [42]. In a study comparing lamotrigine and phenytoin, 43% of lamotrigine-treated patients were seizure-free during the last 24 weeks of treatment compared to 36% treated with phenytoin; this difference was not statistically significant [43]. Lamotrigine is also effective in the treatment of generalized absence, atonic, and generalized tonic-clonic seizures, and in seizures associated with Lennox-Gastaut syndrome [38], although it is probably less effective than valproate in generalized epilepsy [5]. Lamotrigine may lead to exacerbation of myoclonic seizures [39]. Therefore, while it is effective in a variety of seizure types, lamotrigine should be used with caution in patients with myoclonic seizures as a prominent seizure type.

Levetiracetam

Indications, usage, and potential side effects

Levetiracetam is approved for use as adjuvant therapy for partial seizures, and myoclonic and generalized tonic-clonic seizures in patients with primary generalized epilepsy. Levetiracetam is used widely, likely due to its favorable pharmacokinetic and interaction profile, low incidence of major toxicity, and ease of use. Levetiracetam may be associated with hypersomnolence and irritability, both of which may be sufficient to warrant discontinuation. Hypersensitivity rashes occur but are rare.

Dosage, pharmacokinetics, and potential interactions

Levetiracetam is available in standard and extended-release tablets, and oral and parenteral solutions. The recommended starting dose in adults is 250–500 mg b.i.d. in patients with normal renal function. The dose can be increased in 250–500 mg b.i.d. increments every one to two weeks to a maximum dose of 1500–2000 mg b.i.d. Levetiracetam is excreted largely unchanged in the urine, but about a third undergoes enzymatic hydrolysis by a mechanism independent of the cytochrome P450 system. Since levetiracetam is predominantly renally excreted, the dose must be adjusted in patients with renal insufficiency. Levetiracetam does not affect hepatic enzyme activity and exhibits little protein binding, so is not generally associated with pharmacokinetic drug–drug interactions. However, postmarketing experience has led to reports of a pharmacodynamic interaction when coadministered with carbamazepine leading to symptoms characteristic of carbamazepine toxicity [12].

Efficacy

The clinical trials leading to approval of levetiracetam for the treatment of partial epilepsy showed a statistically significant response at a dose of 1000 mg per day. There was no significant increase in response associated with higher dosages in these trials. One study comparing doses of 1000 and 3000 mg/day found responder rates of 37.1 and 39.6% respectively [44]. Another study comparing doses of 1000 and 2000 mg/day found 50% responder rates of 22.8% in the 1000-mg group and 31.6% in the 2000-mg group [45]. In a study comparing daily dosages of 2000 and 4000 mg per day, a 50% responder rate of 43% was found without a significant difference between the dosage groups [46]. Despite widespread use, there is no clear evidence that levetiracetam has superior efficacy over other AEDs. Both a meta-analysis comparing the efficacy of levetiracetam and carbamazepine, and another comparing levetiracetam and other second generation medications, showed no statistically significant difference in responder rates in the treatment of partial epilepsy [47, 48]. In generalized epilepsy, levetiracetam was found to have a responder rate of 53.3% for patients with juvenile absence epilepsy, 61.0% for juvenile myoclonic epilepsy, and 61.9% for patients with the syndrome of generalized tonic-clonic seizures upon awakening [49].

Oxcarbazepine

Indications, usage, and potential side effects

Oxcarbazepine is approved as adjunctive treatment and monotherapy for partial seizures in children over age four and adults. Oxcarbazepine is rapidly converted to a metabolite known as the 10-monohydroxy derivative, which confers its clinical activity. The main side effects of oxcarbazepine therapy include dizziness, diplopia, asthenia, and nausea. Similar to carbamazepine, oxcarbazepine may lead to hyponatremia and leukopenia in 10% of patients [50]. Although typically not clinically significant, these potential effects warrant periodic monitoring of complete blood cell counts and sodium levels. A third of patients with a history of hypersensitivity to carbamazepine will show cross-sensitivity to oxcarbazepine [51].

Dosage, pharmacokinetics, and potential interactions

Oxcarbazepine is completely absorbed and metabolized to MHD. The parent drug has no significant antiepileptic effect. A steady-state plasma concentration of MHD is reached in two to three days. Carbamazepine, phenytoin, phenobarbital, and valproic acid may all decrease the plasma concentration of MHD. Oxcarbazepine may produce increases in phenytoin levels (up to 40%) and a modest increase in phenobarbital levels (approximately 14%). A decrease in the phenytoin dose may be warranted when adding oxcarbazepine. Oxcarbazepine may also result in a lower plasma concentration of the active ingredients in oral contraceptive medications, and can interact with other nonAED medications (see Table 10.7) [52].

Efficacy

Trials comparing oxcarbazepine to phenytoin, carbamazepine, and valproate showed no differences in seizure control [53–55]. In a Cochrane analysis of clinical trials, the overall odds ratio (OR) for 50% or greater reduction in seizure frequency compared to placebo was 2.96 (2.20,4.00) [56]. Oxcarbazepine has not been studied extensively in the treatment of the generalized epilepsies. However, some have reported exacerbation of seizures and inducement of new seizure types in patients with generalized epileptiform abnormalities on EEG suggesting that it is not likely to be helpful in this population [57].

Pregabalin

Indications, usage, and potential side effects

Pregabalin is approved for adjunctive use in the treatment of partial epilepsy, but not for generalized epilepsy. Pregabalin was associated with the following side effects in clinical trials: somnolence 11% (0.07–0.15), dizziness 22% (0.16–0.28), ataxia 10% (0.06–0.14), and fatigue 4% (0.01–0.08) [58]. Weight gain has also been reported [37]. Pregabalin is classified in the US as a controlled substance, which complicates prescribing.

Dosage, pharmacokinetics, and potential interactions

Pregabalin is available in capsular form in multiple dosage strengths. Pregabalin is best initiated at low doses, typically 25 mg b.i.d. The dose is then titrated in 25 mg b.i.d. increments weekly to a target dose of 300–600 mg per day. Pregabalin is rapidly absorbed, has ≥90% oral bioavailability, shows linear and predictable pharmacokinetics across the usual dose range (150–600 mg/day), and is not bound by plasma proteins. It is excreted virtually unchanged in urine. There are no known pharmacokinetic interactions with pregabalin. It does not affect the plasma concentrations of other AEDs, and pregabalin is not affected by other AEDs. There does not appear to be any affect on oral contraceptive pharmacokinetic properties [37].

Efficacy

In a review of pregabalin clinical trials, a 50% or higher seizure reduction was significantly more likely in patients randomized to pregabalin than to placebo (RR 3.56, 95% CI 2.60–4.87) [59]. Greater efficacy may be seen with higher dosages. In a summary of pregabalin clinical trials, the placebo-corrected efficacy rates of pregabalin ranged from 17.4% in patients receiving 150 mg/day to 36.6% in patients receiving 600 mg/day [60]. Unfortunately, the side-effect incidence is also dose related, and many patients are not able to tolerate higher dosages.

Tiagabine

Indications, usage, and potential side effects

Tiagabine is indicated for use in partial seizures. Its mechanism of action involves inhibition of presynaptic GABA reuptake, leading to nonselective enhancement of GABAergic activity [61]. Tiagabine is not widely used in the treatment of epilepsy, likely due to its potential for CNS and behavioral side effects and the risk of nonconvulsive status epilepticus for which it has a black-box warning in its official labeling [62].

Dosage, pharmacokinetics, and potential interactions

Tiagabine is metabolized extensively in the liver but does not induce or inhibit hepatic enzyme activity. The half-life of tiagabine is only 5–8 hours; however, no significant difference in efficacy was found in one trial comparing b.i.d. and q.i.d. dosing [63]. Tiagabine is 96% protein-bound, but no clinically significant drug–drug interactions attributed to competition for protein-binding displacement have been reported. Tiagabine should be initiated gradually and increased slowly over a six to eight week period of time in order to minimize the occurrence of side effects. Multiple dosage strengths are available to facilitate tailoring of the titration schedule for individual patients. While tiagabine serum levels can be affected by hepatic enzyme-altering AEDs, it does not have a reciprocal effect. Although not reported, from a pharmacodynamic standpoint, one should probably be cautious when prescribing tiagabine in combination with other GABAergic medications such as valproate, benzodiazepines, and vigabatrin given its mechanism of action.

Efficacy

The efficacy in partial epilepsy is similar to that seen with other second generation AEDs. The clinical response was somewhat related to dose: 50% responder rates of 10, 22, and 29% were seen with daily dosages of 16, 32, and 56 mg daily respectively [63–65]. Tiagabine is not effective in the generalized epilepsies [61].

Topiramate

Indications, usage, and potential side effects

Topiramate is approved as monotherapy in the treatment of partial seizures, primary and secondary generalized tonic-clonic seizures, and seizures associated with Lennox-Gastaut syndrome. Side effects include urolithiasis, which was reported in 1.5% of patients in clinical trials [66]. Hydration is recommended in order to decrease this risk. Word-finding difficulties are common, as are dizziness, ataxia, and somnolence. Anorexia, weight loss and paresthesias can also occur. While effective in the treatment of seizures, topiramate was associated with one of the higher drop-out rates in clinical trials due to tolerability when compared to trials of other second generation AEDs [18].

Dosage, pharmacokinetics, and potential interactions

Topiramate comes in tablet and sprinkle formulations in multiple strengths. The tablets are not scored. A slow-dose titration schedule is recommended in order to avoid discontinuation due to side effects. The minimum effective dose in adults is 100 mg b.i.d. Doses of up to 400 mg per day are commonly used in the treatment of epilepsy.

Approximately 70% of topiramate is excreted unchanged in the urine. In patients with moderate to severe renal impairment, lower dosages should be considered. Although only 30% of the dose is metabolized by the liver, clearance may be reduced in patients with hepatic disease as well. Therefore, a modest dose reduction may be necessary in patients with significant liver disease.

Topiramate does not significantly affect the serum levels of other AEDs. However, topiramate clearance is increased by enzyme-inducing AEDs. For example, carbamazepine and phenytoin cause a 40–50% reduction in topiramate concentration [67]. Although it does not generally affect hepatic enzyme pathways, topiramate has been found to affect the pharmacokinetics of other medications through unknown mechanisms (see Table 10.7). Of note, topiramate has been shown to increase the clearance of ethinyl estradiol which may affect efficacy of oral contraceptive therapies containing this ingredient.

Efficacy

In the clinical trials leading to FDA approval, the 50% responder rates for topiramate were more favorable than those observed in the studies of the other second generation AEDs [18]. A dose–response relationship was noted up to a daily dose of 400 mg per day: the responder rate in the 200 mg per day arm in one study was 27%, compared to 45% in the 400 mg per day arm [68]. Doses up to

1000 mg per day were evaluated in one clinical trial and found to be safe; however, the drop-out rates secondary to adverse effects were higher, and the responder rates were not better than those seen at a dose of 400 mg per day (44% at 600 mg, 40% at 800 mg, and 38% at 1000 mg) [69]. A similar responder rate of 46% was seen in patients treated for primary generalized epilepsy [70].

Zonisamide

Indications, usage, and potential side effects

Zonisamide is approved for the treatment of partial epilepsy. Zonisamide has been reported in open-labeled studies to have efficacy in the treatment of seizures seen in the generalized epilepsies, but it does not have FDA approval for use in this epilepsy type at present. Zonisamide is associated with an increased risk of urolithiasis. Urolithiasis was seen in 3.7% of patients in the initial clinical trial of zonisamide in the US [71]. Zonisamide is a sulfonamide and should not be used in patients with a previous history of sulfonamide hypersensitivity. Zonisamide has been associated with oligohidrosis and hyperthermia, and may pose a risk for patients with glaucoma. In clinical trials, the most common side effects associated with zonisamide were ataxia, somnolence, agitation, irritability, and anorexia [72].

Dosage, pharmacokinetics, and potential interactions

Zonisamide is available in capsular form. The dosage is typically titrated over a two to four week period of time. Zonisamide is metabolized in the liver, and enzyme-inducing AEDs increase zonisamide elimination. Zonisamide may lead to an increase in phenytoin and carbamazepine levels, but this effect is inconsistent. The relatively long half-life of zonisamide allows b.i.d. dosing [73].

Efficacy

In a study of partial epilepsy, zonisamide was associated with a median percent reduction in seizure frequency of 51.8% [71]. In another study, a 50% responder rate of 29% was seen [74]. When taking into account all available clinical trials, the OR for a 50% reduction in seizure frequency was found to be 2.07 (1.36,3.15) for a 400 mg/day dose [72].

Zonisamide has shown some efficacy in the treatment of myoclonic seizures in idiopathic and progressive myoclonic epilepsy [75]. In clinical studies, 50% responder rates of 32% were reported for patients with Lennox-Gastaut syndrome, 26–40% for patients with generalized tonic seizures, and 59–67% for patients with primary generalized tonic-clonic seizures [73].

Subspecialty AEDs

Felbamate

Indications, usage, and potential side effects

Felbamate is approved as monotherapy and adjunctive treatment of partial epilepsy and Lennox-Gastaut syndrome. Felbamate is available in tablet and suspension dosage form. Felbamate held promise at its inception due to its efficacy in many seizure types and lack of sedating properties. Its use significantly declined after the risks of fatal hepatotoxicity and aplastic anemia became recognized, and other lower-risk treatment options became available [76]. A "worst case scenario" estimate for rate of aplastic anemia was calculated by Kaufman *et al.* to be 209 per million [77]. More common side effects include insomnia, anorexia, weight loss, and occasionally psychiatric complications [78].

Dosage, pharmacokinetics, and potential interactions

Felbamate is associated with inhibition of both cytochrome P450 and beta-oxidation activity, leading to 20–50% increases in phenytoin, phenobarbital, and valproic acid serum levels. Felbamate is associated with a reduction in carbamazepine levels, but leads to an increase in carbamazepine-9,10-epoxide due to inhibition of epoxide hydrolase [79]. The dosage of phenytoin, phenobarbital, valproic acid, and carbamazepine should be reduced by one-third prior to the addition of felbamate given the potential for these drug–drug interactions.

Efficacy

The efficacy of felbamate was established in several placebo-controlled trials [80]. In an active-controlled monotherapy trial comparing felbamate and valproic acid 15 mg/kg/day, 38/56 (68%) of patients treated with felbamate were able to complete the study without a significant increase in seizure activity compared to 18/55 (33%) treated with valproic acid [81]. In a placebo-controlled trial evaluating the efficacy of felbamate in Lennox-Gastaut syndrome, felbamate was associated with a 34% decrease in frequency of atonic seizures and an overall 19% decrease in total seizure frequency. In this study, felbamate was also associated with a statistically significant improvement in physician and parent global assessment scales [82].

Rufinamide

Indications, usage, and potential side effects

Rufinamide is approved in the US for the treatment of Lennox-Gastaut syndrome. Clinical trials showed modest efficacy in partial seizures in adults, and it is not approved for use in partial seizures at the present time. The most common adverse events associated with rufinamide are somnolence, dizziness, nausea, diplopia, and ataxia [83, 84]. It is contraindicated for use in patients with the Short QT syndrome.

Dosage, pharmacokinetics, and potential interactions

Rufinamide is available in tablet form. Its absorption is increased by 40% when administered with food. Rufinamide exhibits low protein binding ($\sim$34%), and undergoes extensive enzymatic hydrolysis through a process that is independent of the cytochrome p450 pathways; the hydrolyzed end-products are renally excreted. Rufinamide may lead to an increase in phenytoin levels ($<$21%), but has no clinically relevant effect on the pharmacokinetics of other AEDs. Valproate coadministration may lead to elevated rufinamide levels, sometimes necessitating dosage adjustment [37].

Efficacy

In a large trial of patients with Lennox-Gastaut syndrome, the median percentage reduction in total seizure frequency was greater in the rufinamide therapy group than in the placebo group (32.7% vs. 11.7%; p $=$ 0.0015), and a significant reduction in tonic-atonic ("drop attack") seizure frequency with rufinamide versus placebo (42.5% vs. 1.4% increase; p $<$ 0.0001) [83]. In a published trial of rufinamide in partial seizures, rufinamide was associated with a 20.4% median reduction in seizure frequency compared to a 1.6% increase in the placebo arm (p $=$ 0.02) [84].

Vigabatrin

Indications, usage, and potential side effects

Vigabatrin is approved in the US "as adjunctive therapy for adult patients with refractory complex partial seizures who have inadequately responded to several alternative treatments and for whom the potential benefits outweigh the risk of vision loss." It has also become established as an important treatment for infantile spasms, but it does not have a specific approved indication for this in the US at this time. It is particularly useful in the treatment of infantile spasms secondary to tuberous sclerosis [37].

The most significant limiting side effect is the association with progressive bilateral concentric visual field impairment, which was found in 23% of children and 43% of adults treated with vigabatrin for more than six months [85]. The visual field impairment in these cases is often asymptomatic, however visual field monitoring is required for patients treated with the drug. In the US, the prescribing and distribution of vigabatrin are tightly controlled due to this risk. Asymptomatic white matter MRI abnormalities have also been observed in patients receiving vigabatrin as well. The clinical significance of these imaging changes has not been established. Other side effects include hypersomnolence, weight gain, and edema.

Dosage, pharmacokinetics, and potential interactions

Vigabatrin comes in tablet and oral solution dosage forms. Vigabatrin is a "suicide inhibitor" of GABA transaminase, an enzyme involved with GABA degradation, leading to accumulation of GABA in the synaptic cleft. Given this mechanism of action, pharmacokinetic characteristics of vigabatrin such as its half-life and serum concentration are not thought to be important in determining its clinical effect. The duration of activity is likely more dependent on the rate of GABA-transaminase re-synthesis than to serum levels.

Vigabatrin is eliminated in the urine and undergoes minimal enzymatic degradation. The dose therefore needs to be adjusted in the setting of renal insufficiency. While its effect on hepatic enzyme activity is generally considered insubstantial, vigabatrin may be associated with reductions in phenytoin levels, and has been shown to lead to increases and decreases in carbamazepine levels when coadministered [12]. In adults, the dose is usually initiated at 500 mg b.i.d., and increased in 500 mg increments thereafter usually to a maximum dose of 3000 mg per day.

Efficacy

In a Cochrane meta-analysis of 11 clinical trials of vigabatrin in the treatment of partial epilepsy, patients treated with vigabatrin were significantly more likely to obtain a 50% or greater reduction in seizure frequency compared with those treated with placebo (RR 2.58, 95% CI 1.87–3.57) [86]. Vigabatrin has been increasingly used in the treatment of infantile spasms as an alternative to hormonal treatment. In the treatment of infantile spasms in one clinical trial in the UK, the proportion of infants who experienced persistent cessation of spasms was similar in those receiving vigabatrin (19/52 [37%]) and hormonal therapy (prednisolone or tetracosactide) (22/55 [40%]; p = 0·71) [87]. However, in another trial, early ACTH therapy was associated with a better long-term outcome than vigabatrin. In the case study, a normal cognitive outcome was achieved in 100% of the early-ACTH group, and 54% of the vigabatrin group (P = 0.03). Seizures subsequently developed in 54% of the vigabatrin group, 33% of the late ACTH group, and 0% of the early ACTH group (P < 0.05) [88].

References

1. LaRoche, S.M. and Helmers, S.L. (2004) The new antiepileptic drugs: scientific review. *J Am Med Assoc*, **291**, 605–614.

2. Kwan, P. and Brodie, M.J. (2000) Early identification of refractory epilepsy. *N Engl J Med*, **342**, 314–319.

3. Perucca, E., Gram, L., Avanzini, G. *et al.* (1998) Antiepileptic drugs as a cause of worsening seizures. *Epilepsia*, **39**, 5–17.

4. Bourgeois, B.F.D. (2007) Broader is better: the ranks of broad-spectrum antiepileptic drugs are growing. *Neurology*, **69**, 1734–1736.

5. Marson, A.G., Al-Kharusi, A.M., Alwaidh, M. *et al.* (2007) The SANAD study of effectiveness of valproate, lamotrigine, or topiramate for generalised and unclassifiable epilepsy: an unblinded randomised controlled trial. *Lancet*, **369**, 1016–1026.

6. Levy, R.H., Mattson, R.H., Meldrum, B.S. *et al.* (eds.) (2002) *Antileptic Drugs*, 5th edn, Lippincott, Williams & Wilkins, Philadelphia, PA.

7. Lacerda, G., Krummel, T., Sabourdy, C. *et al.* (2006) Optimizing therapy of seizures in patients with renal or hepatic dysfunction. *Neurology*, **67**, S28–S33.

8. de Lacerda, G.C.B. (2008) Treating seizures in renal and hepatic failure. *J Epilepsy Clin Neurophysiol*, **14**, 46–50.

9. Perucca, E. (2006) Clinically relevant drug interactions with antiepileptic drugs. *Br J Clin Pharmacol*, **61**, 2 46–255.

10. Patsalos, P.N., Froscher, W., Pisani, F. *et al.* (2002) The importance of drug interactions in epilepsy therapy. *Epilepsia*, **43**, 365–385.

11. Spina, E., Perucca, E., and Levy, R.H. (2005) Predictability of metabolic antiepileptic drug interactions, in *Antiepileptic Drugs: Combination Therapy and Interactions*, 1st edn (eds. J. Majkowski, B. Bourgeois, P.N. Patsalos, and R.H. Mattson), Cambridge University Press, New York, NY, pp. 57–92.

12. Micromedex® Healthcare Series (2010) *DRUG-REAX® System [Internet Database]*, Thomson Reuters (Healthcare) Inc.

13. Gidal, B.E., French, J.A., Grossman, P. *et al.* (2009) Assessment of potential drug interactions in patients with epilepsy: impact of age and sex. *Neurology*, **72**, 419–425.

14. Harden, C.L., Meador, K.J., Pennell, P.B. *et al.* (2009) Management issues for women with epilepsy—focus on pregnancy (an evidence-based review): II. Teratogenesis and perinatal outcomes: report of the Quality Standards Subcommittee and Therapeutics and Technology Subcommittee of the American Academy of Neurology and the American Epilepsy Society. *Epilepsia*, **50**, 1237–1246.

15. Harden, C.L., Meador, K.J., Pennell, P.B. *et al.* (2009) Practice parameter update: management issues for women with epilepsy—focus on pregnancy (an evidence-based review): Teratogenesis and perinatal outcomes: report of the Quality Standards Subcommittee and Therapeutics and Technology Assessment Subcommittee of the American Academy of Neurology and American Epilepsy Society. *Neurology*, **73**, 133–141.

16. Harden, C.L., Pennell, P.B., Koppel, B.S. *et al.* (2009) Practice parameter update: management issues for women with epilepsy—focus on pregnancy (an evidence-based review): Vitamin K, folic acid, blood levels, and breastfeeding: report of the Quality Standards Subcommittee and Therapeutics and Technology Assessment Subcommittee of the American Academy of Neurology and American Epilepsy Society. *Neurology*, **73**, 142–149.

17. Cramer, J.A., Glassman, M., and Rienzi, V. (2002) The relationship between poor medication compliance and seizures. *Epilepsy Behav*, **3**, 338–342.

18. Marson, A.G., Kadir, Z.A., and Chadwick, D.W. (1996) New antiepileptic drugs: a systematic review of their efficacy and tolerability. *Br Med J*, **313**, 1169–1174 [see comments].

19. Gencarelli, D.M. (2005) *One Pill Many Prices: Variation in Prescription Drug Prices in Selected Government Programs. Forum NHP*, George Washington University, Washington, DC, pp. 1–20.

20. Physician's Desk Reference (2009) *Red Book 2009: Pharmacy's Fundamental Reference*, 113th edn, Thomson Reuters (Healthcare) Inc.
21. FDA (2009) Therapeutic equivalence-related terms, *Approved Drug Products with Therapeutic Equivalence Evaluations*, 29th edn, US Department of Health and Human Services, Washington, DC, pp. 6–23.
22. Oles, K.S., Penry, J.K., Smith, L.D. *et al.* (1992) Therapeutic bioequivalency study of brand name versus generic carbamazepine. *Neurology*, **42**, 1147.
23. Kishore, K., Jailakhani, B.L., Sharma, J.N. *et al.* (1986) Serum phenytoin levels with different brands. *Indian J Physiol Pharmacol*, **30**, 171–176.
24. Andermann, F., Duh, M.S., Gosselin, A. *et al.* (2007) Compulsory generic switching of antiepileptic drugs: high switchback rates to branded compounds compared with other drug classes. *Epilepsia*, **48**, 464–469.
25. Liow, K., Barkley, G.L., Pollard, J.R. *et al.* (2007) Position statement on the coverage of anticonvulsant drugs for the treatment of epilepsy. *Neurology*, **68**, 1249–1250.
26. Knapp, L.E. and Kugler, A.R. (1998) Clinical experience with fosphenytoin in adults: pharmacokinetics, safety, and efficacy. *J Child Neurol*, **13**, S15–S18; discussion S30–S32.
27. Mattson, R.H., Cramer, J.A., Collins, J.F. *et al.* (1985) Comparison of carbamazepine, phenobarbital, phenytoin, and primidone in partial and secondarily generalized tonic-clonic seizures. *N Engl J Med*, **313**, 145–151.
28. Mattson, R.H., Cramer, J.A., and Collins, J.F., The Department of Veterans Affairs Epilepsy Cooperative Study No. 264 Group (1992) A comparison of valproate with carbamazepine for the treatment of complex partial seizures and secondarily generalized tonic-clonic seizures in adults. *N Engl J Med*, **327**, 765–771 [comment].
29. Tomson, T., Perucca, E., and Battino, D. (2004) Navigating toward fetal and maternal health: the challenge of treating epilepsy in pregnancy. *Epilepsia*, **45**, 1171–1175.
30. Baulac, M., Cavalcanti, D., Semah, F. *et al.*, The French Gabapentin Collaborative Group (1998) Gabapentin add-on therapy with adaptable dosages in 610 patients with partial epilepsy: an open, observational study. *Seizure*, **7**, 55–62.
31. McLean, M.J. (1995) Gabapentin. *Epilepsia*, **36**, S73–S86.
32. Perucca, E. (2006) Clinical pharmacokinetics of new-generation antiepileptic drugs at the extremes of age. *Clin Pharmacokinet*, **45**, 351–363.
33. Leiderman, D.B. (1994) Gabapentin as add-on therapy for refractory partial epilepsy: results of five placebo-controlled trials. *Epilepsia*, **35**, S74–S76.
34. The US Gabapentin Study Group No. 5 (1993) Gabapentin as add-on therapy in refractory partial epilepsy: a double-blind, placebo-controlled, parallel-group study. *Neurology*, **43**, 2292–2298.
35. Harris, J.A. and Murphy, J.A. (2009) Lacosamide: an adjunctive agent for partial-onset seizures and potential therapy for neuropathic pain. *Ann Pharmacother*, **43**, 1809–1817.
36. Beydoun, A., D'Souza, J., Hebert, D. *et al.* (2009) Lacosamide: pharmacology, mechanisms of action and pooled efficacy and safety data in partial-onset seizures. *Expert Rev Neurother*, **9**, 33–42.
37. Bialer, M., Johannessen, S.I., Kupferberg, H.J. *et al.* (2007) Progress report on new antiepileptic drugs: a summary of the Eighth Eilat Conference (EILAT VIII). *Epilepsy Res*, **73**, 1–52.
38. Verrotti, A., Greco, R., Giannuzzi, R. *et al.* (2007) Old and new antiepileptic drugs for the treatment of idiopathic generalized epilepsies. *Curr Clin Pharmacol*, **2**, 249–259.
39. Guerrini, R., Dravet, C., Genton, P. *et al.* (1998) Lamotrigine and seizure aggravation in severe myoclonic epilepsy. *Epilepsia*, **39**, 508–512.

40. Faught, E., Morris, G., Jacobson, M. *et al.*, Postmarketing Antiepileptic Drug Survey (PADS) Group (1999) Adding lamotrigine to valproate: incidence of rash and other adverse effects. *Epilepsia*, **40**, 1135–1140.

41. Garnett, W.R. (1997) Lamotrigine: pharmacokinetics. *J Child Neurol*, **12**, S10–S15.

42. Brodie, M.J., Richens, A., and Yuen, A.W., UK Lamotrigine/Carbamazepine Monotherapy Trial Group (1995) Double-blind comparison of lamotrigine and carbamazepine in newly diagnosed epilepsy. *Lancet*, **345**, 476–479 [published erratum appears in *Lancet* 1995 Mar 11, **345** (8950), 662] [see comments].

43. Steiner, T.J., Dellaportas, C.I., Findley, L.J. *et al.* (1999) Lamotrigine monotherapy in newly diagnosed untreated epilepsy: a double-blind comparison with phenytoin. *Epilepsia*, **40**, 601–607.

44. Cereghino, J.J., Biton, V., Abou-Khalil, B. *et al.* (2000) Levetiracetam for partial seizures: results of a double-blind, randomized clinical trial. *Neurology*, **55**, 236–242.

45. Shorvon, S.D., Lowenthal, A., Janz, D. *et al.*, European Levetiracetam Study Group (2000) Multicenter double-blind, randomized, placebo-controlled trial of levetiracetam as add-on therapy in patients with refractory partial seizures. *Epilepsia*, **41**, 1179–1186.

46. Betts, T., Waegemans, T., and Crawford, P. (2000) A multicentre, double-blind, randomized, parallel group study to evaluate the tolerability and efficacy of two oral doses of levetiracetam, 2000 mg daily and 4000 mg daily, without titration in patients with refractory epilepsy. *Seizure*, **9**, 80–87.

47. Brodie, M.J., Perucca, E., Ryvlin, P. *et al.* (2007) Comparison of levetiracetam and controlled-release carbamazepine in newly diagnosed epilepsy. *Neurology*, **68**, 402–408 [see comment].

48. Otoul, C., Arrigo, C., van Rijckevorsel, K. *et al.* (2005) Meta-analysis and indirect comparisons of levetiracetam with other second-generation antiepileptic drugs in partial epilepsy. *Clin Neuropharmacol*, **28**, 72–78.

49. Rosenfeld, W.E., Benbadis, S., Pascal, E. *et al.* (2009) Levetiracetam as add-on therapy for idiopathic generalized epilepsy syndromes with onset during adolescence: analysis of two randomized, double-blind, placebo-controlled studies. *Epilepsy Res*, **85**, 72–80.

50. Ryan, M., Adams, A.G., and Larive, L.L. (2001) Hyponatremia and leukopenia associated with oxcarbazepine following carbamazepine therapy. *Am J Health Syst Pharm*, **58**, 1637–1639.

51. Hirsch, L.J., Arif, H., Nahm, E.A. *et al.* (2008) Cross-sensitivity of skin rashes with antiepileptic drug use. *Neurology*, **71**, 1527–1534.

52. Bialer, M., Johannessen, S.I., Kupferberg, H.J. *et al.* (1999) Progress report on new antiepileptic drugs: a summary of the Fourth Eilat Conference (EILAT IV). *Epilepsy Res*, **34**, 1–41.

53. Bill, P.A., Vigonius, U., Pohlmann, H. *et al.* (1997) A double-blind controlled clinical trial of oxcarbazepine versus phenytoin in adults with previously untreated epilepsy. *Epilepsy Res*, **27**, 195–204.

54. Christe, W., Kramer, G., Vigonius, U. *et al.* (1997) A double-blind controlled clinical trial: oxcarbazepine versus sodium valproate in adults with newly diagnosed epilepsy. *Epilepsy Res*, **26**, 451–460.

55. Dam, M., Ekberg, R., Loyning, Y. *et al.* (1989) A double-blind study comparing oxcarbazepine and carbamazepine in patients with newly diagnosed, previously untreated epilepsy. *Epilepsy Res*, **3**, 70–76.

56. Castillo, S.M., Schmidt, D.B., White, S., Shukralla, A. (2000) Oxcarbazepine add-on for drug-resistant partial epilepsy. *Cochrane Database of Systematic Reviews*, **3**. Art. No.: CD002028. DOI: 10.1002/14651858.CD002028.

57. Vendrame, M., Khurana, D.S., Cruz, M. *et al.* (2007) Aggravation of Seizures and/or EEG features in children treated with oxcarbazepine monotherapy. *Epilepsia*, **48**, 2116–2120.

58. Zaccara, G., Gangemi, P.F., and Cincotta, M. (2008) Central nervous system adverse effects of new antiepileptic drugs: a meta-analysis of placebo-controlled studies. *Seizure*, **17**, 405–421.

59. Lozsadi, D., Hemming, K., and Marson A.G. (2008) Pregabalin add-on for drug-resistant partial epilepsy. *Cochrane Database Syst Rev*, **1**, Art. No.: CD005612.

60. Tassone, D.M., Boyce, E., Guyer, J. *et al.* (2007) Pregabalin: a novel gamma-aminobutyric acid analogue in the treatment of neuropathic pain, partial-onset seizures, and anxiety disorders. *Clin Ther*, **29**, 26–48.

61. Adkins, J.C. and Noble, S. (1998) Tiagabine: a review of its pharmacodynamic and pharmacokinetic properties and therapeutic potential in the management of epilepsy. *Drugs*, **55**, 437–460.

62. Eckardt, K.M. and Steinhoff, B.J. (1998) Nonconvulsive status epilepticus in two patients receiving tiagabine treatment. *Epilepsia*, **39**, 671–674.

63. Sachdeo, R.C., Leroy, R.F., Krauss, G.L. *et al.*, The Tiagabine Study Group (1997) Tiagabine therapy for complex partial seizures: a dose-frequency study. *Arch Neurol*, **54**, 595–601.

64. Uthman, B.M., Rowan, A.J., Ahmann, P.A. *et al.* (1998) Tiagabine for complex partial seizures: a randomized, add-on, dose-response trial. *Arch Neurol*, **55**, 56–62.

65. Kalviainen, R., Brodie, M.J., Duncan, J. *et al.*, Northern European Tiagabine Study Group (1998) A double-blind, placebo-controlled trial of tiagabine given three-times daily as add-on therapy for refractory partial seizures. *Epilepsy Res*, **30**, 31–40.

66. Shorvon, S.D. (1996) Safety of topiramate: adverse events and relationships to dosing. *Epilepsia*, **37**, S18–S22.

67. Johannessen, S.I. (1997) Pharmacokinetics and interaction profile of topiramate: review and comparison with other newer antiepileptic drugs. *Epilepsia*, **38**, S18–S23.

68. Faught, E., Wilder, B.J., Ramsay, R.E. *et al.*, Topiramate YD Study Group (1996) Topiramate placebo-controlled dose-ranging trial in refractory partial epilepsy using 200-, 400-, and 600-mg daily dosages. *Neurology*, **46**, 1684–1690.

69. Privitera, M., Fincham, R., Penry, J. *et al.*, Topiramate YE Study Group (1996) Topiramate placebo-controlled dose-ranging trial in refractory partial epilepsy using 600-, 800-, and 1,000-mg daily dosages. *Neurology*, **46**, 1678–1683.

70. Biton, V., Montouris, G.D., Ritter, F. *et al.*, Topiramate YTC Study Group (1999) A randomized, placebo-controlled study of topiramate in primary generalized tonic-clonic seizures. *Neurology*, **52**, 1330–1337.

71. Leppik, I.E., Willmore, L.J., Homan, R.W. *et al.* (1993) Efficacy and safety of zonisamide: results of a multicenter study. *Epilepsy Res*, **14**, 165–173.

72. Chadwick, D.W., Marson, A.G. (2005) Zonisamide add-on for drug-resistant partial epilepsy. *Cochrane Database of Systematic Reviews*. **4**, Art. No.: CD001416. DOI: 10.1002/14651858.CD001416.pub2.

73. Peters, D.H. and Sorkin, E.M. (1993) Zonisamide: a review of its pharmacodynamic and pharmacokinetic properties, and therapeutic potential in epilepsy. *Drugs*, **45**, 760–787.

74. Schmidt, D., Jacob, R., Loiseau, P. *et al.* (1993) Zonisamide for add-on treatment of refractory partial epilepsy: a European double-blind trial. *Epilepsy Res*, **15**, 67–73.

75. Wallace, S.J. (1998) Myoclonus and epilepsy in childhood: a review of treatment with valproate, ethosuximide, lamotrigine and zonisamide. *Epilepsy Res*, **29**, 147–154.

76. Pellock, J.M. and Brodie, M.J. (1997) Felbamate: 1997 update. *Epilepsia*, **38**, 1261–1264.

77. Kaufman, D.W., Kelly, J.P., Anderson, T. *et al.* (1997) Evaluation of case reports of aplastic anemia among patients treated with felbamate. *Epilepsia*, **38**, 1265–1269.

78. French, J., Smith, M., Faught, E. *et al.* (1999) Practice advisory: the use of felbamate in the treatment of patients with intractable epilepsy: report of the Quality Standards Sub-committee of the American Academy of Neurology and the American Epilepsy Society. *Neurology*, **52**, 1540–1545.

79. Graves, N.M. (1993) Felbamate. *Ann Pharmacother*, **27**, 1073–1081.

80. Leppik, I.E. (1995) Felbamate. *Epilepsia*, **36**, S66–S72.

81. Faught, E., Sachdeo, R.C., Remler, M.P. *et al.* (1993) Felbamate monotherapy for partial-onset seizures: an active-control trial. *Neurology*, **43**, 688–692.

82. The Felbamate Study Group in Lennox-Gastaut Syndrome (1993) Efficacy of felbamate in childhood epileptic encephalopathy (Lennox-Gastaut syndrome). *N Engl J Med*, **328**, 29–33.

83. Glauser, T., Kluger, G., Sachdeo, R. *et al.* (2008) Rufinamide for generalized seizures associated with Lennox-Gastaut syndrome. *Neurology*, **70**, 1950–1958.

84. Brodie, M.J., Rosenfeld, W.E., Vazquez, B. *et al.* (2009) Rufinamide for the adjunctive treatment of partial seizures in adults and adolescents: a randomized placebo-controlled trial. *Epilepsia*, **50**, 1899–1909.

85. Wild, J.M., Chiron, C., Ahn, H. *et al.* (2009) Visual field loss in patients with refractory partial epilepsy treated with vigabatrin: final results from an open-label, observational, multicentre study. *CNS Drugs*, **23**, 965–982.

86. Hemming, K., Maguire, M.J., Hutton, J.L. Marson, A.G. (2008) Vigabatrin for refractory partial epilepsy. *Cochrane Database of Systematic Reviews*, **3**, Art. No.: CD007302. DOI: 10.1002/14651858.CD007302.

87. Lux, A.L., Edwards, S.W., Hancock, E. *et al.* (2005) The United Kingdom Infantile Spasms Study (UKISS) comparing hormone treatment with vigabatrin on developmental and epilepsy outcomes to age 14 months: a multicentre randomised trial. *Lancet Neurol*, **4**, 712–717.

88. Cohen-Sadan, S., Kramer, U., Ben-Zeev, B. *et al.* (2009) Multicenter long-term follow-up of children with idiopathic West syndrome: ACTH versus vigabatrin. *Eur J Neurol*, **16**, 482–487.

Section 4

Generalized epilepsies

11 Idiopathic generalized epilepsies

Raj D. Sheth

Department of Neurology, Division of Epilepsy, Mayo Clinic, FL, USA; Division of Pediatric Neurology, Nemours Children's Clinic, Jacksonville, FL, USA

11.1 Overview of the generalized epilepsies

The generalized epilepsies can be broadly categorized as idiopathic generalized epilepsy and symptomatic generalized epilepsy. The latter category includes "cryptogenic" generalized epilepsy. Cryptogenic refers to the presence of subtle neurological deficits, intellectual deficiency, or motoric and cognitive delays in the absence of an identifiable neurological lesion or disease. The prognosis and management of cryptogenic epilepsy closely follows that of symptomatic epilepsy. The idiopathic epilepsies are usually familial and are presumed to have a genetic basis.

There are several practical reasons to properly classify these disorders since an appropriate diagnosis carries significant prognostic and therapeutic implications. As an example, childhood absence epilepsy would typically be expected to disappear by age 10 years, whereas juvenile absence epilepsy is usually a lifelong condition. Improper classification of staring spells as complex partial epilepsy may result in the use of carbamazepine for the treatment of absence epilepsy, a condition that the medication usually worsens. Furthermore, failure to accurately

Adult Epilepsy, First Edition. Edited by Gregory D. Cascino and Joseph I. Sirven.
© 2011 John Wiley & Sons, Ltd. Published 2011 by John Wiley & Sons, Ltd.

classify epilepsy syndromes may limit the ability to decide on the appropriate timing of medication withdrawal.

11.2 Introduction

The idiopathic generalized epilepsies comprise a diverse group of disorders that include common features of generalized spike-waves on EEG associated with a normal neurological examination and absent cognitive deficits. Although cerebral imaging is not necessary for the diagnosis, the presence of lesions on neuroimaging should suggest either partial epilepsy or symptomatic generalized epilepsy. The idiopathic generalized epilepsies can occur across the life spectrum; although, they usually do not have their onset in the neonatal period or in the mid-life years or in the elderly.

The types of idiopathic generalized epilepsies include: typical absence, atypical absence, myoclonic, generalized tonic-clonic, tonic, and atonic seizures. Generalized seizures often have an age-dependent presentation. The spectrum of generalized seizures distributed over age is shown in Figure 11.1 and demonstrates some overlap.

A generalized epilepsy syndrome encompasses a generalized seizure type associated with the clinical accompaniments, age, EEG and the presence or absence of neurological deficits and imaging findings and helps arrive at a specific generalized epilepsy syndrome. Generalized seizures occurring in the context of a normal neurological and cognitive examination and in the context of normal cerebral imaging are referred to as the idiopathic generalized epilepsies. However, more recently idiopathic generalized have shown some neuropsychological comorbidity [1, 2]. Examples include childhood absence, juvenile absence, and juvenile myoclonic epilepsy. In contrast generalized seizures occurring in the context of cognitive impairment, neurological deficits and/or imaging lesions are referred to

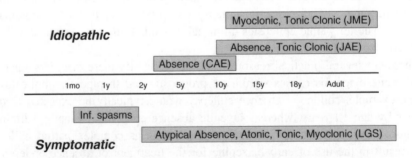

Figure 11.1 Generalized seizures showing age overlap of idiopathic and symptomatic seizures and ages at which they typically appear and disappear. CAE: childhood absence epilepsy; JAE: juvenile absence epilepsy; JME: juvenile myoclonic epilepsy; LGS: Lennox-Gastaut syndrome; Inf. Spasms: infantile spasms (West syndrome).

as the symptomatic generalized epilepsies. An intermediate group referred to as the cryptogenic generalized epilepsies may have normal imaging and laboratory investigations but are associated with developmental, cognitive, and neurological deficits. Examples of symptomatic or cryptogenic epilepsy include West and Lennox-Gastaut syndrome.

Generalized seizures can occur in the context of any of these three broad categories. Differentiating between them carries important therapeutic and prognostic information.

11.3 Differentiating generalized seizures from partial seizures

Generalized seizure implies that the entire cerebrum is electrically involved at the onset of the seizure (Figure 11.2). As such generalized seizures clinically manifest at the onset of the electrographic seizure. In contrast partial seizures evolve, in other words start, in a portion of the cerebrum and propagate to involve expanding areas of brain until clinical manifestations become obvious.

Generalized seizures manifest in several distinct manners: as a convulsive seizure involving all extremities at onset (generalized tonic-clonic seizures), as

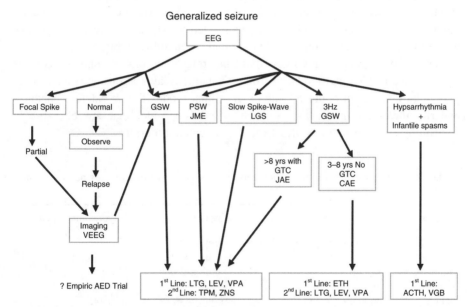

GSW: generalized spike-wave, PSW: polyspike-wave, JME: juvenile myoclonic epilepsy, JAE: juvenile absence epilepsy, CAE: childhood absence epilepsy, LGS : Lennox-Gastaut syndrome, ETH: ethosuccimide, LTG: lamotrigene, LEV: levetiracetam, VPA: valproate, TPM: topiramate, VGB: vigabatrin, ZNS: zonesamide

Figure 11.2 Diagnostic and treatment algorithm for generalized seizures.

a sudden brief whole body jerk (myoclonic seizures), as staring spells (absence seizures), as a slump (atonic seizures) or as a propulsive movement that drops the patient to the ground (tonic seizures). Consciousness is almost always impaired at the onset and typically returns instantaneously after seizure offset. The exception is generalized tonic-clonic convulsive seizures where there is often a pronounced postictal period.

11.4   Clinical and EEG characteristics of generalized seizures

Typical absence seizures

About 5–10% of all childhood epilepsy involves the presence of absence seizures. Typical absence seizures involve an impairment of consciousness associated with a 2.5 to 4 Hz generalized spike-and-slow-wave discharge. Impairment of consciousness may be mild and is often missed and may require special testing to demonstrate. In addition to a blank stare, there are often other associated clinical manifestations, such as automatisms, eyelid myoclonia, and autonomic disturbances. Absence seizures are often induced by hyperventilation, which may be elicited in the clinic by having the patient blow on a pin-wheel. Differentiating absence seizures from complex partial seizures and daydreaming spells is important (Table 11.1). Epileptic syndromes that include typical absence in their spectrum include the idiopathic epilepsies: childhood absence epilepsy, juvenile absence epilepsy, and juvenile myoclonic epilepsy. Myoclonic absence epilepsy is a component of the cryptogenic/symptomatic generalized epilepsies.

Generalized epilepsy involves thalamic relay neurons, thalamic reticular neurons, and cortical pyramidal neurons. Thalamic relay neurons activate cortical pyramidal neurons in either a tonic or in a burst mode. T-type calcium channels underlie the burst mode. Drugs, such as ethosuximide, that are effective in controlling absence seizures affect the T-type calcium currents.

Table 11.1 Seizure types: differentiation between absence seizures, complex partial seizures, and daydreaming spells

Features	Complex partial seizures	Absence	Daydreaming spells
Onset	May have simple partial onset	Abrupt	Variable
Duration	Usually >30 s	Usually <30 s	Variable
Automatisms	Present	Duration-dependent	None
Awareness	No	No	Partial
Ending	Gradual postictal	Abrupt	Variable
State	Active or passive	Active or passive	Always in passive state

Atypical absence seizures

Atypical absence seizures are much less common then typical absence seizures. They are often seen in the Lennox-Gastaut syndrome where they may accompany atonic and tonic seizures. Clinically, atypical absence is associated with developmental delay or mental retardation whereas mental function in typical absence is normal. The EEG is useful in differentiating atypical absence from typical absence seizures by the presence of diffuse slow (<2.5 Hz) spike-and-wave on EEG. In addition to this, the backgrounds compared to normal background frequencies seen in typical absence are slow and disorganized.

Generalized tonic-clonic seizures

A generalized convulsion may result from the culmination of partial complex seizures as it propagates to involve the entire cerebrum, when it is referred to as secondarily generalized tonic-clonic seizures. Primary generalized tonic-clonic seizures are by definition generalized right at onset of the seizure.

Complications associated with generalized tonic-clonic seizures include, oral and head trauma, stress fractures during the tonic phase, aspiration pneumonia, pulmonary edema, and sudden unexpected death in epilepsy (SUDEP). The interictal EEG shows either a normal background or runs of occipital delta activity and may show either fragmented diffuse spike-wave or polyspike-wave discharges or frank generalized spike-wave discharges. Ictal EEG findings at onset include high amplitude anteriorly dominant generalized spike-wave discharges, diffuse fast frequencies that evolve to generalized spike-wave discharges or polyspike-wave discharges. Once the seizure is clinically manifest muscle activity prevents determination of EEG changes. Postictally the EEG often demonstrates diffuse slowing and slow spike-wave discharges.

Myoclonus and myoclonic seizures

Myoclonus, a sudden involuntary brief shock-like muscle contraction originating in the CNS, is a nonepileptic phenomenon and unassociated with epileptiform discharges. Myoclonic seizures on the other hand are similar movements but associated with epileptiform discharges (often fast polyspike-and-wave discharge) and arise from the cerebral cortex. Consciousness may be impaired but is often preserved. They often precede generalized tonic-clonic seizures, commonly a series of myoclonic seizure jerks are followed by a generalized convulsive seizure. When present in the context of a normal exam and imaging, they are strongly suggestive of juvenile myoclonic epilepsy. However, myoclonic seizures may be an accompaniment of the more ominous Lennox-Gastaut syndrome. In young children they may occur in the context of myoclonic-astatic epilepsy of Doose syndrome. Clinically, they can be separated from sleep myoclonus in that they often occur with awakening or randomly throughout the day while the patient is awake.

Tonic and atonic seizures

Both tonic and atonic seizures are typically seen in the symptomatic generalized epilepsies, occurring in up to 90% of patients with Lennox-Gastaut syndrome. They most characteristically result in a drop attack, where the patient is either propelled to the ground head first in tonic seizures, or slumps to the ground with atonic seizures. The duration of both seizure types is usually under one minute and can be associated with autonomic changes, including facial flushing, tachycardia, hypertension, and papillary changes. The EEG correlates of the seizures typically involve a sudden interruption of the slow background for the duration of the seizures. This activity is somewhat similar to the electrodecremental response seen on EEG in infantile spasms.

11.5   Generalized epilepsy syndromes

Childhood absence epilepsy

Childhood absence epilepsy accounts for up to 10% of children with epilepsy. Absence seizures usually have an onset around 3–4 years and often disappear by age 10 years [3]. The absence seizures are associated with normal intelligence and neurological function, although there is concern that subtle learning and attentional disorders are associated comorbidities. The cause is predominantly genetic, with about one-third of the families of children reporting a family history of similar seizures [4]. Siblings of children have about a 10% chance of developing epilepsy. Typical childhood absence is not associated with generalized tonic-clonic seizures.

The pathogenic mechanisms of absence epilepsy are unknown; although animal models suggest activation of the thalamo-cortical pathways in a rhythmic manner resulting in hypersynchronous discharges [5]. Response to antiepileptic medication is usually excellent with over 70% of patients achieving complete control of absence seizures with the first medication used. A recently completed childhood absence study indicated that valproate has been reported to be equally efficacious to ethosuximide in the treatment of absence seizures, although it may have more side effects [6–8]. Lamotrigine had the least side effects but was not as effective in controlling absence seizures [9]. Ethosuximide has undergone a number of studies as adjunct therapy and first-line treatment and has been found to have the best balance between efficacy and adverse effects. A common side effect is gastrointestinal upset. In rare instances, it can cause aplastic anemia, and hepatic or renal failure. Second-line agents include topiramate and zonisamide. Levetiracetam may be effective for juvenile absence with some data demonstrating efficacy for absence seizures per se [10, 11].

There are patients with typical childhood absence who do not respond to maximal doses of monotherapy and there is some evidence that a combination of valproate and ethosuximide or lamotrigine may be effective. Possibly 10% of childhood absence epilepsy does not respond to polytherapy.

The EEG is not only helpful in diagnosing absence but is also useful in evaluating the effectiveness of treatment. Typically, medication is increased until clinical seizures disappear and then increased until the EEG no longer demonstrates 3 Hz generalized spike-wave discharges. Fragmented discharges during sleep that last less than three seconds and occurring during sleep may be considered as acceptable control by some.

Juvenile absence epilepsy

Juvenile absence epilepsy is relatively common, with seizures beginning around puberty. Typically, onset is between 10 and 17 years of age with intelligence, neurologic function, EEG background, and cerebral imaging being normal. The EEG shows generalized spike-and-wave discharges with normal background activity. The generalized spike-and-wave are often 3 Hz or occur at a slightly faster rate with typical bursts lasting 4–15 seconds. Juvenile absence epilepsy was first distinguished from childhood absence in the 1950s when Janz and Christian identified the occurrence of generalized tonic-clonic seizures as a differentiating feature. Furthermore, unlike childhood absence which shows a female preponderance, juvenile absence occurs equally in males and females. The absence seizures may not be noticed until the occurrence of a generalized tonic-clonic seizure which leads to an EEG and to the diagnosis. Absence seizures usually occur sporadically compared to childhood absence where they occur multiple times a day.

Response to anti-absence medication is good, with 80% of patients becoming seizure-free. Ethosuximide is effective against the absence seizures, but is not effective in controlling generalized tonic-clonic seizures. As such ethosuximide is rarely used. Valproate, lamotrigine, and levetiracetam are usually effective agents.

Juvenile myoclonic epilepsy

This syndrome is the most common primary generalized idiopathic epilepsy with important implications for prognostication and treatment [12]. Typically, patients experience a series of myoclonic jerks that may at times be asymmetric. These myoclonic jerks may occur in clusters in the morning while awake, or randomly throughout the day. They may be activated by flickering lights or sleep deprivation. Attention is sought when the patient experiences a first generalized tonic-clonic seizure, often after sleep deprivation. The neurological exam and cerebral imaging studies if obtained are normal. The EEG demonstrates generalized polyspike-and-wave discharges. Often these discharges are activated by photic light stimulation, or can occur during sleep. They may be associated with a myoclonic jerk. Myoclonic seizures should be differentiated from sleep myoclonus which occurs as normal phenomena during drowsiness. Sleep myoclonus is not associated with polyspike-and-wave discharges on EEG.

Treatment is most effective with valproate, although more recently other medications such as levetiracetam or lamotrigine have been shown to be effective. Lamotrigine, although initially thought to exacerbate myoclonic seizures, has not been shown to do this in randomized studies, although it may not be as effective as valproate in controlling myoclonic seizures. Carbamazepine and phenyotin are effective against the generalized tonic-clonic seizures, although as in absence seizures, they may exacerbate myoclonic seizures.

11.6   Treating generalized seizures

While there are several treatment options for generalized seizures, as indicated earlier, there are medications that should be avoided. Absence epilepsy is not effectively treated with phenyotin, gabapentin, and carbamazepine. Exacerbations of absence following the initiation of carbamazepine have been well documented. Typically, myoclonic seizures do not respond well to phenyotin, carbamazepine, or lamotrigine. As with absence epilepsy some patients may have their myoclonic seizures exacerbated by these medications. While not effective generally against absence and myoclonic seizures these medications are effective in controlling the generalized tonic-clonic seizures that may accompany the primary generalized epilepsies.

11.7   Treatment algorithm

There is a paucity of well-designed, randomized clinical trials for patients with generalized seizures. The American Academy of Neurology has issued broad recommendations for the treatment of generalized seizures. Generally, wherever possible monotherapy should be used.

A diagnostic and treatment algorithm for treating generalized seizures is presented in Figure 11.2. A starting point in the treatment algorithm is an EEG. The EEG is usually essential to appropriately classify seizures, including avoiding the misidentification of secondarily generalized seizures as being primarily generalized seizures. The EEG may show focal spikes in which case the diagnosis of true generalized epilepsy needs to be questioned. A normal EEG does not rule out a generalized seizure and in this case it may be appropriate to observe the patient. If there is a relapse in seizures then a video-EEG and an imaging study may be useful. If the video-EEG shows generalized spike-waves then the diagnosis is confirmed and treatment proceeds from there. If the video-EEG including capturing sleep fails to show epileptiform discharges then the diagnosis may be questioned or an empiric antiepileptic medication trial considered.

If the EEG shows a traditional pattern thereby confirming a primary generalized seizure then the next step is to differentiate between generalized polyspike-waves (usually seen in juvenile myoclonic epilepsy), 3 Hz generalized spike-waves (usually seen in either childhood or juvenile absence epilepsy), or slow spike-waves (usually less than 2.5 Hz, seen in symptomatic Lennox-Gastaut syndrome). The EEG may show hypsarrythmia, which in the presence of infantile spasms is diagnostic of West syndrome.

Cerebral imaging is not usually required if an epilepsy syndromic diagnosis is arrived at. However, imaging should be considered if there are focal epileptiform discharges on EEG, atypical features, or if a definitive epilepsy syndrome cannot be arrived at. Other indications for imaging include the presence of either cognitive deficits or focal deficits seen on neurological examination.

First-line agents for the treatment of generalized epilepsy, especially those associated with generalized spike-wave, polyspike-wave, and slow spike-wave, include levetiracetam, lamotrigine, or valproate. Valproate is the most effective agent in treating the spectrum of generalized seizures. However, the potential for neural tube defects should be considered when considering its use in females of childbearing age. Second-line agents include topiramate and zonisamide. Medications to be avoided include carbamazepine, phenyotin, and oxcarbazepine. These agents are effective against convulsive generalized tonic-clonic seizure, although as mentioned earlier they may exacerbate absence or myoclonic seizures.

If the EEG shows typical 3 Hz generalized spike-wave then a diagnosis of absence epilepsy can be made. Childhood absence is usually not associated with convulsive seizures and ethosuximide is usually a first-line agent that can be used. If the child has a diagnosis of juvenile absence epilepsy then there is an increased risk of accompanying generalized convulsive seizures against which ethosuximide has not been shown effective. In these situations a first-line agent is as for the treatment of primary generalized seizures as discussed above. The presence of hypsarrythmia in an infant raises suspicion for West syndrome with accompanying infantile spasms. Agents that are effective against West syndrome include ACTH and vigabatrin. The academy has also indicated the use of vigabatrin as a first-line therapy for the treatment of infantile spasm. This presents an added option to the long-established use of ACTH. ACTH has many adverse effects associated with its use, including weight increase, hyperglycemia, hypertension, and the possibility of associated cerebral atrophy. Vigabatrin has been reported to constrict visual fields and be associated with reversible MRI white matter changes. Felbamate has a broad spectrum of activity in generalized seizures, but rare reports of fatal aplastic anemia and hepatic failure limit its use to a third-line agent where other treatment alternatives have failed.

11.8   Prognosis/outcomes

The EEG can help guide treatment. When seizures are effectively controlled clinically, an EEG showing residual generalized epileptiform discharges usually indicates the need for an increased dose of medication. Juvenile myoclonic epilepsy and juvenile absence epilepsy typically do not remit with age, whereas childhood absence epilepsy usually remits by age 10 years. Infantile spasms often transition to Lennox-Gastaut syndrome associated with slow spike-and-wave discharges.

References

1. Hermann, B.P., Jones, J.E., Sheth, R. *et al.* (2008) Growing up with epilepsy: a two-year investigation of cognitive development in children with new onset epilepsy. *Epilepsia*, **49** (11), 1847–1858.
2. Hermann, B.P., Jones, J., Sheth, R., and Seidenberg, M. (2007) Cognitive and magnetic resonance volumetric abnormalities in new-onset pediatric epilepsy. *Semin Pediatr Neurol*, **14** (4), 173–180.
3. Wirrell, E.C., Camfield, C.S., Camfield, P.R., Gordon, K.E., and Dooley, J.M. (1996) Long-term prognosis of typical childhood absence epilepsy: remission or progression to juvenile myoclonic epilepsy. *Neurology*, **47** (4), 912–918.
4. Delgado-Escueta, A.V., Medina, M.T., Serratosa, J.M. *et al.* (1999) Mapping and positional cloning of common idiopathic generalized epilepsies: juvenile myoclonus epilepsy and childhood absence epilepsy. *Adv Neurol*, **79**, 351–374.
5. Pulsipher, D.T., Seidenberg, M., Guidotti, L. *et al.* (2009) Thalamofrontal circuitry and executive dysfunction in recent-onset juvenile myoclonic epilepsy. *Epilepsia*, **50** (5), 1210–1219.
6. Montouris, G. and Abou-Khalil, B. (2009) The first line of therapy in a girl with juvenile myoclonic epilepsy: should it be valproate or a new agent? *Epilepsia*, **50** (Suppl 8), 16–20.
7. Sheth, R.D., Wesolowski, CA., Jacob, J.C. *et al.* (1995) Effect of carbamazepine and valproate on bone mineral density. *J Pediatr*, **127** (2), 256–262.
8. Sheth, R.D. and Montouris, G. (2008) Metabolic effects of AEDs: impact on body weight, lipids and glucose metabolism. *Int Rev Neurobiol*, **83**, 329–346.
9. Coppola, G., Licciardi, F., Sciscio, N. *et al.* (2004) Lamotrigine as first-line drug in childhood absence epilepsy: a clinical and neurophysiological study. *Brain Dev*, **26** (1), 26–29.
10. Abou-Khalil, B. (2008) Levetiracetam in the treatment of epilepsy. *Neuropsychiatr Dis Treat*, **4** (3), 507–523.
11. Noachtar, S., Andermann, E., Meyvisch, P. *et al.* (2008) Levetiracetam for the treatment of idiopathic generalized epilepsy with myoclonic seizures. *Neurology*, **70** (8), 607–616.
12. Camfield, C.S. and Camfield, P.R. (2009) Juvenile myoclonic epilepsy 25 years after seizure onset: a population-based study. *Neurology*, **73** (13), 1041–1045.

12 Symptomatic generalized epilepsies

Katherine C. Nickels and Elaine Wirrell

Child and Adolescent Neurology, Mayo Clinic, Rochester, MN, USA

12.1 Introduction

An "epilepsy syndrome" has been defined by the ILAE as "a complex of signs and symptoms that define a unique epileptic condition" [1]. Epilepsy syndromes denote specific constellations of clinical seizure type(s), EEG findings, other characteristic clinical features such as age at onset, course of epilepsy, associated neurological and neuropsychological finding, and underlying pathophysiologic or genetic mechanisms [2]. Categorization of epilepsy into a specific "syndrome" provides important information to guide therapeutic decision making and accurately prognosticate long-term outcome.

The term *symptomatic* refers to an epilepsy syndrome in which there is either a known underlying etiology, or there is a presumed etiology, based on other evidence of brain dysfunction, such as developmental delay. Symptomatic epilepsy syndromes are further classified into those with generalized seizures and those with localization-related seizures. This chapter will focus on symptomatic generalized epilepsy syndromes (Figure 12.1 and Table 12.1).

Adult Epilepsy, First Edition. Edited by Gregory D. Cascino and Joseph I. Sirven.
© 2011 John Wiley & Sons, Ltd. Published 2011 by John Wiley & Sons, Ltd.

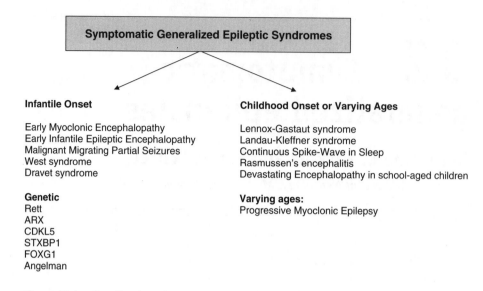

Figure 12.1   Classification of symptomatic generalized epileptic syndromes.

12.2   Infantile onset syndromes

Early myoclonic encephalopathy

Early myoclonic encephalopathy is an exceedingly rare syndrome, initially described in 1978 [3–5]. It usually begins in the first hours after birth with erratic myoclonus, which characteristically involves the face and limbs, present during both wakefulness and sleep, and may be nearly continuous. Additionally, subtle partial seizures with eye deviation and autonomic signs occur. Several months into the course, tonic spasms may develop. These infants have profound psychomotor delay, decreased alertness, and hypotonia.

The characteristic EEG shows a suppression burst pattern (Figure 12.2) and there is usually no electrographic correlate seen with the erratic myoclonus. Over time, the EEG pattern often evolves, and either an atypical hypsarrhythmia or multifocal pattern is seen by three to five months of age.

This syndrome responds poorly to therapy. No effective antiepileptic therapies exist and these infants remain profoundly delayed. Most children with early myoclonic encephalopathy die in the first few years of life from respiratory complications of their profoundly impaired neurological status.

In most cases, no etiology can be identified. However, treatable conditions such as pyridoxine or pyridoxal phosphate dependency should be ruled out. Additionally, metabolic disorders, including nonketotic hyperglycinemia, molybdenum cofactor deficiency, organic acidurias, and aminoacidopathies should be considered. Structural brain disorders are an exceedingly rare cause of this syndrome.

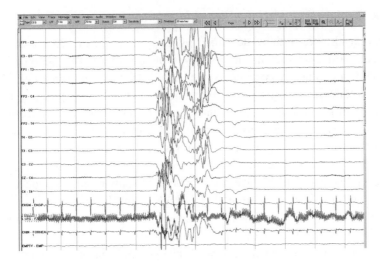

Figure 12.2 Two-week-old child with multifocal myoclonus, global hypotonia, and marked lethargy since birth. Metabolic studies were unremarkable and no response was seen with either pyridoxine, pyridoxal phosphate, or folinic acid. EEG shows a suppression-burst pattern in keeping with early myoclonic encephalopathy.

Early infantile epileptic encephalopathy (Ohtahara's syndrome)

Early infantile epileptic encephalopathy presents characteristically with clusters of tonic spasms in the first three months of life, most commonly in the first 10 days [6]. These spasms are seen both during wakefulness and sleep. Up to half of cases also develop partial motor seizures. However, myoclonic seizures are rare. Neurodevelopmental status is usually severely abnormal, with profound developmental delay from birth. The EEG also shows a burst-suppression pattern during wakefulness and sleep, which may be either widespread and synchronous, or lateralized, in cases with focal cortical malformations. Video-EEG has shown clinical symptoms at the time of the bursts [7]. The most common etiology of early infantile epileptic encephalopathy is malformations of cortical development, and, in particular, hemimegalencephaly. Conversely, inborn metabolic errors are infrequent in this syndrome.

Outcome is often very poor. Epilepsy is typically refractory to medical treatment and infants are often left severely delayed. Mortality is high in the first few years, due to underlying profound neurological impairment. Antiepileptic therapies including valproate, felbamate, vigabatrin, zonisamide, ACTH, and the ketogenic diet have been helpful in rare cases. In infants with a more localized malformation of cortical development, surgical resection should be strongly considered early on to avoid the neurodevelopmental consequences of ongoing, intractable seizures and maximize developmental potential. Evolution to either West syndrome or refractory partial seizures is common.

Malignant migrating partial epilepsy in infancy

This rare syndrome, initially described by Coppola *et al.* in 1995 presents with multifocal, partial seizures in the first seven months of age that become increasingly frequent and nearly continuous over time [8]. The initial semiology consists of focal motor seizures, along with autonomic features such as apnea, cyanosis, or flushing. With increasing age, secondary generalization may occur. Occasionally, seizures may appear to arise from a single focus initially, and in some cases, up to two months have elapsed prior to the appearance of other foci. Characteristically, seizures tend to cluster over several days, followed by seizure-free periods lasting up to several weeks. Infants have been reported to show progressive developmental delay and hypotonia, and mortality is high in the first few years due to the profound neurological impairment, although a more recent case series suggests a slightly more optimistic outcome in some cases [8, 9].

Background slowing and multifocal discharge are seen on the interictal EEG recording. Ictally, rhythmical theta activity arising from multifocal regions of the brain is seen and several focal seizures may be ongoing at any one time. Brief subclinical discharges are also reported.

The underlying etiology is not known and imaging, neuropathologic studies, and metabolic investigations are unremarkable. Familial recurrence has not been reported. No effective treatment has been identified, although isolated successes with a combination of stiripentol and clonazepam, with vigabatrin, bromides, or the ketogenic diet have been described.

West syndrome

West syndrome refers to the triad of infantile spasms, hypsarrhythmia, and psychomotor delay. However, psychomotor delay is not necessary for diagnosis and may be absent, particularly at presentation. It is the most common epileptic encephalopathy, with an incidence of 1/1900–1/3900 infants, and presents at a peak age of four to seven months [10].

Spasms characteristically occur in clusters lasting several minutes and occur only a few times to several hundreds of times per day [11]. They are most frequent shortly after waking. Semiologically, the epileptic spasm consists of a transient contraction of the trunk, neck, and extremities, often followed by a brief second tonic component. Spasms may be flexor, extensor, or mixed. However, asymmetric spasms or coexistent partial seizures should suggest a focal cortical lesion [12]. During the cluster, the child may become irritable and cry, often leading to a misdiagnosis of infantile colic.

The most common EEG pattern seen in children with West syndrome is hypsarrhythmia, a pattern of disorganized, paroxysmal, high-voltage slowing, multifocal epileptiform discharge and a lack of synchrony (Figure 12.3a). While this pattern is often seen on routine EEG, it may occur during non-REM sleep only, emphasizing the importance of a sleep recording. During REM sleep, hypsarrhythmia is reduced or disappears. With age, the EEG evolves to show greater interhemispheric synchronization, focal or multifocal sharp waves, or high-voltage generalized slow activity or slow spike-wave. Not all children with West syndrome show a typical hypsarrhythmia pattern—if the clinical history is suggestive of spasms but the

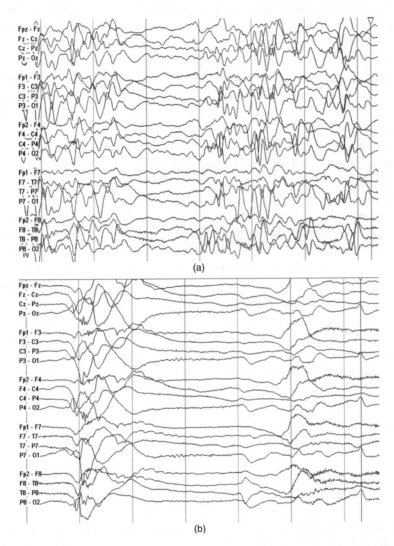

Figure 12.3 (a,b) This six-month-old child had a history of perinatal hypoxic-ischemic brain injury. Over the last month, he has had clusters of flexor spasms lasting several minutes each. His interictal sleep EEG (a) is abnormally high voltage and shows diffuse slowing and multifocal spikes, in keeping with a diagnosis of hypsarrhythmia. During the EEG, a cluster of typical infantile spasms were captured, showing a high-voltage generalized sharp wave (b).

EEG fails to show hypsarrhythmia, a brief admission to record spasms should be considered. During the spasm, the EEG typically shows a high-voltage generalized sharp wave, often followed by a brief electrodecrement (Figure 12.3b). Ictal focal discharges that are seen before, during, or after the spasms should suggest the possibility of a localized area of cortical dysplasia [13].

Most cases of West syndrome are *symptomatic*. An underlying etiology can often be identified, which includes malformations of cortical development, neurocutaneous disorders such as tuberous sclerosis, preexisting brain injury due to ischemia, infection, or trauma, genetic causes including Down syndrome, ARX, or CDKL5 mutations or less commonly, inborn metabolic disorders such as mitochondrial disease, phenylketonuria or Menkes disease [14, 15]. However, in 15–30%, no underlying etiology is found. A small proportion of this latter group is truly *idiopathic*, with a possible hereditary predisposition and normal development prior to spasm onset, symmetric spasms and EEG changes, disappearance of hypsarrhythmia between spasms and rapid control of seizures, and without significant past medical history. The remainder are *cryptogenic*, where there is a presumed underlying etiology that cannot be identified [16, 17].

Developmental delay frequently precedes onset of spasms in cases with symptomatic etiology. However, with seizure onset, further regression and visual disinterest is seen. Outcome is often poor, with over 75% exhibiting motor delay and/or mental retardation [14, 18–20]. Autism develops in between 13 and 33%, and is more prevalent in cases with tuberous sclerosis and temporal lobe tubers. Outcome is strongly related to etiology, with up to 40–50% of truly idiopathic cases having a normal outcome [14, 19, 20].

Partial or generalized seizures predate or coexist with spasms in 12–42% of cases, and two-thirds ultimately develop other seizure types [14, 19, 20]. Focal or multifocal seizures or a mixed generalized seizure syndrome, such as Lennox-Gastaut syndrome (LGS), are most common. Spasms usually disappear in the first two years, but can rarely persist or reappear later in childhood [21].

Once the diagnosis of spasms has been made, an MRI should be strongly considered to rule out a malformation of cortical development or prior brain insult. If this study is noninformative, further metabolic and genetic studies should follow. There is some evidence that early initiation of effective treatment correlates with improved long-term developmental outcome, particularly in cryptogenic or idiopathic cases [22]. First-line therapies used include intramuscular ACTH, high-dose oral steroids, or vigabatrin, with the goal of treatment being resolution of both spasms and hypsarrhythmia. There is little consensus regarding the dose and duration of steroid therapy [23].

While ACTH has been reported to be superior to oral corticosteroids [24, 25], these findings may reflect the dose of prednisone used. One study comparing very high-dose oral prednisolone (40 mg/day) to ACTH found no significant difference between these therapies [26]. If one chooses to use ACTH, the optimal dose and duration remain controversial. While one single-blind study comparing high-dose (150 U/m²/day × 3 weeks followed by a 9-week taper) and low-dose ACTH (20–30 U/day × 2–6 weeks), found no significant difference in response or relapse rates [27], some epileptologists believe that high-dose ACTH is superior. Adverse effects of ACTH or oral corticosteroids are significant, and more common with high-dose regimens and synthetic formulations of ACTH. They include hypertension, hypertrophic cardiomyopathy, gastric ulceration, immunosuppression, electrolyte disturbances, hyperglycemia, irritability, weight gain, and transient brain "shrinkage."

Vigabatrin suppresses spasms in up to two-thirds of infants, but appears most effective in cases of cortical dysplasia or tuberous sclerosis [28]. Side effects include irreversible peripheral visual field constriction (which appears minimal if the duration of treatment is kept at six months or less) [29], reversible T2 hyperintensities on MRI in the brainstem, cerebellum, basal ganglia, and thalamus [30], and sedation, hypotonia, insomnia, and irritability.

Pyridoxine (100 mg IV or 100–200 mg by mouth daily × 14 days) is commonly tried in cryptogenic or idiopathic West syndrome to rule out pyridoxine dependency. Pyridoxine should probably be started along with one of the first-line therapies. Surgical resection should be considered with medically intractable spasms and focal cortical lesions [31].

Other therapies which are usually considered second line in the treatment of West syndrome include the ketogenic diet [32], topiramate, valproate, benzodiazepines.

Dravet syndrome

Dravet syndrome is a rare syndrome with a reported incidence of 1/20 000–1/30 000, but is likely under-recognized [33]. While the diagnosis is clinical, approximately 80% have a mutation in the sodium channel α-1 subunit gene (SCN1A), which can be frameshift or nonsense mutations leading to truncating of the protein, missense mutations (usually of the pore region or the N or C terminus), or splice site or deletions [34]. The vast majority of mutations are sporadic. However, close relatives of children with Dravet syndrome have a higher rate of seizures than the general population, particularly generalized epilepsy with febrile seizures plus (GEFS+). The clinical picture of SCN1A mutations is variable, and not all mutations will lead to a Dravet syndrome phenotype.

Dravet syndrome begins in the first year of life in a previously well infant, initially presenting as a generalized or focal clonic seizure that is often prolonged and frequently triggered by fever, infection, vaccination, or bathing [35]. A diagnosis of atypical febrile seizure is frequently made at the time of initial presentation. However, children then have recurrent, prolonged focal seizures, which often change sides and occur both with and without fever. From the end of the second year through age 5, nonconvulsive seizures emerge. Myoclonic jerks may be frequent but variable in intensity. They may be aggravated shortly after waking, just prior to a convulsive seizure, or with photic stimulation. Atypical absence and complex partial seizures with prominent autonomic symptoms occur in over half of cases but tonic seizures are rare. With age, prolonged convulsive seizures become less frequent but seizures remain refractory to treatment.

The initial EEG is typically normal, excepting postictal slowing [35]. Over time, there is background slowing and emergence of multifocal and generalized polyspike-and-wave discharges, frequently activated by photic stimulation and drowsiness (Figure 12.4a,b). Neuroimaging studies are also unrevealing early on. Later in the course, mild atrophy, and, less commonly, hippocampal sclerosis are seen. The term "borderline or borderland" has been used for cases that lack a number of the key features (myoclonus, generalized spike-wave discharges, limited number, or atypical seizure types). However, the prognosis seems similar [34].

Although development prior to seizure onset is normal, infants demonstrate regression or lack of progression between one and four years, with stabilization after that at a lower level of function [36]. Visuomotor skills are more impacted than is language. Ultimately, most children manifest ataxia and corticospinal tract signs of exam, along with a peculiar crouched gait. Hyperactivity and behavior problems are common. The mortality rate of Dravet syndrome is 16–18%, with deaths predominantly due to status epilepticus, drowning, and SUDEP [37].

Therapy is suboptimal and seizures remain medically intractable [37]. Lamotrigine, carbamazepine, and phenytoin should be avoided as they aggravate seizures. Therapies with some efficacy include valproate, benzodiazepines, topiramate, levetiracetam, zonisamide, and the ketogenic diet. Stiripentol, a medication with orphan drug status in the US and which is an inhibitor of the cytochrome p450 system, has been helpful when used in combination with valproic acid and/or clobazam. A randomized, placebo-controlled study showed a greater than 50% reduction in the frequency of tonic-clonic seizures in 71% of the stiripentol-treated group versus only 5% of those on placebo, and 43% of the stiripentol group were free of tonic-clonic events [38].

12.3   Childhood onset syndromes

Lennox-Gastaut syndrome (LGS)

LGS typically presents in preschool-aged children with frequent falls or head nods. The children are also found to have recurrent myoclonic and atypical absence seizures. The syndrome evolves over months to comprise a triad of symptoms including: (i) multiple generalized seizure types, including tonic, atonic, myoclonic, and atypical absence; (ii) an interictal EEG pattern of diffuse slow spike-and-wave complexes; and (iii) cognitive dysfunction.

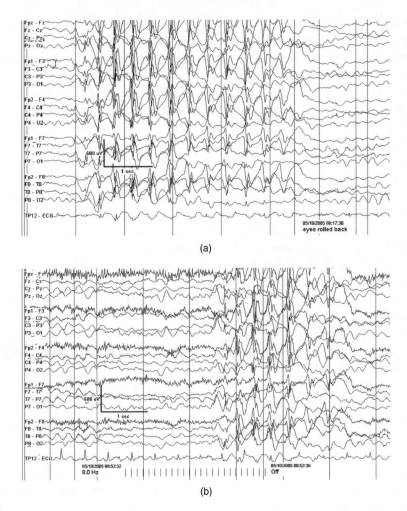

(a)

(b)

Figure 12.4 (a,b) This three-year-old girl presented with a history of multiple prolonged focal and generalized seizures in infancy, the first one occurring after her four-month immunization. Recently she has also developed myoclonus and staring spells. She has mild delay. An exhaustive workup including neuroimaging and metabolic studies were normal; however, she has a nonsense mutation affecting the SCN1A gene. The EEG shows one of her typical staring spells with generalized spike-wave (a). Her background was slow for age and photosensitivity was documented (b).

The most common seizures are tonic seizures. They are usually, but not always, symmetric and can cause the patient to fall forward or backward. They are commonly associated with autonomic manifestations, including facial flushing, tachycardia, and pupillary dilation. Nocturnal tonic events are characteristic of LGS, but are often subtle and difficult to recognize without video-EEG recording. Nonconvulsive status epilepticus is also common, and its frequency and duration appears predictive of poorer long-term developmental outcome [39]. Furthermore, nonconvulsive status epilepticus is frequently difficult to detect, particularly in children with moderate to severe cognitive impairment, resulting in delay in diagnosis. Tonic status epilepticus may be provoked by benzodiazepines [40].

The seizures in LGS are frequently medically intractable, with incomplete response to antiseizure medications. Valproate is commonly used, and lamotrigine, topiramate, felbamate, and rufinamide have been shown to be superior to placebo in randomized, controlled studies [41, 42]. Felbamate is often effective in refractory epilepsies, but should not be used first line due to the potential risks of aplastic anemia and hepatotoxicity. Benzodiazepines, levetiracetam, or zonisamide may reduce all seizure types, but rarely provide complete control. Carbamazepine may lessen tonic seizures, but worsen atypical absences. Ethosuximide may be helpful for refractory atypical absences. Given the poor response to AEDs, the ketogenic diet should be considered early in the course of LGS. Approximately half of children experience significant seizure reduction with some achieving seizure freedom.

Corpus callosotomy is a possible treatment for patients with intractable drop seizures, but not for other seizure types. Section of only the anterior two-thirds limits adverse effects compared to complete callosotomy, but is less effective. Retrospective studies have demonstrated vagal nerve stimulation to reduce seizures by approximately 50% in nearly half of children [43].

The interictal EEG in LGS shows 1.5–2.5 Hz polyspike and spike-and-wave discharges on a slow background with increased activation during sleep recordings (Figure 12.5). However, this pattern may take months to evolve and is present in less than 30% of patients when they initially present. Early on, the EEGs may be normal or show only mild background slowing or infrequent bursts of generalized spike-wave discharges. Low-voltage, frontally predominant, >10 Hz generalized paroxysmal fast activity is seen in slow-wave sleep and is suggestive of the diagnosis of LGS, even if other EEG features have not yet fully evolved.

Developmental delay is common in children with LGS, but may not be obvious early in the course. Ultimately over 80% of children are mentally handicapped [44]. Factors predictive of poorer cognitive outcome include delayed development prior to seizure onset, history of infantile spasms, and onset of symptoms before three years, frequent seizures, and recurrent nonconvulsive status epilepticus. Hyperkinetic behaviors, autistic features, and perseverative behaviors are common.

LGS is a relatively rare epilepsy syndrome with an incidence of 1.9–2.1 per 100 000 children but accounts for approximately 6–7% of patients with intractable pediatric epilepsy. Onset is between the ages of one and eight, with typical onset in the preschool years. The majority of patients are males. Two-thirds of cases are "symptomatic," affecting children with preexistent brain abnormalities, which include malformations of cortical development, neurocutaneous disorders, metabolic or genetic conditions, or pre-, peri-, or postnatal insults due to ischemia,

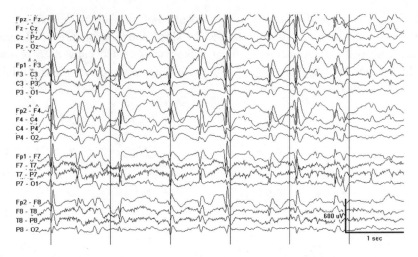

Figure 12.5 This eight-year-old boy has a history of neonatal hypoxia and hypoglycemia with developmental delay. He developed generalized tonic-clonic seizures at age two years. He subsequently developed multiple seizure types, including atonic, complex partial, myoclonic, and atypical absence seizures in addition to rare generalized tonic-clonic seizures. His awake interictal EEG demonstrates high-amplitude generalized slow spike-and-wave discharges, characteristic of Lennox-Gastaut syndrome.

infection, or trauma. One third of these "symptomatic" cases have a history of infantile spasms. However, an underlying etiology frequently is not elucidated, even in those with developmental delay at the onset of seizures. Approximately 30% of LGS cases are "cryptogenic," affecting children who are neurologically and developmentally normal prior to the onset of their epilepsy. Forty-eight percent of this group has a positive family history of epilepsy or febrile seizures, and LGS has been reported to be a phenotype of GEFS+ [45, 46].

LGS should be differentiated from myoclonic astatic epilepsy (MAE), which presents at a similar age with frequent drop seizures and frontally predominant slow spike-wave. Children with MAE typically have normal development before seizure onset, a positive family history of epilepsy, and myoclonic-astatic or prominent generalized tonic-clonic seizures. An EEG demonstrating parietal theta rhythms is also suggestive of MAE. Drop seizures may also be seen in continuous spike-wave in sleep (CSWS). However, the EEG shows CSWS and tonic seizures do not occur. A transient LGS-like picture can also be seen in children with mesial frontal or hemispheric seizures, but tonic seizures are rare.

Electrical status epilepticus in slow sleep (ESES)

ESES is an EEG finding in which there is nearly continuous activation of spike-wave discharges in slow-wave sleep. Early EEG may demonstrate diffuse spikes and slow waves, predominantly in centrotemporal or frontotemporal regions. However, with time, the EEG in non-REM sleep shows a picture of electrical status, with diffuse, unilateral, or focal spike-waves that occupy 85% or more of slow sleep. The discharges resolve upon awakening and are without clinical accompaniment (Figure 12.6a,b).

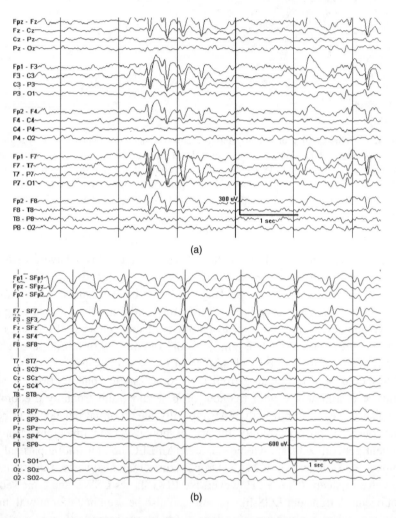

(a)

(b)

Figure 12.6 (a,b) This 10-year-old boy has a history of a left-sided grade 4 intraventricular hemorrhage as a term neonate. He had mild developmental delay until age nine, when his parents noted a global regression in skills. His expressive language was most affected. His awake interictal EEG demonstrates infrequent bursts of generalized atypical spike-and-wave discharges that are maximal over the left hemisphere, consistent with his prior intraventricular hemorrhage (a). During sleep he had nearly continuous spike-wave discharges that were without clinical symptoms, consistent with electrical status epilepticus in slow-wave sleep (ESES) (b).

This EEG finding is seen in two related clinical syndromes: CSWS and Landau-Kleffner syndrome (LKS). In both syndromes, children present in the preschool or early school years with regression and a sleep EEG demonstrating ESES [47]. The clinical symptoms of these two syndromes reflect the localization of the EEG discharge. The EEG discharges in CSWS are maximal over the frontal head regions. This correlates with a global regression in CSWS, including decreased learning, expressive language difficulties, poor memory, hyperactivity and inattentiveness, psychosis, and motor impairment. The EEG discharges in LKS predominantly affect the temporal regions, correlating the regression in receptive language, or acquired auditory agnosia. The majority of children with CSWS present with seizures, which may consist of tonic-clonic, absence, atonic, clonic, complex partial, and simple motor seizures. Tonic seizures are not seen. Seizures are also commonly seen in children with LKS, but they are rarely frequent or intractable. The usual semiology is that of a nocturnal hemiclonic seizure.

Some cases of CSWS are symptomatic of a prior brain insult. However, in others, particularly LKS, no etiology is found and prior psychomotor development was normal. These cases may represent the severe end of the spectrum of "benign partial epilepsy of childhood."

Antiseizure medications may be helpful in treating the seizures in CSWS and LKS, but most drugs have little impact on the electrical status and cognitive impairment. Some medications, such as phenobarbital, carbamazepine, or phenytoin may worsen this condition. Valproic acid or benzodiazepines are most likely the best choices for seizure control. Ethosuximide and levetiracetam have also been shown to be beneficial in small studies [48, 49]. Corticosteroids are often considered the first-line treatment in CSWS but their efficacy has only been shown in several unblinded studies [50]. Other clinicians have reported efficacy with short three- to four-week cycles of high-dose diazepam (0.5 mg/kg) following a rectal diazepam bolus of 1 mg/kg [49]. Case reports have also claimed efficacy for intravenous immune globulin (IVIG), methylprednisolone, ACTH, sulthiame (for cryptogenic cases), ketogenic diet, and multiple subpial transection [51–56].

Seizures and electrical status do spontaneously resolve in later childhood. However, although some improvements in language and cognition are usually also seen, most children do not return to normal levels of functioning.

Devastating epileptic encephalopathy in school-aged children (DESC)

Devastating epileptic encephalopathy in school-aged children (DESC) occurs in previously healthy school-aged children, without a prior history of epilepsy. It is also known as febrile infection responsive epileptic (FIRE) encephalopathies of school age [57]. The children develop a nonspecific febrile illness, followed by refractory convulsive multifocal status epilepticus. The seizures may last for weeks, in spite of all therapies, including general anesthesia. Although there is a febrile prodrome, no infectious etiology can be elucidated. The cerebrospinal fluid (CSF) often does not demonstrate any significant abnormalities that would suggest encephalitis [58]. The MRI findings are often nonspecific. There is no effective treatment and no known etiology [59]. Unfortunately, those that survive continue to have frequent intractable seizures with status epilepticus and profound cognitive dysfunction. The death rate is high [58].

12.4   Symptomatic generalized epilepsy syndromes of known cause

Specific genetic disorders leading to refractory seizures in infancy

Several genetic disorders, which may have characteristic associated findings, can be associated with symptomatic generalized epilepsy that is usually severe (Table 12.2).

Metabolic disorders

Metabolic disorders should be considered in children with symptomatic epilepsy without clear etiology. A history of developmental plateau or regression, a family history of similar symptoms in other family members or consanguinity, or other systemic pathology is suggestive of metabolic disease. Seizures occur due to storage of abnormal material within the neurons, deficits in energy production, or interference with neurotransmitter synthesis and metabolism. Some of these conditions may be treatable (Table 12.3).

Progressive myoclonic epilepsies

The progressive myoclonic epilepsies represent multiple rare degenerative disorders that present with the combination of progressive myoclonus epilepsy with multiple seizure types, cerebellar impairment, and cognitive regression (Table 12.4). The EEG demonstrates diffuse background slowing. The myoclonus is associated with a generalized spike-wave discharge. Occipital discharge may also be present in Lafora disease. Photosensitivity is often present. Unfortunately, there is no specific therapy available for most underlying disorders. However, antiepileptic agents, such as valproic acid, zonisamide, benzodiazepines, and levetiracetam, may substantially reduce the myoclonus. Piracetam is of particularly benefit. Phenytoin and carbamazepine should be avoided as they may worsen these disorders (Table 12.4).

Table 12.1   Symptomatic epilepsy syndromes in infants and children

Epilepsy syndrome	Age at presentation	Clinical features	EEG characteristics	Etiology	Therapy	Outcome
Early myoclonic encephalopathy	Birth to first few weeks	Prominent myoclonus. Partial seizures often with eye deviation and autonomic signs. Tonic spasms may develop later in the course. Infant is hypotonic and poorly responsive	Suppression burst without EEG correlate to myoclonus	Usually unknown. Rarely an underlying metabolic disorder is found	No effective therapies	Very poor. High mortality in first few years of life
Early infantile epileptic encephalopathy	Several weeks to several months of age	Tonic spasms. Partial seizures	Suppression burst	Malformation of cortical development. Some unknown	Vigabatrin, zonisamide or ACTH may be helpful, many intractable to AEDs. Epilepsy surgery if child has a focal malformation	Poor with high mortality in first few years
Malignant migrating partial seizures in infancy	First seven months	Focal motor seizures often with apnea, cyanosis, flushing. Often cluster. May become secondarily generalized with increasing age	Slow background with multifocal discharge. Ictal EEG shows rhythmic theta from multiple sites	Unknown	Poor response to AEDs. Bromides or stiripentol and clonazepam may rarely help	Very poor with significant mortality in early years

(Continued)

Table 12.1 (*Continued*)

Epilepsy syndrome	Age at presentation	Clinical features	EEG characteristics	Etiology	Therapy	Outcome
West syndrome	Peak age at onset 4–7 months	Epileptic spasms in clusters, particularly on awakening	Hypsarrhythmia	Multiple— see text	First line: ACTH, steroid or vigabatrin. Second line: valproate, topiramate, benzodiazepines, ketogenic diet	Depends on etiology. Most are symptomatic and do poorly
Dravet syndrome	First year of life	Prolonged focal or generalized tonic clonic seizures, often triggered by fever, infection, immunizations or bathing. Myoclonic seizures and absences later in course	Usually normal initially. Later, slow background, multifocal or generalized polyspike-wave discharge	SCN1A gene mutation on chromosome 2 detected in 80%	Effective agents include stiripentol with valproate and clobazam, topiramate, levetiractam, zonisamide or the ketogenic diet	Often poor. High mortality—16–18%—due to SUDEP, status epilepticus, and drowning
Lennox Gastaut syndrome	2–8 years, peak age 3–5 years	Multiple types of generalized seizures including tonic, atonic, atypical absence, myoclonic. Most children have preexisting neurological disability and have lack of normal development progress after onset	Frontally predominant slow spike-wave. In sleep, see fast, frontally predominant 10 Hz rhythmic spike activity	Multiple	Valproate, topiramate, lamotrigine, felbamate, rufinamide. Early use of the ketogenic diet should be considered. First line AEDs: valproate, lamotrigine, topiramate	Seizures often refractory. Mental handicap in 80%

Landau-Kleffner syndrome	3–8 years	Acquired auditory agnosia Nearly three-quarters have seizures—partial motor seizures affecting lower face and upper extremity most common	Centrotemporal sharp waves which markedly increase in sleep	Usually idiopathic	Oral steroids, high-dose diazepam	EEG changes and seizures resolve in mid-late childhood but children may be left with language impairment
Continuous spike-wave in sleep	3–8 years	Global regression with partial and generalized (atypical absence, atonics, generalized tonic-clonic, but not tonic) seizures	Frontal and multifocal sharp waves which become nearly continuous in sleep	Often symptomatic of underlying brain insult	Oral steroids or high-dose diazepam	EEG changes and seizures improve or resolve in mid-late childhood but children are often left with cognitive impairment
Rasmussen's encephalitis	18 months to young adulthood	Focal seizures which progressively increase in frequency over time, epilepsia partialis continua, progressive hemiparesis and atrophy of affected hemisphere	Hemispheric slowing, multifocal epileptiform discharges are widespread over affected hemisphere and may be bilateral	Immune-mediated but remains poorly understood	Immunotherapy can be tried but most children ultimately require hemispherectomy	After hemispherectomy, two-thirds are seizure-free, cognitive deterioration stabilizes but hemiparesis is permanent (although children can ambulate)

(Continued)

Table 12.1 (*Continued*)

Epilepsy syndrome	Age at presentation	Clinical features	EEG characteristics	Etiology	Therapy	Outcome
Devastating encephalopathy in school age children (DESC)	4–11 years	Intractable convulsive status epilepticus with fever but without intracranial infection. Followed by intractable temporal lobe epilepsy	Recurrent, often multifocal seizures with status epilepticus	Unknown	No effective therapies reported	Very poor. Children are left with intractable partial epilepsy and cognitive delay
Progressive myoclonic epilepsy	Infancy to adulthood	Progressive myoclonus, generalized tonic-clonic and other seizures, mental deterioration, cerebellar dysfunction	Slow background with generalized spike- and polyspike-and-wave discharge	Multiple metabolic and neurode-generative conditions	AEDs may help but do not provide complete control. Valproate, clonazepam, zonisamide, levetiracetam	Progressive but rapidity depends on etiology

Table 12.2   Genetic disorders which can be associated with symptomatic generalized epilepsy

Syndrome	Chromosome	Other features	Semiology of seizures	EEG	Course
Angelman	Partial monosomy 15q	Ataxia, tremor, minimal speech, severe delay, happy demeanor	Atypical absence, myoclonic, tonic-clonic, unilateral clonic complex partial	High-amplitude, symmetrical, synchronous notched 2 Hz polyphasic slow waves or slow and sharp waves, particularly during slow-wave sleep	VPA + BZDs helpful. Seizure severity decreases over time
Wolf-Hirschhorn	Partial monosomy 4p	Prenatal growth failure, severe delay, cleft lip or palate, beaked nose, hypertelorism, low-set ears	Partial, myoclonic, generalized tonic-clonic or atypical absence seizures	High-voltage spike-wave or slow waves or sequences of sharp waves in the centroparietal or occipital regions	Severity decreases with time
Ring chromosome 20	20	Mild-moderate delay, restlessness, aggression, nondysmorphic	Runs of atypical absence or myoclonic status epilepticus	Ictal: high-voltage, 2–3 Hz slow activity with superimposed spikes maximal over frontal regions. Interictal: normal or mild slowing/sharp waves	Seizures are refractory and do not remit with age
Miller Dieker	17p13.3 deletion	Four-layered lissencephaly, microcephaly, bitemporal narrowing, small, anteverted nose, micrognathia, high forehead, cardiac, renal, and sacral anomalies	In first weeks to months, massive myoclonus and epileptic spasms are seen. Over time, partial and tonic seizures emerge as predominant seizure types	Prominent fast activity, although slowing is common in the first year of life	Seizures are refractory

(Continued)

Table 12.2 (Continued)

Syndrome	Chromosome	Other features	Semiology of seizures	EEG	Course
CDKL5		Severe developmental delay with hypotonia. Acquired microcephaly in some cases. Impaired eye contact and gaze avoidance	Generalized tonic seizures beginning in first 10 wks, followed by spasm, atypical absences and myoclonic seizures	Interictal EEG normal early on, then see slowing of background and modified hypsarrhythmia	Intractable generalized seizures
Rett syndrome	MECP2 mutation on X chromosome	Normal early development followed by acquired microcephaly, autistic features, lack of purposeful hand movement with characteristic hand wringing	Genereralized tonic-clonic seizures, other generalized and partial seizures	Slowing of background with multifocal and generalized epileptiform discharge	Often refractory
ARX	Xp22.13	Severe developmental delay and seizures in boys. Often associated cerebral malformations including lissencephaly, agenesis of corpus callosum. May have dystonia, spasticity	Spasms, other generalized seizures	Suppression-burst, hypsarrhythmia	Usually refractory

FOXG1	14q	Severe delay without microcephaly "congenital Rett"	Partial and generalized seizures	Slowing of background, focal and multifocal discharge	Often refractory
POLG1	DNA polymerase in mitochondria	Cerebral atrophy, liver dysfunction	Myoclonic, other partial and generalized seizures	Multifocal discharge with slowing	Refractory
Trisomy 12p	12	Severe delay, short neck, prominent forehead, flat occiput, hypertelorism, micrognathia, low-set ears	Myoclonic or myoclonic absence, generalized tonic-clonic	3 Hz spike and polyspike	Seizures often respond to AEDs
Ring chromosome 14	14	Severe delay, microcephaly, narrow face, high-arched palate, short palpebral fissures, flat nasal bridge, retrognathia, ocular anomalies	Symptomatic generalized epilepsy with onset in first year of life; Occasionally complex partial seizures; Ictal apnea	Slow spike-wave	Seizures are usually refractory
Inversion-duplication 15 syndrome	15	Moderate to severe delay, autism, microcephaly, mild occasional dysmorphic features	Symptomatic generalized epilepsy resembling West or Lennox-Gastaut syndrome, occasional focal seizures	Hypsarrhythmia, slow spike-wave	Often refractory

Table 12.3 Metabolic disorders associated with symptomatic epilepsy

Metabolic disorder	Age at onset	Clinical	Prognosis
Pyridoxine dependency	Birth to one year	Multiple seizure types refractory to antiseizure medications, often beginning before birth, with progressive encephalopathy, clinical and EEG response to pyridoxine	Variable, depending on duration of symptoms prior to supplementation
Pyridoxal phosphate dependency	Neonatal	Multiple seizure types refractory to antiseizure medications, encephalopathy, clinical and EEG response to pyridoxal phosphate and pyridoxine	Variable, depending on duration of symptoms prior to supplementation
Folinic acid responsive seizures	Neonatal	Multiple seizure types refractory to antiseizure medications, encephalopathy, clinical and EEG response to folinic acid, incomplete pyridoxal phosphate and pyridoxine	Variable, depending on duration of symptoms prior to supplementation
Serine deficiency	Neonatal	Congenital microcephaly, cognitive disability, epilepsy	Variable, depending on duration of symptoms prior to supplementation
Creatine deficiency	Neonatal and infancy	Variable developmental delay, seizures, autistic behavior, gastrointestinal disturbances, decreased growth	Poor, majority with moderate to severe mental retardation
Untreated phenylketonuria	Neonatal and infancy	Growth failure, microcephaly, seizures, mental retardation	Good if diagnosed and treated early
Urea cycle disorders	Neonatal, later if partial enzyme deficiency	Vomiting, lethargy, coma, seizures, developmental delay, protein avoidance	Variable, depending on severity and duration of symptoms
Nonketotic hyperglycinemia	Neonatal	Lethargy, hypotonia, hiccups, intractable seizures, apnea	Poor, death usually within the first year
GABA transaminase deficiency	Neonatal	Intractable neonatal seizures, lethargy, irritability, severely delayed development	Poor, death usually within the first five years

Syndrome	Age of onset	Clinical features	Outcome
Sulfite oxidase deficiency	Neonatal	Intractable seizures, progressive neurocognitive decline, acquired microcephaly, MRI demonstrating leukoencephalomalacia and atrophy	Poor
Peroxisomal disorders	Neonatal	Hepatic disease, developmental delay, retinopathy, deafness, seizures	Variable, depending on phenotype
Glutaric acidemia type 1	Infancy and childhood	Macrocephaly, acute neurologic decompensation with hypotonia, opisthotonic posturing, dystonia, dyskinesia, seizures, encephalopathy, often triggered by infection or fever	Poor, although detection and treatment prior to decompensation may improve outcome
Biotinidase deficiency	Neonatal through childhood	Seizures, hypotonia, mental retardation, ataxia, dermatitis, hair loss, autistic behavior	Outcome can be good if diagnosed and treated early
Vitamin B6 (pyridoxine) dependency	Infancy and childhood	Multiple seizure types, possible prenatal onset, that are refractory to medications	Outcome can be good if diagnosed and treated early
Succinic semialdehyde dehydrogenase deficiency	Infancy and childhood	Developmental delay, ataxia, hypotonia, seizures, hyperactivity, behavior problems	Variable, treatment targeted at symptoms
Disorders of serine metabolism	Infancy and childhood	Microcephaly, seizures, mental retardation, spasticity	Poor, although outcome may be improved with early detection and treatment
Tetrahydrobiopterin deficiencies	2–12 months	Cognitive regression, microcephaly, generalized seizures, irritability	Outcome can be good if diagnosed and treated early
Glucose transporter deficiency	Birth to early childhood	Seizures, developmental delay, acquired ataxia, hypoglycorrhachia on CSF exam	Variable, depending on duration of symptoms prior to treatment with ketogenic diet
Myoclonic epilepsy with ragged red fibers	3–65 years	Partial or generalized seizures, deafness, myopathy, lactic acidosis, ataxia, optic atrophy	Variable, depending on severity
Menkes disease	Infancy	Developmental regression, seizures, hypopigmentation of skin and hair, hypothermia, characteristic "kinky" hair	Poor with progression to death typically within five years

Table 12.4 Progressive myoclonic epilepsy syndromes

Syndrome	Age at onset	Clinical	Investigations	Prognosis
Tay-Sachs and Sandhoff diseases	4–9 months	Exaggerated startle reflex, developmental regression, visual loss, cherry-red spot	Hexosaminidase A (Tay-Sachs) and A and B (Sandhoff)	Death in two to four years
Tetrahydrobiopterin deficiencies	2–12 months	Cognitive regression, microcephaly, generalized seizures, irritability	Urine for pterins	May respond to tetrahydrobiopterin
Alper's disease	0–5 years	Progressive cognitive deterioration, peripheral neuropathy, recurrent status epilepticus and epilepsia partialis continua, hepatic failure	Genetic—POLG1 mutation	Death, usually due to hepatic failure or status epilepticus
Juvenile Huntington disease	5–20 years	Myoclonic tremor, chorea, cognitive regression, behavior change	Genetic—expanded trinucleotide CAG repeat on chromosome 4p16.3	Slow progression to death in 10–20 years
Neuronal ceroid lipofuscinosis	Infancy to adulthood, depending on subtype	Progressive seizures, ataxia, myoclonus, dementia, visual loss with some subtypes, cerebral atrophy, pyramidal and extrapyramidal signs	Skin, rectal, conjunctival or brain biopsy demonstrating characteristic ultrastructural pathology. Genetic diagnosis available for many subtypes	Death within 1–15 years, depending on subtype
Sialidosis type 1	8–15 years	Decreased vision, cherry-red spots, burning extremity pain, progressive myoclonus, cognition mildly impaired	A-Neuraminidase. Urine oligosaccharides	Profound impairment from myoclonus, death in third or fourth decade

Sialidosis type 2	0–10 months (infantile form) or adolescence (juvenile form)	Course features, visual deficits, cherry-red spot, generalized seizures, burning extremity pain, dementia	A-Neuraminidase. Urine oligosaccharides	Often severe
Unverricht-Lundborg disease	6–18 years	Ataxia, mild cognitive deterioration, generalized tonic-clonic seizures	Genetic—EPM1 (21q22.3)	Slow progression with tendency to stabilize in adulthood
Lafora disease	6–19 years	Generalized tonic-clonic and occipital seizures, rapid cognitive regression	Genetic—EMP2A or EMP2B. Axillary skin biopsy	Rapidly progressive to death within 2–10 years
Myoclonus epilepsy with ragged red fibers	3–65 years	Partial or generalized seizures, deafness, myopathy, lactic acidosis, ataxia, optic atrophy	Genetic testing of mitochondrial DNA, muscle biopsy for ragged red fibers	Variable
Gaucher's disease	Childhood to early adulthood	Supranuclear gaze palsy, generalized or partial seizures, rigidity, ataxia, cognitive regression, splenomegaly	Glucocerebrosidase deficiency	Variable but often more severe if younger onset
Dentato-rubral-pallido-luysian atrophy (DRPLA)	6–69 years	Choreoathetosis, dementia, psychosis, ataxia	CAG expansion at 12p13	Variable

References

1. Engel, J. Jr. (2001) A proposed diagnostic scheme for people with epileptic seizures and with epilepsy: report of the ILAE Task Force on Classification and Terminology. *Epilepsia*, **42**, 796–803.
2. Engel, J. Jr. (2006) Report of the ILAE classification core group. *Epilepsia*, **47**, 1558–1568.
3. Oka, E., Ishida, S., Ohtsuka, Y., and Ohtahara, S. (1995) Neuroepidemiological study of childhood epilepsy by application of international classification of epilepsies and epileptic syndromes (ILAE, 1989). *Epilepsia*, **36**, 658–661.
4. Aicardi, J. and Goutieres, F. (1978) Encephalopathie myoclonique neonatale. *Rev EEG Neurophysiol*, **8**, 99–101.
5. Cavazzuti, G.B., Nalin, A., Ferrari, F. *et al.* (1978) Encefalopatia epilettica ad insorgenza neonatale. *Clin Pediatr*, **60**, 239–246.
6. Aicardi, J. and Ohtahara, S. (2002) Severe neonatal epilepsies with suppression-burst pattern, in *Epileptic Syndromes in Infancy, Childhood and Adolescence*, 3rd edn (eds. J. Roger, M. Bureau, Ch. Dravet *et al.*), John Libbey & Co. Ltd, London, pp. 33–44.
7. Fusco, L., Pachatz, C., Di Capua, M., and Vigevano, F. (2002) Video-EEG aspects of early-infantile epileptic encephalopathy with suppression-bursts (Ohtahara syndrome). *Brain Dev*, **23**, 708–714.
8. Coppola, G., Plouin, P., Chiron, C. *et al.* (1995) Migrating partial seizures in infancy: a malignant disorder with developmental arrest. *Epilepsia*, **36**, 1017–1024.
9. Marsh, E., Melamed, S.E., Barron, T., and Clancy, R.R. (2005) Migrating partial seizures in infancy: expanding the phenotype of a rare seizure syndrome. *Epilepsia*, **46**, 568–572.
10. Hurst, D.L. (1994) Epidemiology, in *Infantile spasms and West syndrome* (eds. O. Dulac, B.D. Bernardina, and H.T. Chugani), WB Saunders, London, pp. 12–22.
11. Kellaway, P., Hrachovy, R.A., Frost, J.D., and Zion, T. (1979) Precise characterization and quantification of infantile spasms. *Ann Neurol*, **6**, 214–218.
12. Fusco, L. and Vigevano, F. (1993) Ictal clinical electroencephalographic findings of spasms in West syndrome. *Epilepsia*, **34**, 671–678.
13. Dalla Bernardina, B. (1984) Epileptic syndromes and cerebral malformations in infancy: multicentric study. *Boll Lega It Epil*, **45/46**, 65–67.
14. Riikonen, R. (1982) A long-term follow-up study of 214 children with the syndrome of infantile spasms. *Neuropediatrics*, **13**, 14–23.
15. Dalla Bernardina, B. and Dulac, O. (1994) Introduction to etiology, in *Infantile Spasms and West Syndrome* (eds. O. Dulac, B.D. Bernardina, and H.T. Chugani), WB Saunders, London, pp. 166–171.
16. Dulac, O., Plouin, P., and Jambaque, I. (1993) Predicting favorable outcome in idiopathic West syndrome. *Epilepsia*, **34**, 747–756.
17. Vigevano, F., Fusco, L., Cusmai, R. *et al.* (1993) The idiopathic form of West syndrome. *Epilepsia*, **34**, 743–746.
18. Glaze, D.G., Hrachovy, R.A., Frost, J.D. Jr. *et al.* (1988) Prospective study of outcome of infants with infantile spasms treated during controlled studies of ACTH and prednisone. *J Pediatr*, **112**, 389–396.
19. Jeavons, P.M., Bower, B.D. and Dimitrakoudi, M. (1973) Long-term prognosis of 150 cases of "West syndrome". *Epilepsia*, **14**, 153–164.
20. Matsumoto, A., Watanabe, K., Negoro, T. *et al.* (1981) Long-term prognosis after infantile spasms: a statistical study of prognostic factors in 200 cases. *Dev Med Child Neurol*, **23**, 51–65.

21. Camfield, P., Camfield, C., Lortie, A., and Darwish, H. (2003) Infantile spasms in remission may reemerge as intractable epileptic spasms. *Epilepsia*, **44**, 1592–1595.

22. Lombroso, C.T. (1983) A prospective study of infantile spasms: clinical and therapeutic correlations. *Epilepsia*, **24**, 135–158.

23. Mackay, M.T., Weiss, S.K., Adams-Webber, T. *et al.* (2004) Practice parameter: medical treatment of infantile spasms: report of the American Academy of Neurology and the Child Neurology Society. *Neurology*, **62**, 1668–1681.

24. Hrachovy, R.A., Frost, J.D., Kellaway, P., and Zion, T.E. Jr. (1983) Double-blind study of ACTH vs prednisone therapy in infantile spasms. *J Pediatr*, **103**, 641–645.

25. Baram, T.Z., Mitchell, W.G., Tournay, A. *et al.* (1996) High-dose corticotropin (ACTH) versus prednisone for infantile spasms: a prospective, randomized, blinded study. *Pediatrics*, **97**, 375–379.

26. Lux, A.L., Edwards, S.W., Hancock, E. *et al.* (2004) The United Kingdom Infantile Spasms Study comparing vigabatrin with prednisolone or tetracosactide at 14 days: a multicentre, randomised controlled trial. *Lancet*, **364** (9447), 1773–1778.

27. Hrachovy, R.A., Frost, J.D. Jr., and Glaze, D.G. (1994) High-dose, long-duration versus low-dose, short-duration corticotropin therapy for infantile spasms. *J Pediatr*, **124** (5 Pt 1), 803–806.

28. Hancock, E. and Osborne, J.P. (1999) Vigabatrin in the treatment of infantile spasms in tuberous sclerosis: literature review. *J Child Neurol*, **14**, 71–74.

29. (a) Willmore, L.J., Abelson, M.B., Ben-Menachem, E. *et al.* (2009) Vigabatrin: 2008 update. *Epilepsia*, **50**, 163–173; (b) Chiron, C., Marchand, M.C., Tran, A. *et al.*, STICLO Study Group (2000) Stiripentol in severe myoclonic epilepsy in infancy: a randomised placebo-controlled syndrome-dedicated trial. *Lancet*, **356**, 1638–1642.

30. Pearl, P.L., Vezina, L.G., Saneto, R.P. *et al.* (2009) Cerebral MRI abnormalities associated with vigabatrin therapy. *Epilepsia*, **50**, 184–194.

31. Jonas, R., Asarnow, R.F., Lo Presti, C. *et al.* (2005) Surgery for symptomatic infantile-onset epileptic encephalopathy with and without infantile spasms. *Neurology*, **64**, 746–750.

32. Kossoff, E.H., Hedderick, E.F., Turner, Z., and Freeman, J.M. (2008) A case-control evaluation of the ketogenic diet versus ACTH for new-onset infantile spasms. *Epilepsia*, **49**, 1504–1509.

33. Yakoub, M., Dulac, O., Jambaque, I. *et al.* (1992) Early diagnosis of severe myoclonic epilepsy in infancy. *Brain Dev*, **14**, 299–303.

34. Harkin, L.A., McMahon, J.M., Iona, X. *et al.* (2007) The spectrum of SCN1A-related infantile epileptic encephalopathies. *Brain*, **130** (Pt 3), 843–852.

35. Dravet, C., Bureau, M., Oguni, H. *et al.* (2002) Severe myoclonic epilepsy in infancy (Dravet syndrome), in *Epileptic Syndromes in Infancy, Childhood and Adolescence*, 3rd edn (eds. J. Roger, M. Bureau, Ch. Dravet *et al.*), John Libbey & Co. Ltd, London, pp. 81–103.

36. Wolff, M., Casse-Perrot, C., and Dravet, C. (2006) Severe myoclonic epilepsy in infants (Dravet syndrome): natural history and neuropsychological findings. *Epilepsia*, **47** (suppl 2), 45–48.

37. Dravet, C., Bureau, M., Oguni, H. *et al.* (2005) Severe myoclonic epilepsy in infancy: Dravet syndrome. *Adv Neurol*, **95**, 71–102.

38. Chiron, C., Marchand, M.C., Tran, A. *et al.*, STICLO Study Group (2000) Stiripentol in severe myoclonic epilepsy in infancy: a randomised placebo-controlled syndrome-dedicated trial. *Lancet*, **356** (9242), 1638–1642.

39. Hoffmann-Riem, M., Diener, W., Benninger, C. *et al.* (2000) Nonconvulsive status epilepticus—a possible cause of mental retardation in patients with Lennox-Gastaut syndrome. *Neuropediatrics*, **31** (4), 169–174.

40. Tassinari, C.A., Dravet, C., Roger, J., Cano, J.P., Gastaut, H. *et al.* (1972) Tonic status epilepticus precipitated by intravenous benzodiazepine in five patients with Lennox-Gastaut syndrome. *Epilepsia*, **13** (3), 421–435.

41. Hancock, E. and Cross, H. (2003) Treatment of Lennox-Gastaut syndrome. *Cochrane Database Syst Rev*, 3 (Art. No.: CD003277).

42. Glauser, T., Kluger, G., Sachdeo, R. *et al.* (2008) Rufinamide for generalized seizures associated with Lennox-Gastaut syndrome. *Neurology*, **70** (21), 1950–1958.

43. Frost, M., Gates, J., Helmers, S.L. *et al.* (2001) Vagus nerve stimulation in children with refractory seizures associated with Lennox-Gastaut syndrome. *Epilepsia*, **42** (9), 1148–1152.

44. Oguni, H., Hayashi, K., and Osawa, M. (1996) Long-term prognosis of Lennox-Gastaut syndrome. *Epilepsia*, **37** (Suppl 3), 44–47.

45. Boniver, C., Dravet, C., and Bureau M.E.A. (1987) Idiopathic Lennox-Gastaut syndrome, in *Advances in Epileptology: XVIth Epilepsy International Symposium* (eds. P. Wolf, M. Dam, and D.E.A. Janz), Raven Press, New York, pp. 195–200.

46. Singh, R., Andermann, E., Whitehouse, W.P. *et al.* (2001) Severe myoclonic epilepsy of infancy: extended spectrum of GEFS+? *Epilepsia*, **42** (7), 837–844.

47. Nickels, K. and Wirrell, E. (2008) Electrical status epilepticus in sleep. *Semin Pediatr Neurol*, **15** (2), 50–60.

48. Kramer, U., Sagi, L., Goldberg-Stern, H. *et al.* (2009) Clinical spectrum and medical treatment of children with electrical status epilepticus in sleep (ESES). *Epilepsia*, **50** (6), 1517–1524.

49. Marescaux, C., Hirsch, E., Finck, S. *et al.* (1990) Landau-Kleffner syndrome: a pharmacologic study of five cases. *Epilepsia*, **31** (6), 768–777.

50. De Negri, M., Baglietto, M.G., Battaglia, F.M. *et al.* (1995) Treatment of electrical status epilepticus by short diazepam (DZP) cycles after DZP rectal bolus test. *Brain Dev*, **17** (5), 330–333.

51. Mikati, M.A., Saab, R., Fayad, M.N., Choueini, R.N. *et al.* (2002) Efficacy of intravenous immunoglobulin in Landau-Kleffner syndrome. *Pediatr Neurol*, **26** (4), 298–300.

52. Tsuru, T. (2000) Effects of high-dose intravenous corticosteroid therapy in Landau-Kleffner syndrome. *Pediatr Neurol*, **22** (2), 145–147.

53. Lerman, P. (1991) Effect of early corticosteroid therapy for Landau-Kleffner syndrome. *Dev Med Child Neurol*, **33** (3), 257–260.

54. Wirrell, E., Ho, A.W., and Hamiwka, L. (2006) Sulthiame therapy for continuous spike and wave in slow-wave sleep. *Pediatr Neurol*, **35** (3), 204–208.

55. Nikanorova, M., Miranda, M.J., Atkins, M., *et al.* (2009) Ketogenic diet in the treatment of refractory continuous spikes and waves during slow-wave sleep. *Epilepsia*, **50** (5), 1127–1131.

56. Morrell, F., Whisler, W.W., Smith, M.C. *et al.* (1995) Landau-Kleffner syndrome. Treatment with subpial intracortical transection. *Brain*, **118** (Pt 6), 1529–1546.

57. Van Baalen, A. and Stephani, U. (2009) *FIRES*: Febrile infection responsive epileptic (FIRE) encephalopathies of school age. *Brain Dev*, **31**, 91.

58. Mikaeloff, Y., Jambaque, I., Hertz-Pannier, L. *et al.* (2006) Devastating epileptic encephalopathy in school-aged children (DESC): a pseudo-encephalitis. *Epilepsy Res*, **69**, 67–79.

59. Baxter, P., Clarke, A., Cross, H. *et al.* (2003) Idiopathic catastrophic epileptic encephalopathy presenting with acute onset intractable status. *Seizure*, **12**, 379–387.

Section 5

Partial epilepsies

13 Overview of diagnosis and medical treatment of partial epilepsies

Joseph I. Sirven

Department of Neurology, Division of Epilepsy, Mayo Clinic Arizona, Mayo Clinic Hospital, Phoenix, Arizona, USA

13.1 Diagnosis and evaluation

Epilepsy is a clinical diagnosis based on the history of having more than one unprovoked event. Few patients have seizures witnessed by physicians personally and therefore the history is either provided by the patient or family members as oftentimes memory is not completely reliable from individuals who provide it. The only way to positively identify epilepsy is to record an EEG during a seizure. However, recording a seizure on a routine outpatient EEG is relatively uncommon so other measures are needed to make a diagnosis (Table 13.1).

The neurological examination is often normal in patients with epilepsy although an abnormal one is more often associated with partial seizures. The diagnosis is aided when a focal or generalized neurologic deficit can be demonstrated suggesting a symptomatic epilepsy syndrome. A focal or lateralized feature can help distinguish partial epilepsies from generalized ones. Examination during the immediate postictal period can reveal lateralized neurological deficits that help to provide some anatomic clues as to the location of the seizure.

Adult Epilepsy, First Edition. Edited by Gregory D. Cascino and Joseph I. Sirven.
© 2011 John Wiley & Sons, Ltd. Published 2011 by John Wiley & Sons, Ltd.

Table 13.1   Diagnostic studies used to confirm partial epilepsy

Clinical history
Neurological examination
Electroencephalogram (EEG)
Magnetic resonance imaging (MRI)
Computed tomography (CT)
Positron emission tomography (PET)
Single-photon emission tomography (SPECT)

The neurological examination often shows memory impairment in partial epilepsies, particularly those arising from the temporal lobe. Memory disturbances result from the underlying lesion and can be due to Antiepileptic Drug (AED) effects or can reflect a reversible dysfunction induced by seizures. Oftentimes one can see subtle abnormalities such as asymmetries in nasal labial fold or other cranial nerves. At other times, the presence of a Todd's paralysis defined as a postictal focal weakness can help elucidate potential lateralizing anatomic clues to underlying lesions that may be responsible for seizures.

A number of procedures are used in the process of evaluating people with epilepsy. The purpose of these tests is to help classify the epilepsy syndrome and then seek remediable causes. Further diagnostic testing is often needed to confirm or classify the cause of a seizure-like spell. Depending on the history, assessing for metabolic derangements, cardiac disease, cerebrovascular disorders, neoplasms, and infections may be considered as appropriate causes for seizures. Investigations are often geared to uncover these etiologies.

For partial epilepsy evaluations, the EEG and neuroimaging are routine and considered standard of care. The value and limitations of these studies are discussed in the following sections.

13.2   Electroencephalography (EEG)

The EEG is the single most informative diagnostic test in patients with partial epilepsy. It should nearly always be performed. The EEG aids in classifying the seizure types and helps distinguish between partial seizures and generalized syndromes.

The characteristic interictal abnormality in epilepsy is a spike or sharp wave. Focal or localized spikes are seen in partial epilepsy, whereas generalized spikes occur in the generalized epilepsies. The interictal EEG in partial epilepsy shows a spike in approximately 90–95% of patients with this type of epilepsy, although up to four recordings may be necessary to demonstrate the abnormality [1]. Recording the EEG during sleep in the laboratory or overnight with an ambulatory EEG device increases the yield of this procedure.

It is important to note that interictal spikes are often seen in a small percentage of normal individuals (i.e., patients without epilepsy), in less than 2% of the time [2]. Therefore, finding a spike in the EEG does not necessarily confirm the diagnosis of epilepsy. The diagnosis can only be absolutely verified if a clinical seizure is recorded during the session. Otherwise the clinical history is the ultimate means in determining the diagnosis. Nevertheless, the EEG remains one of the most important tests that can be done to aid the diagnosis of partial epilepsy.

13.3   Imaging

Magnetic resonance imaging (MRI) and computed tomography (CT) should be performed as part of the initial evaluation of all patients with epilepsy to identify and treat common causes of epilepsy such as central nervous system hemorrhage, tumor, and abscess. Areas of encephalomalacia from trauma can also be readily identified. In the case of temporal lobe epilepsy, mesial temporal sclerosis is a diagnosis that is almost strictly based on imaging characteristics. MRI is the procedure of choice and it is superior to the CT scan in detecting all pathological processes except perhaps subarachnoid hemorrhage. CT scan is helpful in emergent situations or when MRI is contraindicated.

MRI is the preferred imaging modality and it is highly sensitive and identifies nearly all macroscopic lesions including tumors, dysplasias, vascular malformations, encephalomalacia, and atrophy. Finding a focal disturbance leads one toward a diagnosis of partial epilepsy, provided the history is consistent with this lesion. MRI should be performed in all individuals who do not have an inherited epilepsy syndrome. Patients whose seizure types change or who are refractory to medication often merit a repeat study. Epilepsy centers often have specialized MRI protocols and if referral to such a center is contemplated it may be appropriate to defer the MRI until it can be performed there.

Although MRI is clearly superior, the CT is still useful. Tumors larger than 1 or 2 cm in size can usually be identified. However, lesions in the temporal lobe can be missed with CT scans because of bony artifacts. The CT scan is better at identifying calcifications than the MRI scan. However, if the CT scan is normal it cannot be considered adequate and an MRI should be performed as standard of care. Consequently CT is useful only if MRI is not available and imaging needs to be performed immediately.

Positron emission tomography (PET) and single-photon emission computed tomography (SPECT) are often performed in presurgical evaluation processes for patients with epilepsy. These particular studies do not have a common role in the routine diagnosis of patients with partial epilepsy. They do, however, have an important function in the management of patients with refractory epilepsy where surgical therapy is being considered.

13.4   Treatment and management

Once a diagnosis of partial epilepsy has been made the next question that emerges is whether therapy with AEDs is necessary. It is important to consider a number of factors in making that determination. The decisions of whether to start a medication or not will likely depend on a risk-benefit assessment of whether the risk of further seizures is high enough that medication therapy should be initiated. Because medications are not entirely risk free and there is still potential for risk of serious reaction to medications, it is important to demonstrate to the patient that the benefit of therapy outweighs the risk in order to assure compliance. It is important to remember that the main goal of epilepsy treatment is to enable affected individuals to live as normal a life as possible. Therapy is not only directed at seizures but should remediate any psychosocial impairments as well.

13.5   Which patient should be treated with antiseizure drugs?

Nearly all patients who have had more than one partial seizure should be treated with antiseizure medications. The risk of recurrence after two or more partial seizures is 80–90% and is even higher in those individuals with an overt lesion on neuroimaging studies or interictal spike or sharp waves on an EEG [3].

There are very few groups of individuals where initiating seizure medications could be avoided (Table 13.2). Potential caveats could be made for children with rolandic epilepsy given that this condition occurs principally at night. Individuals with simple partial seizures where there is no loss of consciousness and minimal impact on quality of life may be exempted from therapy. Other groups may include those who have a symptomatic cause of their seizures, including alcohol and drug abuse, acute illness, postimpact seizures from head trauma, and seizures from excessive sleep deprivation. It follows that managing the environmental issue or avoiding the offending agent that precipitated the seizure is a better choice of therapy than proceeding with long-term seizure medications.

The AEDs currently available in the US have been presented in other chapters in this text. Currently there are 18 different AEDs that are available for the management of epilepsy. Table 13.3 lists the medications approved for partial epilepsy. Of these, phenytoin, carbamazepine, phenobarbital, gabapentin, pregabalin, tiagabine, oxcarbazepine, vigabatrin, lacosimide, zonisamide, levetiracetam, valproic acid, lamotrigine, and felbamate are all approved for the management of partial seizures. The question that emerges is how does one select between these various choices?

There are a number of factors that play into making a decision between seizure medications. These include both patient- and drug-specific factors. With regards to patient-related factors identifying the right drug for the seizure diagnosis is

Table 13.2 Partial epilepsy patients that may not require medications

Benign rolandic epilepsy
Recurrent symptomatic seizures
Simple partial seizures

Table 13.3 Medications approved for use in partial epilepsy

Carbamazepine
Felbamate
Gabapentin
Lacosamide
Lamotrigine
Levetiracetam
Oxcarbazepine
Phenobarbital
Phenytoin
Pregabalin
Tiagabine
Topiramate
Valproic acid
Vigabatrin
Zonisamide

essential. Because efficacies of most seizure drugs are relatively similar to one another, other factors take on a greater importance in making a choice. The age, gender of the patient, potential drug interactions, and the duration of treatment may all be important factors for the individual making that decision. With regards to drug factors, the titration schedule, whether the drug is metabolized renally versus hepatically, pharmacokinetic profile, available dosage forms, preparations, as well as cost all factor into the equation.

For some physicians, mechanisms of action may play a role in the decision process for choice of seizure agent (Table 13.4). Common mechanisms of action for the treatment of partial epilepsies include agents that modulate repetitive activation of the sodium channel, such as phenytoin, carbamazepine, oxcarbazepine, and lamotrigine. Other sodium channel modulators include lacosamide. GABA enhancers include phenobarbital and benzodiazepines. Increased GABA also may occur via the blockage of reuptake or catabolism of the enzymes responsible for GABA such as tiagabine and vigabatrin respectively. Other mechanisms that may be of importance in partial epilepsy include blockage of unique binding sites exemplified by gabapentin, levetiracetam, and pregabalin. Carbonic anhydrase inhibitors such as topiramate and zonisamide may also be useful.

Table 13.4   Putative mechanisms of action by which AEDs prevent partial seizures

Blockade of repetitive activation of the sodium channel	Other sodium channel modulation	GABA-binding	Increased GABA by blocking reuptake or catabolism of enzymes	Unique binding sites	Carbonic anhydrase inhibition and pH changes
Carbamazepine	Lacosamide	Phenobarbital	Tiagabine	Gabapentin	Topiramate
Felbamate	—	—	Vigabatrin	Levetriracetam	Zonisamide
Lamotrigine	—	—	—	Pregabalin	—
Oxcarbazepine	—	—	—	—	—
Phenytoin	—	—	—	—	—

13.6   Evidence-based guidelines

The American Academy of Neurology published guidelines for new onset and refractory epilepsy with regards to the choice of seizure medications in these various seizure groups [4]. For new onset epilepsy there was evidence to support the use of gabapentin, lamotrigine, topiramate, oxcarbazepine, and levertiracetam [4]. For refractory epilepsy, gabapentin, lamotrigine, pregabalin, topiramate, tigabine, oxcarbazepine, levertiracetam, and zonisamide are useful for adjunctive, partial epilepsy management [4]. In pediatric patients with partial seizures gabapentin, lamotrigine, topiramate, oxcarbazepine, and levertiracetam were also found to be effective.

In older adults, the Veterans' Administration Cooperative Study on Geriatric Epilepsy compared lamotrigine, gabapentin, and carbamazepine for management of older patients with partial epilepsy [5]. Investigators found that adverse effects were a common problem in older adults with epilepsy. More importantly lamotrigine and gabapentin were recommended as initial therapy for older patients with epilepsy as compared to carbamazepine based on adverse effects [5].

McCorry and colleagues have also performed systematic reviews of various medication options for partial epilepsy [6]. The choice of seizure medication varied by gender. For women of childbearing years, lamotrigine is recommended as the first-line agent with topiramate and valproic acid as alternative choices [6]. For women with unclassified seizures who are not potentially childbearing and all other patient groups, first-line AEDs include valproic acid but alternative choices include lamotrigine and topiramate [6].

13.7   How well do seizure medications work?

This question was addressed in a seminal study by Brodie and Kwan in 2002 [7]. Using newer agents Brodie and Kwan investigated 523 untreated patients with epilepsy. Of those 523 patients, 470 were drug naive, 47% responded to their first AED and 13% were seizure-free on the second AED [7]. Of the individuals who failed to respond to the first two agents, only 1% responded to the third choice [7].

The study uncovered that there are two groups of epilepsy patients [7]. There are those that can be managed with literally any type of seizure medication and will likely respond to the first or second agent presented to them in monotherapy. However, there is another group of individuals who are more difficult to identify at an early point and fail to respond to any drug. These cases are defined as refractory epilepsy patients who may need to be assessed for surgical intervention at an earlier point in their evaluation process as opposed to committing them to multiple medication trials. Thus, after failure of two seizure medications one should consider the possibility of refractory epilepsy and refer the patient to an epilepsy specialist for an epilepsy surgery evaluation.

13.8 Conclusion and summary

There are a number of therapeutic options available for the management of patients with epilepsy. There are 18 different seizure medications with unique pharmacokinetic and efficacy characteristics that are suitable for almost any type of patient who presents with partial epilepsy. It is essential to make an early and accurate diagnosis of partial epilepsy so that patients can be appropriately managed with medication, and if they fail medication then with epilepsy surgery. It is only by an accurate diagnosis, history, and appropriate use of confirmatory tests which include EEG and MRI that an individual's quality of life can be maintained and the psychosocial burden of disease prevented.

References

1. Salinsky, M., Kanter, R., and Dashieff, R. (1987) Effectiveness of multiple EEGs in supporting the diagnosis of epilepsy. *Epilepsia*, **28**, 331–334.
2. Zivin, L. and Ajmone-Marson, C. (1968) Incidence and prognostic significance of epileptiform activity in the EEG of nonepileptic subjects. *Brain*, **91**, 751–778.
3. Hauser, W.A., Rich, S.S., and Annegers, J. (1990) Seizure recurrence after a first unprovoked seizure. *Neurology*, **40**, 1163–1170.
4. French, J.A., Kanner, A.M., and Bautista, J. (2004) Efficacy and tolerability of the new antiepileptic drugs II: treatment of refractory epilepsy: report of the Therapeutics and Technology Assessment Subcommittee and Quality Standards Subcommittee of the American Academy of Neurology and the American Epilepsy Society. *Neurology*, **62** (8), 1261–1273.
5. Rowan, A., Ramsay, R.E., Collins, J.F. *et al.* (2005) New onset geriatric epilepsy: a randomized study of gabapentin, lamotrigine and carbamazepine. *Neurology*, **64**, 1868–1873.
6. McCorry, D., Chadwick, D., and Marson, A. (2004) Current drug treatment of epilepsy in adults. *Lancet Neurol*, **3** (12), 729–735.
7. Kwan, P. and Brodie, M.J. (2000) Early identification of refractory epilepsy. *N Engl J Med*, **343** (19), 1369–1377.

14 Medial temporal lobe epilepsy

William O. Tatum IV

Department of Neurology, Division of Epilepsy, Mayo Clinic, Jacksonville, FL, USA

14.1 Introduction

Temporal lobe epilepsy (TLE) is the most common form of localization-related epilepsy (LRE) in adults accounting for approximately 60% of all patients with epilepsy [1]. Medial temporal lobe epilepsy (mTLE) is much more common than neocortical TLE, and represents a heterogeneous spectrum of focal seizures that are clinically expressed by structures of the medial temporal lobe. mTLE with hippocampal onset accounts for at least 80% of all temporal lobe seizures [2]. However, mTLE is a syndrome due to a variety of pathologies and manifestations that have been classified based upon the site of suspected neuroanatomic origin by the International Classification of Epilepsies and Epileptic Syndromes in 1985 [3]. Previous terminology for the focal seizures of temporal lobe origin have included *psychomotor seizures*, *limbic seizures*, and *temporal lobe seizures* and their use has varied over the years with newer classification proposals that have included a shift from complex partial seizures of temporal lobe origin to focal seizures with dyscognitive (or other) characteristic semiologic features [4] though the working definition is continuing to undergo evolution. While mTLE is not only the most

Adult Epilepsy, First Edition. Edited by Gregory D. Cascino and Joseph I. Sirven.
© 2011 John Wiley & Sons, Ltd. Published 2011 by John Wiley & Sons, Ltd.

common human adult epilepsy syndrome that is diagnosed, it is also the one that is most frequently refractory treatment and highly associated with hippocampal sclerosis (HS) [1] making it a frequent medical challenge and common surgical substrate. While it is a well-characterized and relatively homogeneous clinical syndrome, a differential diagnosis exists and overlap between psychiatric and behavioral counterparts have been identified and defined primarily through clinical information that has been obtained from surgical series comprised of patients requiring temporal lobectomy [5]. The overall prognosis for patients with drug-resistant mTLE is often associated with a higher rate of morbidity and impaired health-related quality of life (HRQOL) [6]. In addition, a greater mortality rate is evident that is more often observed among the more severely affected patients who often have ongoing seizures and have failed epilepsy surgery.

14.2   Functional neuroanatomy of the temporal lobe

The temporal lobe is the most epileptogenic region of the brain. The medial temporal lobe is part of the limbic system concerned with the affective aspects of behavior. Focal seizures may arise from one or both mesial temporal lobes including the amygdalae, hippocampus, and parahippocampal gyrus. When activated during an aura, the amygdalae in humans often produce a sense of fear or create a sense of impending doom. The amygdalae may also be involved in defensive behavior that involves pupillary dilation, aggressive posturing, and autonomic effects including piloerection, tachycardia, and tachypnea, and rarely, a sense of anger or rage. Hypersexuality and hyperactivity, and oral exploration may be present following bilateral amygdala lesions. The medial temporal lobe is also highly involved with episodic (information that is tied to the time and place of occurrence) and declarative memory (explicit memory for facts that can be verbalized) involving new memories for experienced events. The hippocampal formation (HF) is composed of the dentate gyrus (DG), hippocampus, and subiculum. It is a three-layered allocortex with pyramidal cells in the subiculum and hippocampus that have the potential for neural plasticity through long-term potentiation [7]. Divided into the head, body, and the tail, the hippocampus ranges in length from 4 to 4.5 cm and is important for memory functions and for spatial navigation. It is divided into subfields of the cornu ammonis (CA): CA1–CA4 are surrounded by the DG that is crucial for transfer of short-term memory to long-term storage in the association cortices. The parahippocampal gyrus has two-way connections between the hippocampus and all of the major cortical association areas and with the primary olfactory cortex [8]. Patients with extensive damage to the mesial temporal lobes may become amnestic with an inability to form and retain new memories. Neuropsychological testing and the intracarotid amobarbital test have allowed us to assess the memory functions of the hippocampus and other cognitive functions in patients with epilepsy [9]. Memory dysfunction has been exemplified by H.M., a man who underwent aggressive bilateral resection of the temporal mesial structures for refractory epilepsy resulting in severe anterograde and retrograde amnesia [10].

The left temporal lobe typically functions as the dominant temporal lobe to govern verbal memory. In one longitudinal study when resective surgery was performed for mTLE a decline in 30% was noted after right temporal resection and 51% after left temporal resection; however, if successful surgery was able to be performed then cessation or reversal of the decline in memory function was noted [11]. The dominant lateral temporal neocortex is involved in auditory comprehension and may become involved with medial temporal dysfunction. Language function within the dominant temporal lobe is involved in both comprehension and naming. Confrontational naming and delayed memory has been shown to be reduced by up to 40% in patients with TLE compared with <5% of controls [12]. The nondominant temporal lobe structures are more involved in visual memory. The basal aspect of the temporal lobes appear to be more involved in visual processing of faces and scenes that reflect activity in the fusiform and parahippocampal gyrus. Cognitive decline is commonly associated with mTLE and may be an effect of progressive hippocampal formation atrophy (HFA) from continued seizures or a cause of seizures. The consequences of HFA remain to be proven because the differences in etiology may have a substantial impact on memory and cognition [13].

14.3   Pathology

mTLE is most often an acquired form of LRE and is highly associated with the pathophysiology of HS especially in patients with drug-resistant seizures also referred to as mesial temporal lobe epilepsy. Other temporal and extratemporal regions are known to be affected in patients with mTLE mainly those areas with anatomic and functional connections to the hippocampus [14]. HS is the most common pathology in surgical series and may be readily detected by brain MRI as mesial temporal sclerosis (MTS). Less frequently gliomas, angiomas, caveromas, or traumatic or infectious lesions may occur and dual pathology occurs in 5–30%. While lesional mTLE is associated with a lesion of the temporal lobe, nonlesional mTLE is distinguished based upon neuroimaging and the absence of identifiable pathological substrate. A normal-appearing hippocampus occurs in 30–40% with the remaining 60–70% of patients with HS on histopathology [15]. HS is comprised of a combination of atrophy and astrogliosis of the amygdala, hippocampus, parahippocampal gyrus, and the entorhinal cortex. Postmortem studies have revealed that the synaptic reorganization in the hippocampus in patients with HS is frequently a bilateral finding that appears to be a permanent feature in patients with mTLE [16]. Other pathological findings include loss of internal HF architecture, atrophy of the ipsilateral amygdalae, mammillary bodies, fornix, and white matter. The hippocampus consists of several functional subfields including the DG, CA 1–3, and the subiculum. Initial recognition of hippocampal atrophy in TLE revealed ipsilateral heterogeneous cytoarchitectural alteration and neuronal loss within the DG and the CA1 subfield with relative preservation of CA2 [17]. Four different patterns of hippocampal atrophy have been described in mTLE due to HS: end folium sclerosis (atrophy of DG); atrophy of CA1; atrophy of CA1 + DG; and global atrophy [18]. Postsurgical pathological series appear to demonstrate more widespread involvement with either global atrophy or atrophy of the CA1, CA3, and DG in those patients with successful seizure outcome following temporal lobectomy [19]. If isolated subfield involvement is encountered alone then the presence of total HFA may appear to be absent using neuroimaging techniques. A specific pathophysiologic mechanism may underlie drug-resistance in mTLE. Cell counts and immunohistochemical staining have been used to identify different cell populations in the dentate in mTLE [15]. Neuronal loss in the hippocampus is accompanied by selective loss of somatostatin and neuropeptide Y interneurons and sprouting and reorganization of surviving synaptic connections that in essence rewires the hippocampal connections [20]. Dynorphin and neuropeptide Y immunohistochemistry demonstrates mossy fiber sprouting into the inner one-third of the granule cell of the dentate molecular layer which facilitates synaptic reorganization and recurrent excitation that leads to epileptogenicity and recurrent seizures [15, 20].

Certain molecular mechanisms are associated with drug-resistant mTLE such as low brain GABA levels [21]. In addition, glutamate levels and changes in neuronal glutamate transporters are another mechanism that is disordered [22]. Vesicular glutamate transporters are responsible for loading presynaptic vesicles with glutamate and are used as a marker for glutamatergic synapses in human hippocampus. In HS, vesicular glutamate transporters have been decreased in the hippocampal subfields (increased in non-HS patients compared with autopsy controls) with severe neuronal loss, but were strongly up-regulated in the DG reflected by synaptophysin, neuropeptide Y, and Timm's staining that indicate additional glutamatergic synapses possibly formed by mossy fiber sprouting [23]. The excitation incurred from seizures propagation, deafferentation from loss of hippocampal connections, or the chronic effects of AEDs may explain an extrahippocampal distribution of atrophy that has been reported in patients with mTLE with HS [24].

Genetic influences have also been notable in mTLE. A familial form of TLE has been reported with autosomal dominance although it is rare and generally not associated with HFA [25]. Additional familial forms have been reported where mTLE was observed in families but not associated with an autosomal dominant transmission. Furthermore, HFA may present in first-degree relatives who do not manifest clinical seizures further confusing the cause-and-effect relationship between HFA and mTLE [26]. HFA has been associated with the APOe4 allele and may be seen with an earlier age of expression of mTLE [27]. TLE phenotypes may be associated with SCN1B mutations as a subtype of cryptogenic generalized epilepsies with febrile seizures [28]. Other genetic markers have been reported to be more common in mTLE associated with HFA [29]. The role of pharmacogenetics in contributing to AED resistance has most closely examined the genetic polymorphisms in the ABCB1 gene [30]. This multiple drug resistance gene and receptor polymorphism has been suggested to facilitate drug efflux transport and reduce the brain–drug response with a greater risk for developing drug-resistant mTLE [31]. The membrane drug transporter P-glycoprotein found in tissue removed at surgery from patients with refractory mTLE due to HS affects drug protein products that can alter AED pharmacokinetics or pharmacodynamics, though there may well be several factors involved in drug resistance [32].

14.4 Differential diagnosis

Reasonable certainty should exist based upon the clinical evaluation alone to establish the diagnosis of mTLE [33]. However, a definitive diagnosis is not always readily established when a direct historical account is lacking, or when nonepileptic seizures mimic TLE [33]. Video-EEG monitoring is the gold standard for refining a differential diagnosis in patients with mTLE and "spells" (see

Table 14.1 "Petit mal" seizures and the clinical differences: mTLE versus absence epilepsy

Clinical features	mTLE	Absence epilepsy
Age of onset	Usually early adolescence	4–8 years (Childhood absence)
Risk factors	Febrile seizures or early childhood "injury"	Family history may be present
Aura	Yes	No
Clinical seizures	**STARING**	**STARING** ± eyelid fluttering
Consciousness	Impaired	Brief interruption to impaired
Automatisms	Often; oral and complex	Occasionally
Duration	>30 s to 2 min	Brief: 10–20 s
Postictal	Yes may be variable	No
MRI	Often lesional/MTS^a	Normal
EEG	(Anterior) temporal IEDs	3 Hz generalized spike-waves
Pathology	HS or focal cortical lesion	None/presumed genetic
Response to AEDs	One-third refractory to AED	Excellent but 15% resistant. Some AEDs may worsen
Course	Often progressive	Remission in 50%

^{a}Lesion status (MTS) is dependent upon the quality of neuroimaging and interpretation.

Table 14.1). Neurologists appear to be more accurate than non-neurologists in arriving at a correct diagnosis with mistake rates of 5.6% versus 18.9% for generalists in one study [34]. Psychogenic nonepileptic attacks (PNEAs) are "seizures" that represent the majority of misdiagnosed TLE. The rate of misdiagnosis ranges from a low of 5% to over 30% in patients with intractable seizures undergoing video-EEG monitoring [35]. The "emotional" changes with temporal partial seizures may involve a feeling of fear that can mimic the psychological appearance of panic attacks though the duration is brief (usually seconds to 1–2 minutes), consciousness is impaired, and other features (such as shortness of breath, chest pain, diaphoresis) are typically absent [36]. Psychic auras that involve experiential symptoms to include "butterflies," fear, déjà vu, jamais vu, or other indescribable symptoms may mimic psychiatric complaints and lead to misinterpretation. Perceptual changes of visual, auditory, or olfactory ictal phenomenon may suggest psychotic symptoms. The diagnostic specificity is less accurate when these symptoms occur as auras or as a part of brief complex partial seizures [33]. Cognitive changes of depersonalization, derealization ("dreamy states"), out-of-body experiences ("autoscopy"), feeling of a presence, or forced thinking may masquerade as dissociative symptoms [37]. Focal seizures involving a broad range of emotions such as crying (dacrocystic), laughing (gelastic), and distress (fear, anxiety, panic) may occur and suggest a primary psychiatric diagnosis or PNEA. Sexual automatisms may also occur and inappropriate behavior such as disrobing, rubbing and scratching the genital area makes nonepileptic behavior suspect.

The overemphasis on MRI and EEG may be a pitfall to the correct diagnosis of mTLE. HS has been identified in PNEA patients without epilepsy [38]. Similarly, wicket waves on the interictal EEG may occur as a normal physiological variant that is misidentified in patients with PNEA [39]. Physiologic nonepileptic seizures are less frequently confused with mTLE though syncope is an important "episode" to recognize given their implication and the prolonged exposure to AEDs prior to recognition [40]. Behavioral misidentification due to nonepileptic attacks, incorrect drug selection, and patient failure to comply with medical recommendations may all contribute to a refractory state. When epilepsy does exist, a differential diagnosis to classify and localize the seizures also occurs. Video-EEG is crucial to correctly classify and characterize those with "pseudotemporal" lobe epilepsy. Misidentification of extratemporal lobe epilepsy such as occipital or orbitofrontal epilepsy that propagates to the temporal lobe may demonstrate mTLE semiology. Similarly, patients with "petit mal" seizures and staring episodes may be quickly differentiated into focal seizures of mTLE or absence seizures of generalized epilepsy with EEG [41] (see Table 14.1).

14.5 Diagnosis

Historical features

The historical features of mTLE are fairly consistent; however, precise knowledge of the natural history is still incompletely available [5, 42]. The birth, labor, delivery, and development are typically normal. Early risk factors are often evident on retrospective studies and report early injury as a common substrate in childhood for patients with mTLE. Most have a history of at least one seizure in early childhood with the majority experiencing febrile seizures (FS) though other symptomatic causes such as head trauma, perinatal injuries, congenital brain malformations, CNS infection, and indolent tumors may also occur.

FS represent the most common risk factor that occurs during infancy and early childhood. Approximately two-thirds of patients with TLE in one series had FS without an infection involving the CNS prior to the onset of complex partial seizures [5]. Nearly 75% of these FS were complex with prolonged or focal features that occurred to distinguish them from simple febrile convulsions. Complex FS are seizures associated with fever for 15 minutes or longer, have focal clinical signs during the seizure, or recur within a 24-hour period. A history of childhood prolonged FS is often present in patients with refractory mTLE and suggests HS as the underlying pathophysiology for recurrent seizures [43]. However, a history of FS does not increase the risk of epilepsy substantially above the general population rates. Whether there is a cause-and-effect relationship between FS and mTLE due to HFA is unclear. However, when complex febrile convulsions are prolonged, hippocampal swelling may be observed and progress to HS when serial MRIs are performed prospectively [44]. While the association FS with TLE and HS remains unresolved, a subset of children with complex FS appear to be at risk for developing mTLE later in life.

The onset of mTLE characteristically occurs at the end of the first or second decade in most people after a latency following an FS or an early cerebral "injury." Hormonal influences during menses and ovulation in women may lead to reports of catamenial exacerbation. Focal seizures without (auras) and with (complex partial) impairment in consciousness are the most common seizure types in mTLE and may exhibit a wide degree of clinical heterogeneity. The ictal semiology of the aura at the initial onset of behavioral symptoms frequently appears in isolation when seizures begin early in life [45]. More than 80% of patients report an aura [5] with experiential and viscerosensory symptoms comprising the most characteristic forms in mTLE. Psychic phenomenon including fear, anxiety, déjà vu, and autoscopy commonly occur with mTLE in addition to viscerosensory auras, and a nausea, "butterflies," or rising epigastric sensation are commonly reported. Sensory and autonomic auras also occur but are less characteristic than an indescribable feeling that many patients with mTLE volunteer. Olfactory auras may raise the possibility of a tumor as opposed to HS [46] and may prompt gadolinium use when neuroimaging.

Clinical features

Focal seizures with impaired consciousness (complex partial) in mTLE are the primary seizure type with a behavioral semiology that reflects its anatomic site of origin in the mesial temporal structures. Men and women are equally affected. The clinical and semiologic differences between patients with TLE exist not only with respect to mesial and lateral distinction but the evolution of semiology is also stratified with respect to the age of onset with greater motor manifestations occurring in those <6 years of age [45, 47]. Epilepsy occurs in all age groups, but the elderly represent the group with the highest prevalence with seizures that are often under-recognized because they may be subtle and associated with unawareness, or present as confusion or memory lapses to suggest a nonepileptic source [48]. The clinical semiology of focal seizures has been best defined through epilepsy surgery referrals that validate the origin of behavior with seizure freedom after resection [49]. Focal seizures with impaired consciousness in mTLE typically occur with a fixed stare, impaired consciousness, and oral or manual automatisms over 30–60 seconds. Ipsilateral automatisms and contralateral dystonic posturing during the seizure are very useful lateralizing signs that reflect seizure onset; however, propagation to symptomatic regions limit use of seizure semiology alone [50]. Semiologies that suggest nondominant lateralization include "ictal speech," vomiting, and intermittent "responsiveness." Postictal aphasia is predictive of epilepsy from the dominant temporal lobe. Tonic or clonic jerking and postictal Todd's paresis lateralize to the contralateral hemisphere and indicate propagation and involvement of the ipsilateral motor extratemporal or neocortical structures. Pupillary dilatation, hyperventilation, piloerection, and tachycardia are autonomic features that may occur. Seizure semiology does not appear to be clearly distinct with different pathologies though HS may be more characteristically associated with ipsilateral limb automatisms and contralateral dystonic posturing. Whether the person with mTLE begins with a first seizure and then follows the course toward intractability or whether the disorder evolves over time with the possibility of intervention remains to be determined [42]. Secondarily generalized seizures are relatively infrequent and are usually controlled with AEDs and do not occur as the exclusive or predominant seizure type [5]. Prolonged seizures and status epilepticus are infrequent but may occur.

Neuroimaging

Brain MRI is the gold standard for neuroimaging when patients are evaluated for focal anatomic pathology in mTLE [51]. MTS can be readily visualized on qualitative high-resolution brain MRI with the characteristic features of HFA (Figure 14.1a) and increased signal on fluid attenuated inversion recovery (FLAIR) or T-2 weighted sequences that are best noted on coronal sections with special

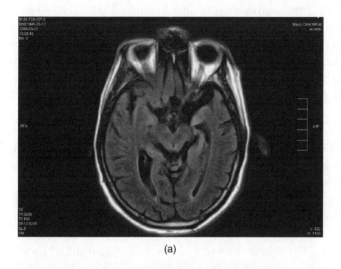

(a)

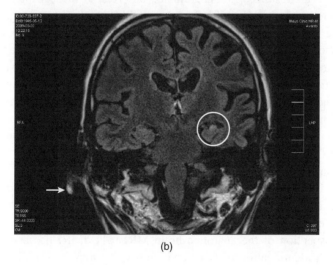

(b)

Figure 14.1 (a) Sagittal high-resolution brain MRI with left HFA. (b) Coronal FLAIR brain MRI showing left MTS.

protocols that include anatomical orientation, thin sections, and imaging sequences to augment visualization (Figure 14.1b). Quantitative volumetric analysis demonstrates normal hippocampal volumes ranging from 2660 to 5180 mm^3 with a standard deviation of <10% from normal volumes in normal young adults [42]. New onset epilepsy typically does not demonstrate HFA when compared with adult controls [52]. When prospectively evaluated, decline in hippocampal volume may begin before 1 year [53] and by 3.5 years demonstrate a volume decline of up to 10% from individual baseline volumes [54]. HFA when visualized is seen to progress over time in patients with refractory mTLE [55]. In addition, the progression of white and gray matter atrophy using voxel-based morphometry was greater in patients with left mTLE when compared to right mTLE and was more pronounced when seizure control was poorer and a longer duration of epilepsy was evident [14]. One study demonstrated that patients with right mTLE are more likely to present bilateral hippocampal abnormalities [56].

The sensitivity of the MRI signal on a 1.5 T magnet is usually too low to achieve a significant resolution to identify individual subfields though higher field strength MRI and alternative sequences may provide greater detail [57]. Higher resolution imaging allows for greater resolution of internal structures of the mesial temporal lobe including visualization of Amon's horn of the hippocampus. Neuroimaging techniques for subfield analysis require brain MRI with high field strength magnets. Regions that are able to be identified include the CA subfields, DG, and global atrophy [57]. About 30% of patients with drug-resistant focal seizures harbor foreign tissue lesions with an estimated 60–70% of those with "nonlesional" MRI suspected to harbor HS [58], though with 30% that are MRI-negative for HS and may be able to be identified by focal or regional cerebral hypometabolism using positron emission tomography (PET) [59]. The anatomic distribution of changes that may be encountered in mTLE have been reported to extend outside the hippocampus and include a network of extrahippocampal gray matter loss that has been detected using voxel-based morphometry to study diffuse abnormalities [24]. These prospective data provide evidence that mTLE can be a progressive disorder characterized by developing atrophy in both the hippocampus and neocortex compared to age-matched controls over a few years time [24, 60].

Other neuroimaging techniques may be useful in mTLE when a lack of concordant or discordant information exists in the presurgical evaluation. Among quantitative MRI techniques, a prolonged T2 relaxation time (T2 relaxometry) is a sensitive technique to identify hippocampal abnormalities that are not obvious on visual inspection of the anatomic brain MRI [61]. fMRI has become used in assisting with identification of functional cortex and may be useful in helping to define language areas [62]. Proton magnetic resonance spectroscopy (MRS) may be useful in patients with congenital malformations to detect significant changes in chemical ratios of neuronal N-acetyl-L-aspartate to choline and total creatine, and to highlight the relationship between gray and white matter. Diffusion MRI enhances neuronal fibers that are operational in water diffusion to permit further functional definition of white matter networks.

Among functional neuroimaging 18F-fluorodeoxyglucose PET (FDG-PET) has been most frequently applied clinically to demonstrate ipsilateral regional cerebral hypometabolism and metabolic rates that are reduced in 60–90% of patients with mTLE when compared with contralateral regions [63]. Ictal single-photon emission computed tomography (SPECT) and subtraction ictal SPECT coregistered with MRI (SISCOM) may assist with localization, operative strategies, and even in predicting surgical outcome [64].

Electrophysiology

The interictal features of mTLE on the EEG are often associated with anterior temporal spikes or sharp waves (Figure 14.2) with maximal voltage over the temporal

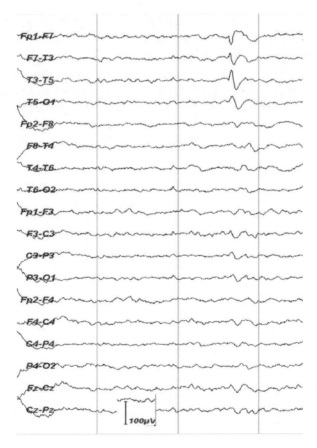

Figure 14.2 Characteristic left anterior temporal sharp-and-slow wave during routine interictal EEG.

basal electrodes. During video-EEG monitoring >90% of patients with mTLE will demonstrate anterior temporal electrode or sphenoidal interictal epileptiform discharges (IEDs) [5, 65]. Intermittent focal slowing is commonly associated with IEDs with localizing value when appearing as temporal intermittent rhythmic delta activity. Special electrodes to record from the mesial-basal temporal regions help facilitate definition of the polarity and field of spread. Mid-temporal epileptiform discharges may occasionally occur in mTLE, but this finding should prompt consideration of a larger or extramesial generator. Approximately one-third of patients demonstrate bilateral temporal IEDs [5, 65, 66] and when not seen are usually the effect of a shorter duration of recording. Temporal IEDs in wakefulness or REM sleep most often are concordant with the site of seizure onset [67]. The strong localizing ability of unilateral temporal IEDs on EEG and ipsilateral hippocampal atrophy has led some to question the need for ictal recordings in patients with mTLE due to the high concordance with seizure onset [68].

The characteristic ictal EEG pattern associated with focal seizures of medial temporal lobe origin is a unilateral regular 5–9 Hz rhythmic ictal theta or alpha discharge maximal in the anterior temporal scalp electrodes (Figure 14.3) that occurs after the onset of clinical symptoms [69]. This finding has been reported to occur in up to 94% of patients with mTLE and correctly lateralize the seizure onset in >95% of patients. Less commonly, a similar vertex and parasagittal positive rhythm or a combination of morphologies may be recorded in mTLE that is coincident with the negativity observed at the temporal basal electrodes [70]. However, this pattern may also occur at some point during the ictal discharge in those

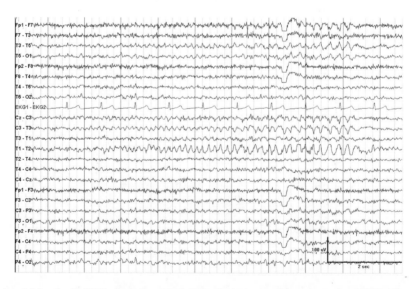

Figure 14.3 Scalp EEG depicting a brief focal electrographic seizure in mTLE. Note the characteristic evolving left regional anterior temporal rhythmic ictal theta discharge.

without hippocampal TLE [71]. Partial seizures propagated from extratemporal or neocortical structures to the mesial structures may explain the reduced specificity seen in patients without HFA. Nevertheless, patients with normal brain MRI and a rhythmic ictal theta discharge at seizure onset may still be able to predict a favorable response to temporal lobectomy [72]. TLE has also been subdivided by means of continuous EEG source imaging using multiple fixed dipole analysis of scalp EEG. Ictal rhythms with a predominant basal source component had hippocampal onset seizures while those with anterior temporal source maximum had entorhinal onset and those with lateral source maximum had neocortical onset [73]. Scalp EEG patterns of temporal lobe seizures are not a direct reflection of ictal activity at seizure onset but rather a reflection of the differences in seizure development, propagation, and synchrony of the direct cortical discharges [74]. Using simultaneous intracranial and surface ictal EEG recordings (64 total channels) obtained from a combination of subdural strip (Figure 14.4), intracerebral

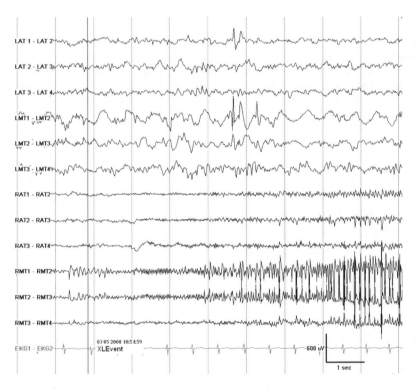

Figure 14.4 Invasive EEG represented by bitemporal subdural strips to lateralize a patient with right mTLE. Note the right regional temporal onset during second 2. L/RAT: L/R anterior temporal; L/RMT: L/R mesial temporal. Reproduced with permission from Tatum W.O., Husain A.M., Benbadis S.R., and Kaplan P.W. (2008) *Handbook of EEG Interpretation*. New York: Demos Medical Publishing, p. 114.

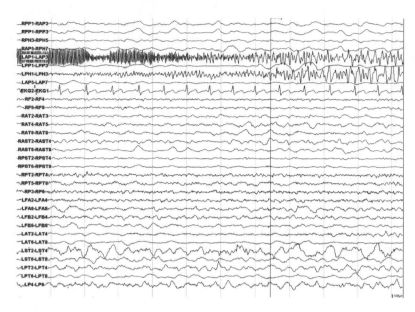

Figure 14.5 Invasive EEG with combined depth and subdural strips to localize left medial temporal onset focal seizures. Note seizure onset in the left depth demonstrating left anterior pes hippocampus onset manifest as rhythmic ictal fast activity. Depth electrodes are denoted by R/L (right/left)AP: R/L anterior pes; R/LPP: R/L posterior pes; R/LPH: R/L parahippocampal while subdural strips are identified as R/LAT: R/L anterior temporal; R/LST: R/L subtemporal; R/LPT: R/L posterior temporal; R/LF: R/L frontal. Courtesy of Michael R. Sperling, MD; Jefferson University Hospital, Philadelphia, PA.

depth (Figure 14.5), and scalp electrodes Pacia and Ebersole reported an ictal EEG classification system for TLE [74]. Discharges initially confined to the hippocampus produce no scalp EEG rhythms but required the recruitment of the inferolateral temporal neocortex before the regular 5–9 Hz subtemporal and temporal EEG pattern was evident on scalp recording. When the ictal discharge was confined to the mesial basal temporal cortex, a vertex dominant rhythm became noted due to the net vertical orientation of the dipole. Widespread bilateral background attenuation (corresponding to 20–40 Hz fast activity on invasive recordings) and irregular 2–4 Hz delta on scalp EEG at onset were more likely to be associated with neocortical seizures with a focal or regional onset on invasive recording. While the conventional range of EEG analysis involves frequencies <100 Hz, depth electrodes and visual analysis have revealed discrete focal high-frequency oscillations (ripples <250 Hz and fast ripples >250 and <500 Hz) that may be present during the immediate preictal period at the region of seizure-onset in mTLE and rarely in the regions of propagated or nonlocalized seizures [75].

Treatment

Most patients with focal seizures will respond to medical treatment with appropriate AEDs. For one-third of patients with continued seizures despite therapy, the sequella may involve a constellation of features. The impact from cumulative AED load, cognitive deterioration, psychosocial dysfunction, restriction in activity of daily living, and compromised quality of life may appear to progress over time [76]. Patients with HS ultimately have a small likelihood of maintaining seizure freedom in surgical series [77] though little is known about the natural history in the community at large.

Consequences of mTLE include morbidity that may be related to the adverse effects of treatment and from recurrent seizures. Soft tissue injuries are the most common type of injury sustained as the result of a seizure. Head injuries are also commonly encountered [78]. Adverse effects on the developing brain may stem from recurrent seizures but may also occur from over-treatment [79]. Increased mortality may occur from many different causes both directly from seizures due to accidents, suffocation, and drowning. In addition, the underlying pathology leading to seizures from head trauma, stroke, infections, and brain tumors may compromise life expectancy independently of the effect from seizures. Sudden unexplained death in epilepsy (SUDEP) is a distinct cause for fatality in epilepsy that is greater in patients with uncontrolled seizures underscoring the need to consider all options including medical and surgical therapy for patients with refractory mTLE. SUDEP requires that there is a diagnosis of epilepsy, that the deceased was in a reasonable state of health, the death was sudden (minutes) and occurred during benign circumstances, and that it was not directly caused by seizures or status epilepticus and was without obvious medical reasons. Patients with mTLE that fail surgery are among the highest risk patients and are at risk for SUDEP occurring with a range between 2.2 and 9.3 per 1000 patient-years compared with 0.5–1.9 in community prevalence samples [6].

Medical

Nearly two-thirds of patients with partial-onset seizures will achieve seizure freedom [80] yet of all etiologies complex partial seizures due to HS have the worst prognosis for medical control with only 11–42% of patients becoming seizure-free [77, 81]. Failure to identify refractory patients early during the course of treatment may be compounded by observing approximately one-quarter of patients with refractory TLE that exhibit a significant period of seizure control before intractability finally becomes evident [82]. Newer generation AEDs hold the promise of similar efficacy but with improved tolerability. However, most AEDs exert their effect by providing a favorable balance between reducing neuronal excitation (by modulating sodium and calcium channels that reduce excitatory amino acids) or enhancing neuronal inhibition (and potentiating the effects of GABA), though some have novel mechanisms that offer the mechanistic rationale for polypharmacy. Suicide is significantly increased in TLE and may have a neurobiological basis from the anatomy that cross-links the limbic system between epilepsy and depression. The effect of AEDs on suicide received attention from the US FDA after demonstrating a small but significant effect that occurred in pooled data taken from the placebo arm of controlled clinical regulatory AED trials compared with placebo. In terms of adjusted risk estimates for the treatment groups, 0.43% of the drug patients experience suicidal behavior or ideation compared to 0.24% of the placebo patients.

Failure of the first AED for reasons of inefficacy has demonstrated to be the most powerful predictor of subsequent successful trials of AED use [80]. A minority of drug-resistant patients are able to achieve seizure freedom even after the failure of two or more AEDs [82, 83]. Still, this minority underscores the need to consider continued AED trials when resective surgery is not feasible. A recent review of over 2734 patients with drug-resistant epilepsy after temporal lobe surgery versus medical treatment found that 12% of patient in the nonoperated pooled controls would become seizure-free without surgery despite a lack of control for many years [84]. In the absence of long-term randomized trials, observational studies have shown that when seizure freedom does occur, the introduction of new AEDs into the maintenance drug regimens to produce seizure freedom may last up to 12 months or longer in a limited number of refractory patients [85]. New AED development will continue to provide a better understanding of the molecular mechanisms that underlie TLE. Still, treatment with a change in medical regimen when necessary, as well as adjunctive treatment with resective epilepsy surgery are both standards of care for eligible patients with drug-resistant TLE [86].

Surgical

When AEDs are ineffective in maintaining seizure freedom, resective epilepsy surgery must be considered. Temporal lobectomy represents two-thirds of the surgical procedures performed for all drug-resistant focal seizures. Surgical outcome is expected to approach 70% or more and is the prototype for surgically remediable epilepsy syndromes [87]. A single one-year randomized controlled trial performed in Canada demonstrated superiority of surgical treatment in TLE over continued medical treatment once pharmacoresistance was established [88]. In this adult trial 40 surgery patients were compared with 40 patients treated medically. Only 3% in the medication-only group were seizure-free at one year; however, after surgery 58% were free of seizures that impaired consciousness. Many other uncontrolled studies are consistent with nearly identical results to the class 1 trial [86]. A multicentered trial found that when HFA was present and generalized tonic-clonic seizures were absent, these were selection criteria that were most predictive of a favorable outcome after epilepsy surgery associated with mTLE [89]. Long-term follow-up studies of medical versus surgical treatment otherwise have been poorly established. A meta-analysis of surgical outcome further demonstrated that two years after surgery 55% of refractory patients are completely seizure-free and 68% are free from complex partial seizures [84]. Though pathological heterogeneity may exist the recognition of HS has dramatically improved our ability to render drug-resistant patients seizure-free after resective epilepsy surgery. Surgery is >4 times more effective than best medical treatment [84, 88]. Early observations of patients with epilepsy and "exploratory" nonresective craniotomies found some influence of surgery on seizure reduction though they did not become seizure-free [90]. This suggests that while an effect from the surgical procedure itself may occur, seizure freedom from successful resection of the medial temporal structures is the only way to definitively validate the origin of the seizures to serve as a "gold standard" for seizure localization. In general, temporal resections (Figure 14.6) are usually more effective than extratemporal or multilobar resections to result in seizure freedom [91]. Additionally, the surgical technique is another crucial factor and even patients with various pathologies may do well with resection of the targeted lesion in its entirety [92]. Quality of life was also shown to be better after epilepsy surgery when compared to continued medical care though was best correlated with those who achieved seizure freedom (P < 0.001) [88]. Additionally imaging evidence has suggested that neuronal dysfunction outside the epileptogenic zone may be reversible after successful surgical treatment [93]. An important minority ranging from approximately 20–50% of seizure-free surgical patients able to discontinue AEDs remained "cured" of refractory mTLE [94]. Similarly, in a minority of patient, risks of intracranial surgery

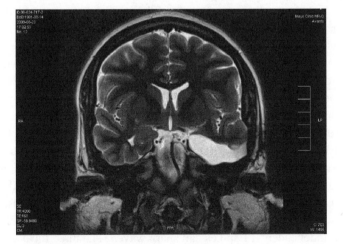

Figure 14.6 Coronal T2-weighted brain MRI showing postoperative changes in the temporal lobe following left anterior-mesial temporal lobectomy.

have included infection, hemorrhage, or focal neurological deficits. Transitory language, "pie in the sky" visual field defects, rare motor deficits, and memory deficits may occur as morbidities with mortality rare in experienced centers.

Neurostimulation is a form of therapy that may be considered when surgery is not an option. Despite the surge of new AEDs, the greater availability of resective epilepsy surgery, and the resurfacing of the ketogenic diet, neurostimulation maintains a unique role in the treatment of refractory mTLE. Vagus nerve stimulation (VNS) is not a curative device with <5% becoming seizure-free with use, though a mean reduction in seizure frequency of 25–28% at three months improving to about 40% by year has been shown [95]. VNS should be considered in patients with mTLE only when craniotomy and resective surgery is undesirable, and after a definitive diagnosis of epileptic seizures. Primary adverse effects of hoarseness, tingling at the electrode site and shortness of breath though are mild. Simultaneous AED reduction appears possible for improved tolerability [96]. Other forms of intracranial neurostimulation including thalamic deep brain stimulation (DBS) and a responsive neurostimulator (RNS) are promising and may benefit more patients in the near future.

Illustrative case

A 33-year-old right-handed white female with a history of depression was self-referred for evaluation of an investigational AED trial. She first experienced a single complex febrile convulsion at 2 years of age and was well until menarche at 12 years of age when a nocturnal "grand mal" seizure was witnessed. A brain MRI and EEG were "negative" and she was treated with carbamazepine (CBZ). Retrospectively, episodes of "déjà vu" were identified where she would "feel as though she had the feeling she had done this before." She would then briefly stare with a brief lapse of awareness for "seconds" while she tried to "fight it" following which she felt fatigue. Others would see her staring and "concentrating" during this time. She was maintained on CBZ monotherapy for 17 years by her primary care physician later with brief trials of lamotrigine and levetiracetam. She continued to experience weekly "déjà vu" without further "seizures" until impaired consciousness intensified leading to her own concerns of driving safety.

The neurological examination was normal. A repeat EEG revealed left anterior temporal IEDs. A high-resolution brain MRI using an epilepsy protocol clearly delineated severe left MTS. Admission for video-EEG monitoring captured three habitual seizures that began with her warning prior to a stare, impaired consciousness, lip smacking, and bilateral hand automatisms for 30–60 seconds, following which she was tired and had trouble with verbal expression. Interictal EEG demonstrated state-independent T1 spikes and sharp waves. The three focal seizures with impaired consciousness were identical and began after an abrupt left regional temporal sharply contoured 7 Hz theta maximal at the T1/F7 derivation with a

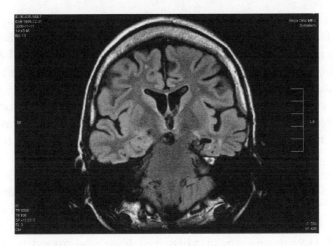

Figure 14.7   Coronal FLAIR sequence brain MRI following amygdalohippocampectomy. Note the small targeted resection margin in the left mesial temporal lobe.

left hemispheric-predominant bilateral field of spread that ceased abruptly with left temporal postictal delta slowing. A brain FDG-PET revealed left temporal hypometabolism. Subsequently, neuropsychological testing revealed a full-scale IQ of 105, mild verbal memory impairment, no psychiatric barriers, and motivation to undergo a surgical procedure. Wada testing demonstrated the left hemisphere to be dominant for language function and 8/8 recognition with left hemispheric injection and 5/8 recognition with right hemispheric injection of sodium methohexital. She subsequently underwent left amygdalohippocampectomy (Figure 14.7) and has been seizure-free for >2 years on tapering doses of CBZ.

This case illustrates a few salient points including the characteristic history of patients with mTLE. Her chronic exposure to AEDs prior to surgical attention is typical of the delays that those with mTLE due to HS incur prior to definitive treatment [86–89]. The caretaker's misinterpretation of "seizure control" as an absence of generalized tonic-clonic seizures is partly responsible for many patients self-referring themselves to an epilepsy center for new treatment options available. In addition, her presurgical evaluation is classic for those with mTLE with a phase 1 that allows her to "skip" directly to surgery as a "slam dunk" straightforward case of surgical mTLE. In the setting of her seizure semiology and concordance of her phase 1 data a >70% likelihood of seizure freedom with a normalized HRQOL was anticipated [97] and realized at two years following surgery.

14.6 Concluding statements

mTLE is a well-recognized, distinct, and prevalent human focal epilepsy syndrome with a well-known clinical, neuroradiographic, electrographic, and pathological profile. Newer neuroimaging techniques are increasingly identifying symptomatic "causes" of acquired mTLE through greater resolution of the medial temporal neuroanatomy. Neurophysiological refinement of macroscopic spatial and temporal resolution may provide more precise seizure localization [98], and advances in seizure prediction allow for earlier recognition to facilitate intervention. Advances in understanding the spectrum of mTLE suggest a continuum from a focal network centered over the medial temporal lobe to a widely extended network that goes beyond the medial temporal structures and even beyond the limits of the temporal lobe [99].

For patients with mTLE, targeting treatment that is aimed at improvement in their health, employment, education, and social activities remains the ultimate goal. The fundamental need for epilepsy classification, definitive diagnosis, and focus on achieving a seizure-free outcome with treatment can not be over-emphasized. Over-treatment with AEDs complicates the risky delay which may introduce serious drug adverse effects and expose the patient to ongoing seizure-related morbidity and mortality. Improvement in the domains of HRQOL is more difficult to achieve the longer mTLE remains uncontrolled and epilepsy surgery remains a standard of care in need of early consideration [100]. In the future other less or non-invasive techniques such as viral vectors that introduce novel genes into the brain and cell grafting may promise a futuristic treatment approach to afford suboptimal surgical candidates with mTLE an alternative to resective surgery [101].

References

1. Hauser, W.A., Annegers, J.F., and Kurland, L.T. (1991) Prevalence of epilepsy in Rochester, Minnesota: 1940–1980. *Epilepsia*, **32**, 429–445.
2. Blume, W.T. (2006) The progression of epilepsy. *Epilepsia*, **47** (Suppl 1), 71–78.
3. Commission on Classification and Terminology of the International League Against Epilepsy (1985) Proposal for classification of epilepsies and epileptic syndromes. *Epilepsia*, **26** (Suppl 3), 268–278.
4. Berg, A.T., Berkovic, S.F., Brodie, M.J. *et al.* (2010) Revised terminology and concepts for organization of seizures and epilepsies: report of the ILAE Commission on Classification and Terminology 2005–2009. *Epilepsia*, **51** (4), 676–685.
5. French, J.A., Williamson, P.D., Thadani, V.M. *et al.* (1993) Characteristics of medial temporal lobe epilepsy: I. Results of history and physical examination. *Ann Neurol*, **34**, 774–780.
6. Hitiris, N., Mohanraj, R., Norrie, J., and Brodie, M.J. (2007) Mortality in epilepsy. *Epilepsy Behav*, **10**, 363–376.
7. Cooke, S.F. and Bliss, T.V. (2006) Plasticity in the human central nervous system. *Brain*, **129**, 1659–1673.
8. http://en.wikipedia.org/wiki/Hippocampus#Role_in_memory (last accessed November 27, 2008).
9. Engel, J. Jr. (2003) A greater role for surgical treatment of epilepsy: why and when? *Epilepsy Curr*, **3**, 37–40.

10. Squire, L.R. (2009) The legacy of patient H.M. for neuroscience. *Neuron*, **61**, 6–9.

11. Helmstaedter, C., Kurthen, M., Lux, S. *et al.* (2003) Chronic epilepsy and cognition: a longitudinal study in temporal lobe epilepsy. *Ann Neurol*, **54**, 425–432.

12. Hermann, B.P., Seidenberg, M., Dow, C. *et al.* (2006) Cognitive prognosis in chronic temporal lobe epilepsy. *Ann Neurol*, **60**, 80–87.

13. Hermann, B.P., Seidenberg, M., Schoenfeld, J., and Davies, K. (1997) Neuropsychological characteristics of the syndrome of mesial temporal lobe epilepsy. *Arch Neurol*, **54**, 369–376.

14. Coan, A.C., Appenzeller, S., Bonilha, L. *et al.* (2009) Seizure frequency and lateralization affect progression of atrophy in temporal lobe epilepsy. *Neurology*, **73**, 834–842.

15. De Lanerolle, N.C., Kim, J.H., Williamson, A. *et al.* (2003) A retrospective analysis of hippocampal pathology in human temporal lobe epilepsy: evidence for distinctive patient subcategories. *Epilepsia*, **44**, 677–687.

16. Thom, M., Martinian, L., Catarino, C. *et al.* (2009) Bilateral reorganization of the dentate gyrus in hippocampal sclerosis: a postmortem study. *Neurology*, **73**, 1033–1040.

17. Bernasconi, N., Bernasconi, A., Caramanos, Z. *et al.* (2001) Entorhinal cortex atrophy in epilepsy patients exhibiting normal hippocampal volumes. *Neurology*, **56**, 1335–1339.

18. Wyler, A.R., Dohan, F.C., Schweitzer, J.B., and Berry, A.D. (1992) A grading system for mesial temporal pathology (hippocampal sclerosis) from anterior temporal lobectomy. *J Epilepsy*, **5**, 220–225.

19. Blümcke, I., Pauli, E., Clusman, H. *et al.* (2007) A new clinico-pathological classification system for mesial temporal lobe sclerosis. *Acta Neuropathol*, **113**, 235–244.

20. Madden, M. and Sutula, T. (2009) Beyond hippocampal sclerosis: the rewired hippocampus in temporal lobe epilepsy. *Neurology*, **73**, 1008–1009.

21. Petroff, O.A.C., Rothman, D.L., Behar, K.L., and Mattson, R.H. (1996) Low brain GABA level is associated with poor seizure control. *Ann Neurol*, **40**, 908–911.

22. Crino, P.B., Jin, H., Shumate, M.D. *et al.* (2002) Increased expression of the neuronal glutamate transporter (EAAT3/EAAC1) in hippocampal and neocortical epilepsy. *Epilepsia*, **43**, 211–218.

23. van der Hel, W.S., Verlinde, S.A.M.W., Meijer, D.H.M. *et al.* (2009) Hippocampal distribution of vesicular glutamate transporter 1 in patients with temporal lobe epilepsy. *Epilepsia*, **50** (1), 1717–1728.

24. Bonilha, L., Rorden, C., Castellano, G. *et al.* (2004) Voxel-based morphometry reveals gray matter network atrophy in refractory medial temporal lobe epilepsy. *Arch Neurol*, **61**, 1379–1384.

25. Cendes, F., Lopes-Cendes, I., Andermann, I., and Andermann, F. (1998) Familial temporal lobe epilepsy: a clinically heterogeneous syndrome. *Neurology*, **50**, 554–557.

26. Berkovic, S.F., McIntosh, A., Howell, R.A. *et al.* (1996) Familial temporal lobe epilepsy: a common disorder identified in twins. *Arch Neurol*, **40**, 227–235.

27. Briellmann, R.S., Torn-Broers, Y., Busuttil, B.E. *et al.* (2000) APOe4 genotype has been associated with an earlier age of onset in temporal lobe epilepsy. *Neurology*, **55**, 435–437.

28. Scheffer, I.E., Harkin, L.A., Grinton, B.E. *et al.* (2006) Temporal lobe epilepsy and GEFS+ phenotypes associated with SCN1B mutation. *Brain*, **130**, 100–109.

29. Kanemoto, K., Kawasaki, J., Miyamoto, T. *et al.* (2000) Interleukin (IL)-1beta, IL-1alpha, and IL-1 receptor antagonist gene polymorphisms in patients with temporal lobe epilepsy. *Ann Neurol*, **47**, 571–574.

30. Siddiqui, A., Kerb, R., Weale, M.E. *et al.* (2003) Association of multidrug resistance in epilepsy with a polymorphism in the drug-transporter gene ABCB1. *N Engl J Med*, **348**, 1442–1448.

31. Gambardella, A., Manna, I., Labate, A. *et al.* (2003) GABA(B) receptor 1 polymorphism (G1465A) is associated with temporal lobe epilepsy. *Neurology*, **60** (4), 560–563.
32. Szoeke, C., Sills, G.J., Kwan, P. *et al.* (2009) Multidrug-resistant genotype (ABCB1) and seizure recurrence in newly treated epilepsy: data from international pharmacogenetic cohorts. *Epilepsia*, **50** (7), 1689–1696.
33. Deacon, C., Wiebe, S., Blume, W.T. *et al.* (2003) Seizure identification by clinical description in temporal lobe epilepsy. How accurate are we? *Neurology*, **61**, 1686–1689.
34. van Donselaar, C.A., Stroink, H., and Arts, W.-F. for the Dutch Study Group of Epilepsy in Childhood (2006) How confident are we of a diagnosis of epilepsy. *Epilepsia*, **47** (Suppl 1), 9–13.
35. Stroink, H., van Donselaar, C.A., Geerts, A.T. *et al.* (2003) The accuracy of the diagnosis of paroxysmal events in children. *Neurology*, **60**, 979–982.
36. Thompson, S.A., Duncan, J.S., and Smith, S.J. (2000) Partial seizures presenting as panic attacks. *Br Med J*, **321**, 1002–1003.
37. So, N.K. (2006) Epileptic auras, in *The Treatment of Epilepsy: Principles and Practice*, 4th edn, (ed. E. Wyllie), Lippincott Williams & Wilkins, Philadelphia, PA, pp. 219–222.
38. Benbadis, S.R., Tatum, W.O., Murtaugh, F.R., and Vale, F.L. (2000) MRI evidence of mesial temporal sclerosis in patients with psychogenic nonepileptic seizures. *Neurology*, **55** (7), 1061–1062.
39. Benbadis, S.R. and Tatum, W.O. (2003) Overinterpretation of EEGs and misdiagnosis of epilepsy. *J Clin Neurophysiol*, **20** (1), 42–44.
40. Spanaki, M.V., Garcia, P., Schuger, C.D., and Smith, B.J. (2006) Vasovagal syncope misdiagnosed as epilepsy for 17 years: prime importance of clinical history. *Epileptic Disord*, **8** (3), 219–222.
41. Tatum, W.O. (2001) Long-term EEG monitoring: a clinical approach to electrophysiology. *J Clin Neurophysiol*, **18** (5), 442–455.
42. Berg, A.T. (2008) The natural history of mesial temporal lobe epilepsy. *Curr Opin Neurol*, **21**, 173–178.
43. Van Landingham, K.E., Heinz, E.R., Cavazos, J.E., and Lewis, D.V. (1998) Magnetic resonance imaging evidence of hippocampal injury after prolonged focal febrile convulsions. *Ann Neurol*, **3**, 413–426.
44. Scott, R.C., King, M.D., Gadian, D.G. *et al.* (2003) Hippocampal abnormalities after prolonged febrile convulsion: a longitudinal MRI study. *Brain*, **126**, 2551–2557.
45. Villanueva, V. and Serratosa, J.M. (2005) Temporal lobe epilepsy: clinical semiology and age of onset. *Epileptic Disord*, **7** (2), 83–90.
46. Acharya, V., Acharya, J., and Luders, H.H. (1998) Olfactory epileptic auras. *Neurology*, **51** (1), 56–61.
47. Fogarasi, A., Jokeit, H., Faveret, E. *et al.* (2002) The effect of age on seizure semiology in childhood temporal lobe epilepsy. *Epilepsia*, **43** (6), 638–643.
48. Tatum, W.O., Ross, J., and Cole, A.J. (1998) Epileptic pseudodementia. *Neurology*, **50**, 1472–1475.
49. Engel, J. Jr. (1993) Update on surgical treatment of the epilepsies: summary of the second International Palm Desert Conference on the Surgical Treatment of the Epilepsies. *Neurology*, **43**, 1612–1617.
50. So, E.L. (2006) Value and limitations of seizure semiology in localizing seizure onset. *J Clin Neurophysiol*, **23** (4), 353–357.
51. Salmenpera, T., Kononen, M., Roberts, N. *et al.* (2005) Hippocampal damage in newly diagnosed focal epilepsy. *Neurology*, **64**, 62–68.
52. Kalviainen, R., Salmenpera, T., Partanen, K. *et al.* (1998) Recurrent seizures may cause hippocampal damage in temporal lobe epilepsy. *Neurology*, **50**, 1377–1382.

53. Van Paesschen, W., Duncan, J.S., Stevens, J.M., and Connelly, A. (1998) Longitudinal quantitative hippocampal magnetic resonance imaging study of adults with newly diagnosed partial seizures: one-year follow-up results. *Epilepsia*, **39**, 633–639.

54. Briellman, R.S., Berkovic, S.F., Syngeniotis, A. *et al.* (2002) Seizure-associated hippocampal volume loss: a longitudinal study of temporal lobe epilepsy. *Ann Neurol*, **51**, 541–644.

55. Bernasconi, N., Natsume, J., and Bernasconi, A. (2005) Progression in temporal lobe epilepsy: differential atrophy in mesial temporal structures. *Neurology*, **65**, 223–228.

56. Garcia-Fiñana, M., Denby, C.E., Keller, S.S. *et al.* (2006) Degree of hippocampal atrophy is related to side of seizure onset in temporal lobe epilepsy. *Am J Neuroradiol*, **27**, 1046–1052.

57. Mueller, S.G., Laxer, K.D., Barakos, J. *et al.* (2009) Subfield atrophy pattern in temporal lobe epilepsy with and without mesial sclerosis detected by high-resolution MRI at 4 Tesla: preliminary results. *Epilepsia*, **50** (6), 1474–1483.

58. Cascino, G.D., Jack, C.R. Jr., Parisi, J.E. *et al.* (1991) Magnetic resonance imaging-based volume studies in temporal lobe epilepsy: pathological correlations. *Ann Neurol*, **30**, 31–36.

59. Carne, R.P., O'Brien, T.J., Kilpatrick, C.J. *et al.* (2004) MRI negative PET positive temporal lobe epilepsy: a distinct surgically remediable syndrome. *Brain*, **127** (10), 2276–2285.

60. Bernhardt, B.C., Worsley, K.J., Kim, H. *et al.* (2009) Longitudinal and cross-sectional analysis of atrophy in pharmacoresistant temporal lobe epilepsy. *Neurology*, **72**, 1747–1754.

61. Bernasconi, A., Bernasconi, N., Caramanos, Z. *et al.* (2000) T2 relaxometry can lateralize mesial temporal lobe epilepsy in patients with normal MRI. *Neuroimage*, **12**, 739–746.

62. Carpentier, A., Constable, R.T., Schlosser, M. *et al.* (2001) Patterns of fMRI activations in association with structural lesions in the central sulcus: a classification of plasticity. *J Neurosurg*, **94**, 946–954.

63. Theodore, W.H., Sato, S., Kufta, C. *et al.* (1992) Temporal lobectomy for uncontrolled seizures: the role of positron emission tomography. *Ann Neurol*, **32**, 789–794.

64. O'Brien, T., So, E., Mullan, B. *et al.* (1998) Subtraction ictal SPECT co-registered with MRI improves clinical usefulness of SPECT in localizing the surgical seizures focus. *Neurology*, **50**, 445–454.

65. Williamson, P.D., French, J.A., and Thadani, V.M. (1993) Characteristics of medial temporal lobe epilepsy: II. Interictal and ictal scalp electroencephalography, neuropsychological testing, neuroimaging, surgical results, and pathology. *Ann Neurol*, **34**, 782–787.

66. Chung, M.Y., Walczak, T.S., Lewis, D.V. *et al.* (1991) Temporal lobectomy and independent bitemporal interictal activity: what degree of lateralization is sufficient? *Epilepsia*, **32**, 195–201.

67. Sammaritano, M., Gigli, G.L., and Gotman, J. (1991) Interictal spiking during wakefulness and sleep and the localization of foci in temporal lobe epilepsy. *Neurology*, **41**, 290–297.

68. Cendes, F., Li, L.M., Watson, C. *et al.* (2000) Is ictal recording mandatory in temporal lobe epilepsy? Not when the interictal electroencephalogram and hippocampal atrophy coincide. *Arch Neruol*, **57**, 497–500.

69. Risinger, M.W., Engel, J. Jr., Van Ness, P.C. *et al.* (1989) Ictal localization of temporal lobe seizures with scalp-sphenoidal recordings. *Neurology*, **39**, 1288–1293.

70. Ebersole, J.S. and Pacia, S.V. (1996) Localization of temporal lobe foci by ictal EEG patterns. *Epilepsia*, **37** (4), 386–399.

71. Gil-Nagel, A. and Risinger, M.W. (1997) Ictal semiology in hippocampal versus extrahippocampal temporal lobe epilepsy. *Brain*, **120**, 183–192.

72. Tatum, W.O. IV, Benbadis, S.R., Hussain, A. *et al.* (2008) Ictal EEG remains the prominent predictor of seizure-free outcome after temporal lobectomy in epileptic patients with normal brain MRI. *Seizure*, **17**, 631–636.

73. Assaf, B.A. and Ebersole, J.S. (1997) Continuous source imaging of scalp ictal rhythms in temporal lobe epilepsy. *Epilepsia*, **38** (10), 1114–1123.

74. Pacia, S.V. and Ebersole, J.S. (1997) Intracranial EEG substrates of scalp ictal patterns from temporal lobe foci. *Epilepsia*, **38** (6), 642–654.

75. Jacobs, J., Zelmann, R., Jirsch, J. *et al.* (2009) High frequency oscillations (80–500 Hz) in the preictal period of patients with focal seizures. *Epilepsia*, **50** (7), 1780–1792.

76. Brodie, M.J. and Kwan, P. (2002) Staged approach to epilepsy management. *Neurology*, **58** (Suppl 5), S2–S8.

77. Sameh, F., Picot, M.C., Adam, C. *et al.* (1998) Is the underlying cause of epilepsy a major prognostic factor for recurrence? *Neurology*, **51**, 1256–1262.

78. Wirrell, E.C. (2006) Epilepsy-related injuries. *Epilepsia*, **47** (Suppl 1), 79–86.

79. Blumer, D. and Adamolekun, B. (2006) Treatment of patients with coexisting epileptic and nonepileptic seizures. *Epilepsy Behav*, **9**, 498–502.

80. Kwan, P. and Brodie, M.J. (2000) Early identification of refractory epilepsy. *N Engl J Med*, **342**, 314–319.

81. Stephen, L.J., Kwan, P., and Brodie, M.J. (2001) Does the cause of localization-related epilepsy influence the response to antiepileptic drug treatment? *Epilepsia*, **42**, 357–362.

82. Kwan, P., Arzimanoglou, A., Berg, A.T. *et al.* (2010) Definition of drug resistant epilepsy: consensus proposal by the ad hoc Task Force of the ILAE Commission on Therapeutic Strategies. *Epilepsia*, **51** (6), 1069–1077.

83. Schiller, Y. and Najjar, Y. (2008) Quantifying the response to antiepileptic drugs: effect of past treatment history. *Neurology*, **70**, 54–65.

84. Schmidt, D. and Stavem, K. (2009) Long-term seizure outcome of surgery versus no surgery for drug-resistant partial epilepsy: a review of controlled studies. *Epilepsia*, **50** (6), 1301–1309.

85. Luciano, A.L. and Shorvon, S.D. (2008) Results of treatment changes in patients with apparently drug-resistant chronic epilepsy. *Ann Neurol*, **62**, 375–381.

86. Engel, J. Jr., Wiebe, S., French, J. *et al.* (2003) Practice parameter: temporal lobe and localized neocortical resections for epilepsy. *Neurology*, **60**, 538–547.

87. Engel, J. Jr. (1996) Surgery for seizures. *N Engl J Med*, **334**, 647–652.

88. Wiebe, S., Blume, W.T., Girvin, J.P., and Eliasziw, M. (2001) A randomized, controlled trial of surgery for temporal lobe epilepsy. *N Engl J Med*, **345**, 311–318.

89. Spencer, S.S., Berg, A.T., and Vickrey, B.G. (2003) Initial outcomes in the multicenter study of epilepsy surgery. *Neurology*, **61** (12), 1680–1685.

90. Penfield, W. and Steelman, H. (1947) The treatment of focal epilepsy by cortical excision. *Ann Surg*, **126**, 740–762.

91. Wyllie, E., Comair, Y.G., Kotagal, P. *et al.* (1998) Seizure outcome after epilepsy surgery in children and adolescents. *Ann Neurol*, **44**, 740–748.

92. Bourgeois, M., Sainte-Rose, C., Lellouch-Tubiana, A. *et al.* (1999) Surgery of epilepsy associated with focal lesions in childhood. *J Neurosurg*, **90**, 833–842.

93. Cendes, F., Andermann, F., Dubeau, F. *et al.* (1997) Normalization of neuronal metabolic dysfunction after surgery for temporal lobe epilepsy: evidence from proton MR spectroscopic imaging. *Neurology*, **49**, 1525–1533.

94. Bien, C.G., Kurthen, M., Baron, K. *et al.* (2001) Long-term seizure outcome and antiepileptic drug treatment in surgically treated temporal lobe epilepsy patients: a controlled study. *Epilepsia*, **42**, 1416–1421.

95. Handforth, A., DeGiorgio, C.M., Schachter, S.C. *et al.* (1998) Vagus nerve stimulation for partial-onset seizures: a randomized active-control trial. *Neurology*, **51**, 48–55.

96. Tatum, W.O., Johnson, K.D., Goff, S. *et al.* (2001) Vagus nerve stimulation and drug reduction. *Neurology*, **56**, 561–563.

97. Radhakrishnan, K., So, E., Silbert, P. *et al.* (1998) Predictors of outcome of anterior temporal lobectomy for intractable epilepsy: a multivariate study. *Neurology*, **51**, 465–471.

98. Staba, R.J., Wilson, D.I., Bragin, A. *et al.* (2002) Quantitative analysis of high-frequency oscillations (80–500 Hz) recorded in human epileptic hippocampus and entorhinal cortex. *J Neurophysiol*, **88**, 1743–1752.

99. Kahane, P. and Bartolomei, F. (2010) Temporal lobe epilepsy and hippocampal sclerosis: lLessons from depth EEG recordings. *Epilepsia*, **51** (Suppl 1), 59–62.

100. Vickrey, B.G., Hays, R.D., and Engel, J. Jr. (1995) Outcome assessment for epilepsy surgery: the impact of measuring health-related quality of life. *Ann Neurol*, **37** (2), 158–166.

101. Vezzani, A. (2004) Gene therapy for epilepsy. *Epilepsy Curr*, **4** (3), 87–90.

15 Substrate-directed epilepsy

Gregory A. Worrell

Department of Neurology, Divisions of Epilepsy and Clinical Neurophysiology, Mayo Clinic, Rochester, MN, USA

15.1 Intractable partial epilepsy

Approximately 30% of all patients with epilepsy will continue to have disabling seizures despite antiepileptic drugs (AEDs). Patients with medically resistant epilepsy are at increased risk for serious morbidity and mortality [1–3]. Most individuals who will respond favorably to AED medication are successfully treated with the initial drug selection. Patients who "fail" two AED medications used appropriately are likely to have drug-resistant seizure disorder and should be investigated for alternative forms of treatment [4, 5].

The World Health Organization estimates that epilepsy is the cause of 1% of the global burden of disease based on productive years lost to disability or premature death [4, 6]. Partial, or localization-related epilepsy, is the most common seizure disorder and 20–40% of patients will experience physically and socially disabling drug-resistant seizures [5, 7–9]. In fact, the majority of studies show that patients who fail to respond to two first-line AED trials, have a low probability of being seizure-free with continued drug trials [5, 8]. The most widely quoted study found less than 3% of patients are rendered seizure-free after failure (due to

Adult Epilepsy, First Edition. Edited by Gregory D. Cascino and Joseph I. Sirven.
© 2011 John Wiley & Sons, Ltd. Published 2011 by John Wiley & Sons, Ltd.

lack of efficacy) of only two AEDs [5, 8]. This study showed that 47% of patients respond to the first AED, 13% respond to the second AED, and only 3% respond to a third drug or multiple drugs. Of those patients who did not respond to the first AED because of lack of efficacy, only 11% subsequently became seizure-free. These results suggest that for a patient who has had adequate trials of two AEDs, i.e. failed because of efficacy and not side effects, the probability of pharmacological seizure remission is low. Generally, after failing two or three AEDs individuals are considered to have drug-resistant epilepsy (DRE) [5, 8]. It should be noted, however, that other recent studies have shown higher seizure remission rates in some populations [10, 11]. French *et al.* [10] found that 32 (16%) of 198 patients with poorly controlled partial epilepsy achieved at least a six-month seizure remission during a three-year period during which they received additional AED trials. Notably, 21 of these patients previously had epilepsy surgery.

When evaluating a patient with DRE it is important to consider and investigate known factors associated with poor seizure control, for example, medication noncompliance, alcohol abuse, and obstructive sleep apnea.

15.2 Epilepsy surgery

Epilepsy surgery is an effective and safe therapy for carefully selected patients with drug-resistant partial epilepsy (DRE) [12–16]. While only one study represents Class I evidence [17] there is now widespread consensus (Neurology consensus practice parameter [18]) that epilepsy surgery should be considered for patients with drug-resistant localization-related partial epilepsy. In particular, many patients with Temporal lobe epilepsy (TLE) or lesional epilepsy have surgically remediable epilepsy syndromes [4, 19]. The majority of these patients will experience a significant reduction in seizure frequency following surgical resection of the region of epileptic brain [13, 18–24]. A recent study using a decision analysis model showed that on average anterior temporal lobe resection provides substantial gains in life expectancy and quality-adjusted life expectancy for surgically treated patients with DRE compared with medical management [16].

Patients with TLE and MRI lesional MRI syndromes are generally the most favorable candidates for surgical resection. The frequency of seizure activity, type of seizure(s), comorbidity, and underlying pathology are important variables to consider when evaluating a patient's candidacy for surgical treatment. The impact of chronic epilepsy on psychosocial, economic, and quality of life should be taken into account [9]. The goals of epilepsy surgery are to eliminate seizures and improve a patient's quality of life, for example, allow individuals to work, attend school, live independently, and drive [16, 25, 26].

The most common operative procedures are focal resection of epileptic brain tissue, for example, focal corticectomy, and anterior temporal lobectomy [18, 19]. The rationale for surgical treatment is that removing the epileptogenic zone

(EZ), that is, site of seizure onset and initial seizure propagation [14, 23, 27], will eliminate seizures (Figure 15.1). The preoperative evaluation is directed at identifying the site of seizure onset, seizure propagation, and the location of functional eloquent cortex. Most patients undergo scalp video-EEG monitoring to record their habitual seizures, MRI to identify possible structural abnormalities, neuropsychological evaluation, visual field testing, and the intracarotid sodium amobarbital procedure, known as the Wada test (named after Canadian neurologist Juhn Wada) (Table 15.1). The high diagnostic yield of MRI to identify pathological substrates, for example, post-traumatic encephalomalcia, vascular malformation, tumor, malformations of cortical development (MCD), mesial temporal sclerosis (MTS), is well established in patients with DRE (Tables 15.2 and 15.3). Selected patients will require functional neuroimaging, that is, PET, SPECT, functional MRI, and possibly chronic intracranial EEG monitoring to localize the region of seizure onset [13, 14, 23, 27–32].

The outcome of epilepsy surgery is dependent on many variables including the age of seizure onset, location of the epileptic brain tissue, underlying pathology,

Table 15.1 Presurgical evaluation

Performed invariably	Performed variably	At selected centers
History and examination	Video-EEG (intracranial)	SISCOM
Routine EEG	Electrocorticography	MRS
MRI head	FDG-PET	PET receptor studies
Video-EEG (scalp)	Interictal-ictal SPECT	Functional MRI
Neuropsychology	Sodium amobarbital study (Wada)	MRI volumetry

Performed invariably: almost always obtained prior to epilepsy surgery; performed variably: available at most epilepsy centers, and used in selected candidates; performed selected centers: not widely available; MRI: magnetic resonance imaging; PET: positron emission tomography; SPECT: single-photon emission computed tomography; SISCOM: subtraction ictal SPECT co-registered to MRI; MRS: magnetic resonance spectroscopy.

Table 15.2 Surgically remediable epileptic syndromes

Selected partial epilepsy syndromes	MRI (%)	SISCOM	Pathology
Substrate-directed			
Medial temporal lobe epilepsy	>90	—	MTS
Lesional epilepsy: tumor	100	—	Ganglioglioma, glioma, DNET
Lesional epilepsy: vascular	100	—	Cavernous hemangioma, AVM
Lesional epilepsy: malformation	80–90	—	FCD
Non-substrate-directed			
Neocortical (extrahippocampal)	0%	75%	Gliosis, focal cell loss, none

FCD: focal cortical dysplasia.
Adapted from Cascino (2001) [33].

Table 15.3 MRI and mesial temporal sclerosis

MRI techniques	Sensitivity (%)
T2-relaxometry	79
IR	86
Visual atrophy	90
IR + visual atrophy	93
Hippocampal volumetry	97

Inversion Recovery (IR).
Reproduced from Kuzniecky *et al.* (1997) [44].

and surgical strategy. Favorable prognostic indicators include an early age of seizure onset, medial temporal lobe seizure onset, and a completely resectable structural lesion on MRI, for example, MTS, cavernous malformation, focal low-grade neoplasms [20, 24, 34]. Approximately 80–90% of patients with TLE secondary to MTS, and the above-listed lesional epilepsy syndromes may be rendered seizure-free or near seizure-free following a total excision of the EZ. Less favorable operative candidates include patients with MCD and normal MRI, that is nonlesional epilepsy [29, 35–38]. Nonlesional extratemporal partial epilepsy remains a very significant challenge [24, 39–43].

The cost of the presurgical evaluation and treatment is considerable. This cost, however, must be considered within the context of the costs of intractable epilepsy that includes AED therapy office visits, laboratory studies, unemployment, and lost productivity [4, 6, 16]. In addition to the psychosocial benefits for individuals the large-scale economic benefits to society of rendering patients seizure-free are well recognized.

15.3   Localization of the epileptogenic zone

The presurgical evaluation for epilepsy surgery is focused on localization of epileptic brain, that is, the region of brain generating the patient's habitual seizures (Figure 15.1). The cornerstones of the presurgical evaluation are (i) the clinical history and neurological exam, (ii) scalp video-EEG to record the patient's habitual seizures, (iii) seizure protocol MRI, and for some patients, (iv) functional neuroimaging (SPECT, PET, MRS, fMRI, magnetoencephalography (MEG)), Wada testing, and chronic intracranial EEG monitoring (iEEG). The surgical treatment is based on the concept that seizures begin in a discrete region of brain, the *seizure onset zone* (SOZ), and then propagate to a critical volume of "susceptible tissue" to generate seizures. In order to obtain seizure freedom, the SOZ and the surrounding EZ must be resected [27]. Unfortunately, in practice the EZ does not have a clear anatomical, imaging, or electrophysiological definition. In patients with a focal lesion on MRI, for example, low-grade tumor or a vascular malformation,

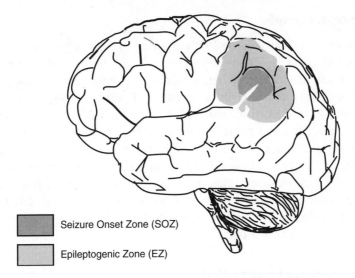

Seizure Onset Zone (SOZ)

Epileptogenic Zone (EZ)

Figure 15.1   The epileptogenic zone is defined as the region that must be resected for the patient to be seizure-free. The seizure onset zone is the region of seizure onset determined by iEEG.

if the SOZ localizes to the MRI lesion then *complete* resection of the MRI lesion will most often eliminate the seizures [19]. The rate of seizure-free outcomes in these selected patients with MRI lesions can approach 80–90%, *demonstrating the efficacy of epilepsy surgery* [4, 14, 19, 23, 24, 34]. However, many patients have a normal MRI, or lesions that extend beyond what is evident on MRI, for example, MCD [38], or into functionally eloquent brain that cannot be safely removed. These patients make up at least 30% of evaluations at major epilepsy centers. For patients with normal MRI scans only 30–50% of those finally deemed surgical candidates will achieve seizure freedom [24, 39–43] (Table 15.4), *demonstrating the current limitation of epilepsy surgery*.

The history and exam

The evaluation of patients with epilepsy requires a careful history and neurological exam [14, 18, 23, 45]. The age of epilepsy onset, history of febrile seizures, family history of epilepsy, history of significant head trauma, meningitis or encephalitis, cognitive deficits and abnormal neurological exam are of particular importance. To establish the likelihood of DRE it is important to establish the history of appropriate AED trials, the reason for AED failure, and history of medication compliance. In addition, lifestyle factors known to exacerbate seizures such as alcohol abuse should be pursued. Additionally, recent studies have identified sleep apnea as exacerbating seizure control [46].

Electroencephalography

Scalp video-EEG emerged in the 1970s as a way to obtain rigorous electroclinical correlation of seizures. Video-EEG is an indispensible tool for characterizing seizure type and identifying the region on onset in partial seizure disorders. Using simultaneous video and EEG the correlation of seizure semiology and EEG is possible [47, 48]. Video-EEG monitoring is performed in these individuals to confirm the diagnosis of a partial seizure disorder, establish the seizure-type, and determine the disabling effect of the ictal behavior.

The practice of EEG and video-EEG has undergone very little change over the past three decades. However, there is emerging data to support that the clinical bandwidth of current clinical EEG may be too restricted, and that activity outside the clinical bandwidth is important [49, 50]. This is discussed further below in the context of intracranial EEG.

Magnetic resonance imaging (MRI)

MRI has been demonstrated to be the most sensitive and specific structural neuroimaging procedure in patients with epilepsy [19, 51, 52]. Importantly, MRI is a noninvasive technique that has no known adverse biological effect. The presence of an MRI-identified structural abnormality often will suggest the location of seizure onset. The high diagnostic sensitivity of MRI for lesions, for example, tumor, vascular malformation, enecephalomalcia, low-grade neoplasm, MCD and MTS, is well established [30, 31, 37, 43, 44, 52–54]. There is a broad consensus that MRI identifies MTS with high sensitivity, one of the most common pathologies encountered in patients with intractable partial epilepsy [44]. The importance of MRI in selection of favorable candidates for epilepsy surgery, tailoring the operative resection, and to confirm the extent of the resection postoperatively is well recognized.

The optimal MRI techniques and magnet strength continue to be advanced [55–60]. In patients with partial epilepsy the MRI should include coronal or oblique-coronal images using T1-weighted and T2-weighted sequences. FLAIR sequences have also been shown to increase the sensitivity of MRI to indicate a signal change.

The MRI seizure protocol at the Mayo Clinic Rochester includes: (i) sagittal T1-weighted imaging with minimum echo time (TE) and 500 ms repetition time (TR) required for whole-head coverage with 5 mm thick contiguous sections, (ii) whole-head coronal three-dimensional volumetric spoiled gradient-echo (SPGR) acquisition is performed with minimum full TE and TR, 192 views, one repetition, 1.5 mm section thickness with 124 partitions, 22 cm field of view, and 45 flip angle, and (iii) coronal spin-echo (SE) imaging is performed with TE of 30 and 80 ms, TR greater than 2000 ms, 20 cm field of view, 4 mm section thickness and

2 mm intersection gap, and 192 views with one repetition. An oblique-coronal FLAIR sequence is also obtained. The FLAIR sequence allows the pathological signal change to be differentiated from the physiological signal alteration related to cerebrospinal fluid. Contrast enhancement study will be performed if a space-occupying lesion is detected [51, 52, 61].

15.4 Lesional MRI (or substrate-directed epilepsy syndromes)

Patients with lesional epilepsy may have a primary brain tumor, vascular anomaly, MCD, encephalomalcia, gliosis, or MTS [13, 24, 34, 38, 40, 44]. The common surgical pathologies encountered in patients with lesional epilepsy include a low-grade neoplasm [62–64], vascular malformations such as cavernous hemangioma [65–67] and focal cortical dysplasia [35, 36, 38, 57]. Individuals with MTS and lesional pathology usually have an abnormal MRI study and the seizure-types are classified as substrate-directed partial epilepsy [13, 19]. The MRI in these individuals suggests the likely site of seizure onset. The goal of the presurgical evaluation is to identify the site of seizure onset and initial propagation [23, 27]. In patients with an MRI-identified lesion or unilateral MTS the purpose of the electroclinical correlation is to confirm that the structural abnormality is consistent with region of seizure onset [19, 44]. The demonstration of concordance between the MRI and the SOZ indicates the potential for a favorable operative outcome. Approximately 80% of patients with unilateral MTS, low-grade glial neoplasm, or a cavernous hemangioma are rendered seizure-free with surgical resection of the entire epileptogenic lesion [4, 13, 17, 18, 20, 24, 55, 68–71]. Unfortunately, the operative outcome is currently less favorable for individuals with focal cortical dysplasia and other MCDs [19, 20, 35, 36, 38, 39, 57, 72].

15.5 Functional neuroimaging and intracranial EEG

Functional neuroimaging procedures may not be necessary in patients with a structural MRI abnormality that is concordant with the presurgical evaluation. Both MRS and PET have a good diagnostic yield in patients with TLE [31, 58, 73]. These techniques may be useful in patients with indeterminate structural MRI studies, for example bilateral hippocampal abnormalities [31, 58, 73]. In patients with normal MRI localization of the EZ is challenging. Chronic intracranial EEG monitoring may be required in these patients, especially patients with extratemporal epilepsy. Identification of a localized subtraction ictal SPECT co-registered to MRI (SISCOM) focus may be a reliable indicator of the SOZ [31, 74–78]. SISCOM may reveal a localized region of cerebral hyperperfusion or hypoperfusion [31, 74–78]. The SISCOM findings are also often predictive of operative

MEG, PET and SISCOM Surgical Outcomes			
Diagnostic value	MEG (CI)	PET (CI)	SISCOM (CI)
Sensitivity (%)	31 (12.0–46.9)	54 (31.6–66.3)	62 (38.8–74.0)
Specificity (%)	79 (61.2–93.6)	86 (65.0–97.3)	86 (64.6–97.3)
PPV (%)	57 (22.4–87.2)	78 (45.6–95.8)	80 (50.4–96.2)
NPV (%)	55 (42.8–65.5)	67 (50.6–75.7)	70.6 (53.2–80.1)

Figure 15.2 Diagnostic value of functional imaging studies. Adapted from Knowlton *et al.* (2008) [79].

outcome (Figure 15.2). Ultimately, a decision regarding surgical treatment must be based on a convergence of the neurodiagnostic evaluation [30].

Positron emission tomography (PET)

PET is a functional neuroimaging study that may be useful in identifying a localization-related abnormality and assist the surgical planning in patients with intractable partial epilepsy [58, 73, 80–82]. The most common study used in the evaluation of intractable partial epilepsy is the FDG-PET. The disadvantages of PET include the difficulty in obtaining ictal studies and the cost of the procedure. A cyclotron is required for the production of the short half-life radiopharmaceuticals. The sensitivity of PET in patients with TLE these individuals is reported to approach 90% [83]. The false lateralization rate for PET in patients with unilateral TLE is reported to be approximately 1–2% [83, 84]. The most common interictal FDG-PET abnormality is a region of focal hypometabolism that corresponds to the localization of the EZ [80, 83]. The anatomical region associated with the interictal hypometabolism is characteristically larger than the pathological findings underlying the EZ. The focal hypometabolism may indicate a functional metabolic alteration related to the underlying pathological network generating partial seizures, and does not correlate with focal cell loss in hippocampus [82]. Unfortunately, PET has been shown to be less useful in patients with neocortical epilepsy [83]. Approximately one-third of patients with extra-temporal epilepspy may have a localized PET abnormality indicating the site of seizure onset [85]. The inability to perform peri-ictal studies in patients and the current lack of sensitivity of FDG-PET in non-substrate-directed extratemporal seizures is a significant limitation of PET in the evaluation of potential operative candidates.

Novel positron emission tomography tracers

Imaging the spatial distribution of neuronal receptors using PET may prove useful in patients with localization-related epilepsy [86]. Benzodiazepine receptors (BZDRs) and central opiate receptors can be identified with (11C) flumazenil PET and (11C) carfentanil PET, respectively [86]. Focal BZDR decreases and increased or decreased selected opiate receptor activity may be present in patients with substrate-directed pathology [86].

The PET tracer alpha [11C] methyl-L-tryptophan (AMT) has also been shown to be potentially useful in the assessment of patients with intractable epilepsy [87]. AMT is selectively taken up by epileptogenic cortical malformation in tuberous sclerosis.

Magnetic resonance spectroscopy (MRS)

Proton (1H) MRS has been shown to be a reliable indicator of the temporal lobe of seizure origin in patients with mesial TLE [88–92]. 1H MRS is highly sensitive in the lateralization of temporal lobe seizures by revealing a reduction in N-acetylated compound (NA) concentrations or abnormalities in the creatine (Cr)/NA or NA/choline ratios. The underlying pathogenesis for the metabolic changes are likely to be complex and may relate to focal neuronal loss, gliosis, or a functional alteration intimately associated with the frequency of seizure activity. The diagnostic yield of MRS is similar to structural MRI in patients with mesial TLE related to MTS [93]. The detection of metabolic abnormalities by 1H MRS also correlates with the outcome following temporal lobectomy for intractable partial epilepsy [89, 93]. Preoperative metabolic abnormalities in the contralateral temporal lobe were predictive of operative failure. 1H MRS may be of particular benefit in patients with TLE and normal structural MRI [89, 93]. Proton spectroscopy may also lateralize the epileptic temporal lobe in patients with bilateral HFA. There is limited information regarding the diagnostic yield of 1H MRS in patients with neocortical, extrahippocampal seizures. The potential benefits of proton spectroscopy in patients with nonlesional extratemporal seizures remain to be determined. At present, 1H MRS is an investigative diagnostic tool that is largely restricted to some epilepsy centers. Despite observations of focal metabolic abnormalities in selected patients with nonlesional extratemporal seizures, it is currently not clear if this technique will have a role in patients with non-substrate-directed extratemporal partial epilepsy.

Single-photon emission computed tomography (SPECT)

A primary advantage of SPECT over other functional imaging techniques is the ability to obtain peri-ictal (interictal/ictal/postictal) imaging in patients with partial epilepsy being considered for epilepsy surgery. There is a broad consensus that ictal SPECT studies are superior to interictal images in localization-related epilepsy [28, 30, 85, 94]. SPECT studies involve cerebral blood flow imaging using radio-pharmaceuticals, principally either technetium-99m-hexamethylpropylene amine oxime (99mTc-HMPAO) or 99mTc-bicisate, which have a rapid first pass brain extraction with maximum uptake being achieved within 30–60 seconds of an intravenous injection [28, 30, 74, 77, 78, 85, 94]. These studies may produce a "photograph" of the peri-ictal cerebral perfusion pattern that was present soon after the injection. The SPECT images can be acquired up to four hours after the termination of the seizure so that the individual patient can recover from the ictus prior to being transported to the nuclear medicine laboratory. SPECT studies have an important clinical application in the potential identification of the epileptic brain tissue when the remainder of the noninvasive presurgical evaluation is unable to lateralize or localize the site of seizure onset [30, 85].

The initial blood flow SPECT studies in patients with intractable partial epilepsy involved interictal imaging that variably detected a focal hypoperfusion in the region of the EZ [30, 85]. Interictal SPECT images have proven to have a relatively low sensitivity and a relatively high false positive rate in TLE [85]. Interictal SPECT has also been shown to have a low diagnostic yield in patients with extratemporal seizures [83]. Ictal SPECT studies have been confirmed to be useful in patients with TLE to identify a region of focal hyperperfusion [85]. The rationale for interictal SPECT imaging at present is to serve as a reference for a baseline study for the interpretation of ictal SPECT images. The diagnostic yield of ictal SPECT has been established to be superior to interictal SPECT in patients being considered for surgical resection [78]. The recent development of stabile radiotracers that do not require mixing immediately before injection has made ictal SPECT more practical [74].

Subtraction ictal SPECT co-registered to MRI (SISCOM)

The imaging paradigm using computer-aided SISCOM has been introduced in patients with intractable partial epilepsy [31, 75–78]. SISCOM represents an innovation in neuroimaging that may be useful in the evaluation of patients with non-substrate-directed partial epilepsy [31, 75–78]. Subtracting normalized and co-registered ictal and interictal SPECT images, and then matching the resultant difference image to the high resolution MRI for anatomical correlation has been shown to be useful for localization of the EZ [77]. SISCOM in a series of 51 patients had a higher rate of localization (88.2% vs. 39.2%, p < 0.0001), better inter-observer agreement, and was a better predictor of surgical outcome than visual inspection of the interictal and ictal images [77]. The study demonstrated the inherent problems with visual interpretation of either peri-ictal or interictal SPECT studies alone. The methodology used for SISCOM at the Mayo Clinic involves co-registering of the interictal to the ictal SPECT study using a surface-matching algorithm [75–78].

The clinical parameters that are significant in determining the diagnostic yield of SISCOM include the duration of the seizure and the length of time of the injection from ictal onset. The seizure should be at least 5–10 seconds in duration and the time from seizure onset should be less than 45 seconds for optimal results [76]. The disadvantages of a SISCOM study include the need for hospitalization and long-term EEG monitoring, the use of radioisotopes for two imaging procedures, and the need to record the patient's habitual seizure. The indications for SISCOM in patients undergoing a presurgical evaluation include: non-substrate-directed partial epilepsy and conflicting findings in the noninvasive evaluation. SISCOM has proven to be useful to identify a "target" for placement on intracranial EEG electrodes [30, 95]. The presence of a SISCOM alteration may obviate the need for intracranial EEG recordings in selected patients. For example, patients with non-substrate-directed partial epilepsy of non-dominant temporal lobe origin may not require chronic intracranial EEG monitoring if the extracranial ictal EEG pattern and peri-ictal SPECT studies are concordant. SISCOM also improves the diagnostic yield of postictal studies in patients with intractable partial epilepsy [78].

SPM-SPECT analysis

The above reviewed SPECT and SISCOM imaging methods do not account for the physiological variations expected in cerebral profusion. In particular, the interictal SPECT is a selected sample that will reflect the cerebral blood flow at that time of isotope injection. Recently, statistical parametric mapping (SPM) has been applied to SPECT and SISCOM imaging methods to address this deficiency. SPM-SPECT techniques show significant improvement in localization of epileptogenic brain [96, 97].

Intracranial EEG (iEEG)

Patients with drug-resistant partial epilepsy undergoing evaluation for epilepsy surgery may require implantation of intracranial electrodes to localize the brain region(s) generating seizures. Intracranial EEG is generally considered the clinical gold standard for localizing the SOZ [13, 14, 23, 27, 72, 98], and is used to guide resective surgery. Without an MRI lesion, however, there is currently *no clear definition beyond the SOZ* and seizure propagation to guide what must be resected for seizure freedom. While interictal epileptiform spikes and sharp-waves are established signatures of epileptic brain [13, 14, 23, 27], and studies demonstrate that iEEG spikes are increased in the SOZ [99], it is well known that the brain regions mapped by interictal spikes generally extend well beyond what must be resected for seizure freedom. For example, the presence of independent bitemporal spikes in unilateral TLE is well known [24]. Clearly, the spikes should not be used to direct surgery to the contralateral temporal lobe. The standard practice in most epilepsy centers is to record a patient's habitual seizures and use the SOZ determined by iEEG to guide surgical resection. Recent studies have demonstrated the importance of seizure onset pattern recorded by iEEG in the localization of the EZ and outcome from resective surgery [100–102].

Despite advances in digital electronics and computing that have revolutionized animal electrophysiology [103, 104], clinical iEEG continues to utilize narrow bandwidth (0.1–100 Hz) recordings from widely spaced (5–10 mm) macroelectrodes (>1 mm^2). The optimal spatial and spectral resolution for recording seizures remains and area of active research. The spatial organization of the human brain extends from submillimeter diameter cortical columns to centimeter scale lobar structures. The activity generated by these neural assemblies ranges from DC to high-frequency oscillations (DC–1000 Hz). This remarkable range of human brain electrophysiology is not probed by current clinical iEEG [103, 105–109].

15.6   Symptomatic partial epilepsy

The three major categories of symptomatic partial epilepsy are as follows: (i) mesial temporal lobe epilepsy (mTLE); (ii) lesional epilepsy; and (iii) nonlesional neocortical epilepsy [21]. Partial seizures disorders account for the majority of epilepsy [110]. In one tertiary center cohort of 2200 patients, partial epilepsy was more than twice as common as symptomatic, cryptogenic, and idiopathic generalized epilepsies combined. Moreover, in that study two-thirds of the partial seizure disorders localized to the temporal lobe [111]. Unfortunately, despite optimal medical therapy many patients continue to experience seizures [110, 112]. As has been discussed above surgery is an established therapeutic option for DRE.

Mesial temporal sclerosis

The EZ in the temporal lobe most often involves the amygdalohippocampal complex. A common pathological substrate of mTLE is MTS [12]. The surgically excised hippocampus in these patients almost invariably shows neuron loss and gliosis [113]. MRI findings in patients with MTS include hippocampal atrophy and an increased mesial temporal T2 signal intensity [44, 61]. Inspection of a seizure protocol MRI will allow detection of 80–90% of the cases of MTS [44, 61]. The hippocampal atrophy is most obvious using the T1-weighted image in the oblique-coronal plane. The signal intensity alteration can be identified using T2-weighted imaging or the FLAIR sequence in the oblique-coronal plane. The oblique-coronal planes are useful for MRI studies in patients with MTS because of the ability to directly compare the two hippocampi for any side to side asymmetry [44, 61]. Potential limitations of visual inspection of the MRI in patients with suspected

MTS includes head rotation, symmetrical bilateral hippocampal atrophy, subtle unilateral atrophy or signal intensity alteration. Most importantly, visual inspection is a subjective determination that is strongly dependent on the inspector's expertise for appropriate interpretation. Three-dimensional SPGR images are helpful since they are reformatted into true anatomic coronal plane.

MRI-based quantitative hippocampal formation volumetric studies have been developed to objectively determine the degree of hippocampal volume loss in patients with MTS [51, 52, 61]. Absolute hippocampal volume measurements are performed using a standardized protocol with the results being compared to age-matched normal controls to assign abnormal values [114]. A unilateral reduction in hippocampal volume has been shown to be a reliable indicator of the temporal lobe of seizure origin in patients with medically refractory partial epilepsy. A history of a neurologic illness in childhood, for example, febrile seizure, head trauma, or meningitis, appears to be important risk factors for the development of MTS [114–116]. The duration of epilepsy and age at the time of surgery have not correlated with volumetric results in most studies.

The identification of MTS in the surgically excised temporal lobe is a favorable prognostic for seizure control following epilepsy surgery [12]. Nearly 90% of patients with unilateral hippocampal atrophy are rendered seizure-free [12, 24]. MRI is also a recognized predictor of neurocognitive outcome in patients undergoing anterior temporal lobectomy [117]. Patients with normal left hippocampal volumes are at significantly greater risk for experiencing a significant decline in cognitive performance following a left medial temporal lobe resection compared to patients with left hippocampal atrophy [118, 119].

Primary brain neoplasms

The epileptogenic potential of primary brain neoplasms has been recognized since the initial work of J. Hughlings Jackson over a century ago. Low-grade, slowly growing tumors are most commonly associated with a chronic seizure disorder [120]. The histopathology commonly associated with seizures includes the following tumors: oligodendroglioma, fibrillary astrocytoma, pilocytic astrocytoma, mixed glioma, ganglioglioma, and dysembroblastic neuroepithelial tumor (DNET). The DNET probably is more closely related to a disorder of cortical development than a primary brain neoplasm [63, 121]. Imaging features common to all these tumors include a typically small size, localization at or near a cortical surface, sharply defined borders, little or no surrounding edema and, with the exception of the pilocytic astrocytomas, little or no contrast enhancement. Most patients with primary CNS tumors and chronic epilepsy do not present with progressive neurological deficits, "changing" neurological examination or evidence for increased intracranial pressure [120].

Vascular malformations

There are four types of congenital cerebral vascular malformations: arteriovenous malformations (AVMs), cavernous hemangiomas, venous angiomas, and telangiectasias [52, 66, 67, 122, 123]. The epileptogenic potential of these pathological lesions is quite different. The common malformations resected for partial epilepsy are cavernous hemangiomas and AVMs. Seizures may in fact be are often the only clinical manifestation with these lesions. Venous angiomas and telangiectasias are often incidental findings in patients with seizure disorders. MRI is essential for the recognition and diagnosis of cavernous hemangiomas and occult AVMs. AVMs may be associated with a flow signal on MRI. Cavernous hemangiomas characteristically have a target appearance on T2-weighted images with a region of increased T2 signal intensity surrounded by an area of decreased signal produced by remote (often occult) hemorrhage with methemoglobin deposition. Resection typically leads to complete or significant improvement in seizure control.

Malformations of cortical development

MCD are an important etiology for symptomatic partial epilepsy [36, 38, 57, 124, 125]. The use of MRI has allowed recognition of these lesions and demonstrated the frequency and importance of cortical developmental malformations in patients with intractable partial epilepsy. A variety of developmental abnormalities have been recognized that are commonly associated with medically refractory seizures and neurocognitive decline [126]. Cerebral developmental malformations could previously only be diagnosed by postmortem examination. MRI is essential for the diagnosis and proper classificiation of these pathological lesions.

A classification of the developmental abnormalities has been introduced by Kuzniecky based on the structural neuroimaging findings [127]. The disorders of cortical development have been classified by localization of the pathological lesions: generalized or diffuse disorders, unilateral disorders, focal disorders, and diffuse disorders [38, 127]. The generalized disorders include lissencephaly, "double cortex" or band heterotopia, subependymal heterotopia, and megalencephaly. Hemimegalencephaly is a unilateral cortical developmental malformation. Focal disorders include the following: focal cortical dysplasia, polymicrogyria, schizencephaly, and focal subcortical heterotopia. Focal cortical dysplasias are the most often considered for surgical resection [38, 127]. Thin section three-dimensional volumetric MRI is extremely useful in evaluating these anomalies. It is difficult to resolve volume-averaged normal cortical infolding from true areas of abnormalities if the spatial resolution of the images is coarser than 1.5 mm. Reformatting of 1.5 mm three-dimensional SPGR MRI sequences is also helpful. Tuberous sclerosis can present as a focal or diffuse developmental abnormality.

15.7 Non-lesional MRI (non-substrate-directed partial epilepsy)

The seizure-types in patients with localization-related seizure disorders and normal MRI studies are classified as non-substrate-directed partial epilepsy [127]. The anatomical localization of the EZ in these individuals commonly involves the neocortex, that is, extrahippocampal [38, 52, 127]. The surgical pathology in these patients includes gliosis, focal cell loss, MCD, or no clear histopathological abnormality [120]. The MRI may be indeterminate in selected lesional pathology, for example, focal cortical dysplasia [127]. The primary determinant of outcome in patients with normal MRI is the origin of seizure onset. Patients with normal MRI and TLE have significantly higher probability of excellent outcome compared to patients with extratemporal lobe epilepsy (Table 15.4).

The reason for the unfavorable operative outcome in patients with non-substrate-directed partial epilepsy is the inherent difficulty identifying the EZ [120]. The potential limitations of interictal and ictal extracranial and intracranial EEG monitoring in patients with partial seizures of extratemporal origin have been well defined [120]. The anatomical region of epileptic brain in these patients is often spatially diffuse making a complete resection of the EZ difficult. A large resection increases the likelihood of rendering the patient seizure-free, but increases the potential for operative morbidity [38, 120, 125]. Advances in peri-ictal SPECT

Table 15.4 Surgical outcomes for localization-related partial epilepsy (surgically remediable syndromes)

Localization-related partial	Outcomes (excellent[a]) (%)
Epilepsy syndrome	
Temporal lobe epilepsy	
Lesional (pathological substrate)	(70–90) [13, 17, 18, 24, 128]
Nonlesional (cryptogenic)	(48–65)
	49–60 [97]
	65 [129]
	48 [130]
Extratemporal epilepsy	
Lesional (pathological substrate)	(66–72)
	72 [131]
	66 [41]
	67 [120]
Nonlesional (cryptogenic)	(25–41)
	41 [131]
	37 [39]
	29 [41]
	25 [120]

[a] There is some variability in definition of excellent outcome across studies.

imaging have assisted the selection of operative candidates with non-substrate-directed partial epilepsy, altered the preoperative evaluation, and tailored the surgical excision. Contemporary neuroimaging studies used to localize the EZ in patients with non-substrate-directed partial epilepsy being considered for surgical treatment include PET, MRS, and SPECT [82, 84–87, 132].

When MRI fails to demonstrate a potentially epileptogenic lesion, the chance of excellent surgical outcome is lowered [12, 20, 28, 101, 133, 134]. Surgical results for extratemporal epilepsy with normal preoperative MRI findings can be particularly poor, likely reflecting the difficulty with accurate localization and resection of the EZ. The reported frequency of excellent surgical outcomes for nonlesional partial epilepsy is 48–65% for the temporal lobe [130], 37% for mixed mesial temporal and neocortical [60, 135, 136], and 25–56% for extratemporal epilepsy [24, 41, 134, 131, 137]. However, the reports of seizure-free outcome in nonlesional extratemporal disease are all based on relatively small case series (Smith *et al.* [41] $n = 17$; Mosewich *et al.* [131] $n = 24$; Chapman *et al.* [39] $n = 10$; Sylaja *et al.* [137] $n = 17$). Without a clear anatomic lesion, localization of the epileptogenic region must rely on scalp and intracranial EEG recording, magnetoencephalography, or functional imaging tests such as SPECT or PET.

15.8   Non-lesional temporal lobe epilepsy (surgically remediable syndrome?)

Temporal lobectomy has been shown to render about 80% of patients seizure-free if a MRI structural abnormality is concordant to the SOZ [13]. On the other hand, patients with TLE and normal MRI have received less attention and physicians may be reluctant to consider surgery for TLE when structural neuroimaging appears normal. Existing research suggests disparate rates of successful surgery in patients with nonlesional MRI [70, 137–140]. Some of these studies were conducted during the 1980s and early 1990s, prior to the widespread use of epilepsy neuroimaging protocols that are more sensitive for detecting MTS. Some studies have used pathologic findings to categorize patients [20, 69], which is not available preoperatively for clinical prognostication. Other studies include heterogeneous patient populations and only small numbers of patients with nonlesional MRI.

We recently examined the efficacy of epilepsy surgery and noninvasive predictors of favorable outcome for patients with drug-resistant TLE and a normal seizure protocol MRI [1]. We identified a cohort of 40 patients with a normal "mayo seizure protocol" MRI who underwent anterior temporal lobectomy. Engel class I outcomes (free of disabling seizures) were observed in 60% (24/40) patients. Preoperative factors associated with Engel class I outcome were: (i) absence of contralateral or extratemporal interictal epileptiform discharges, (ii) SISCOM localized to the resection site, and (iii) subtle nonspecific MRI findings in the mesial temporal lobe concordant to the resection. In conclusion, carefully selected patients with TLE and nonlesional MRI anterior temporal lobectomy often are rendered seizure-free. This favorable rate of surgical success is likely due to the detection of concordant abnormalities indicating unilateral TLE and the use of standard temporal lobectomy that includes anterior temporal neocortex and the amygdala-hippocampal structure.

15.9 Surgical advances

The use of gamma-knife for treatment of DRE is currently under investigation. While the use of gamma-knife for treatment of AVM is widely used, the role of gamma-knife for treatment of substrate-directed epilepsy remains investigational [141, 142]. The current data suggest slightly reduced and delayed efficacy compared to resective surgery for mesial temporal epilepsy. The post-procedure morbidity and mortality are higher, and currently there is no convincing evidence that there are cognitive benefits.

Whether gamma-knife has a role in treatment of seizures that co-localize with eloqent brain or regions that are not safely accessible for resection remains unexplored [142].

References

1. Bell, G.S., Bell, G.S., Gaitatzis, A., Bell, C.L., Johnson, A.L., and Sander, J.W. (2008) Drowning in people with epilepsy: how great is the risk? *Neurology*, **71** (8), 578–582.
2. Hitiris, N., Mohanraj, R., Norrie, J., and Brodie, M.J. *et al.* (2007) Mortality in epilepsy. *Epilepsy Behav*, **10** (3), 363–376.
3. So, E.L., Bainbridge, J., Buchhalter, J.R. *et al.* (2009) Report of the American Epilepsy Society and the Epilepsy Foundation joint task force on sudden unexplained death in epilepsy. *Epilepsia*, **50** (4), 917–22.
4. Engel, J. Jr. (2008) Surgical treatment for epilepsy: too little, too late? *J Am Med Assoc*, **300** (21), 2548–2550.
5. Kwan, P. and Brodie, M.J. (2000) Early identification of refractory epilepsy. *N Engl J Med*, **342** (5), 314–319.
6. Murray, G. and Lopez, A. (1994) Global Comparative Assessments in the Health Sector: Disease Burden, Expenditure, Intervention Packages, World Health Organization, Geneva, Switzerland.
7. Berg, A.T. (2004) Understanding the delay before epilepsy surgery: who develops intractable focal epilepsy and when? *CNS Spectr*, **9** (2), 136–144.
8. Kwan, P. and Brodie, M.J. (2004) Drug treatment of epilepsy: when does it fail and how to optimize its use? *CNS Spectr*, **9** (2), 110–119.
9. Fisher, R.S., Vickrey, B.G., Gibson, P. *et al.* (2000) The impact of epilepsy from the patient's perspective I. Descriptions and subjective perceptions. *Epilepsy Res*, **41** (1), 39–51.
10. Callaghan, B.C., Anand, K., Hesdorffer, D., Hauser, W.A., and French, J.A. (2007) Likelihood of seizure remission in an adult population with refractory epilepsy. *Ann Neurol*, **62** (4), 382–389.

11. French, J.A. (2006) Refractory epilepsy: one size does not fit all. *Epilepsy Curr*, **6** (6), 177–180.
12. Cascino, G., Boon, P., and Fish, D. (1993) Surgically remediable lesional syndromes, in *Surgical Treatment of the Epilepsies* (ed. J.J. Engel), Raven Press, New York, pp. 77–86.
13. Cascino, G.D. (2004) Surgical treatment for epilepsy. *Epilepsy Res*, **60** (2–3), 179–186.
14. Engel, J.J. and Pedley, T.A. (1997) *Epilepsy: A Comprehensive Textbook*, Lippincott-Raven Publishers, Philadelphia, PA.
15. Luders, J.J. and Comair, Y. (eds) (2001) *Epilepsy Surgery*, Lippincott Williams & Wilkins, Philadelphia, PA.
16. Choi, H., Sell, R.L., Lenert, L. *et al.* (2008) Epilepsy surgery for pharmacoresistant temporal lobe epilepsy: a decision analysis. *J Am Med Assoc*, **300** (21), 2497–2505.
17. Wiebe, S., Blume, W.T., Girvin, J.P., and Eliasziw, M. (2001) A randomized, controlled trial of surgery for temporal-lobe epilepsy. *N Engl J Med*, **345** (5), 311–318 [see comment].
18. Engel, J. Jr., Wiebe, S., French, J. *et al.* (2003) Practice parameter: temporal lobe and localized neocortical resections for epilepsy: report of the Quality Standards Subcommittee of the American Academy of Neurology, in association with the American Epilepsy Society and the American Association of Neurological Surgeons. *Neurology*, **60** (4), 538–547.
19. Cascino, G., Boon, P., and Fish, D. (1993) Surgically remedial lesional syndromes, in *Surgical Treatment of the Epilepsies* (ed. J.J. Engel), Raven Press, New York, pp. 77–86.
20. Cohen-Gadol, A.A., Cohen-Gadol, A.A., Wilhelmi, B.G., Collignon, F. *et al.* (2006) Long-term outcome of epilepsy surgery among 399 patients with nonlesional seizure foci including mesial temporal lobe sclerosis. *J Neurosurg*, **104** (4), 513–524.
21. Engel, J., Weiser, H.G., and Spencer, D. (1997) Overview: surgical therapy, in *Epilepsy: A Comprehensive Textbook* (eds J. Engel and T.A. Pedley), Lippincott-Raven Publishers, Philadelphia, PA, pp. 1673–1676.
22. Engel, J.J. (1996) Principles of epilepsy surgery, in *The Treatment of Epilepsy* (eds S. Shorvon, F. Dreifuss, and D. Fish), Blackwell, Oxford, pp. 519–529.
23. Luders, H. (1992) *Epilepsy Surgery*, Raven Press, New York.
24. Radhakrishnan, K., So, E.L., Silbert, P.L. *et al.* (1998) Predictors of outcome of anterior temporal lobectomy for intractable epilepsy: a multivariate study. *Neurology*, **51** (2), 465–471.
25. Spencer, S. and Huh, L. (2008) Outcomes of epilepsy surgery in adults and children. *Lancet Neurol*, **7** (6), 525–537.
26. Tellez-Zenteno, J.F., and Wiebe, S. (2008) Long-term seizure and psychosocial outcomes of epilepsy surgery. *Curr Treat Options Neurol*, **10** (4), 253–259.
27. Luders, H. and Awad, I. (1992) Conceptual Considerations, in *Epilepsy Surgery* (ed. H. Luders), Raven Press, New York, pp. 51–62.
28. Cascino, G.D., Buchhalter, J.R., Mullan, B.P., and So, E.L. (2004) Ictal SPECT in nonlesional extratemporal epilepsy. *Epilepsia*, **45** (Suppl 4), 32–34.
29. Cascino, G.D. and O'Brien, T.J. (2001) Resection for Epilepsy in the setting of a nonlocalizing MRI, in *Treatment of Epilepsy* (ed. E. Wyllie), Lippincott Williams and Williams, Philadelphia, PA, pp. 1135–1145.
30. So, E.L. (2000) Integration of EEG, MRI, and SPECT in localizing the seizure focus for epilepsy surgery. *Epilepsia*, **41** (Suppl 3), S48–S54.
31. So, E.L. (2002) Role of neuroimaging in the management of seizure disorders. *Mayo Clin Proc*, **77** (11), 1251–1264.
32. Spencer, S., Sperling, M., and Shewmon, D. (1997) Intracranial Electrodes, in *Epilepsy: A Comprehensive Textbook* (eds J. Engel Jr. and T. Pedley), Lippincott-Raven Publishers, Philadelphia, PA, pp. 1719–1747.

33. Cascino, G.D. (2001) Advances in neuroimaging: surgical localization. *Epilepsia*, **42**, 3–12.

34. Awad, I.A. *et al.* (1991) Intractable epilepsy and structural lesions of the brain: mapping, resection strategies, and seizure outcome. *Epilepsia*, **32** (2), 179–186.

35. Alonso-Nanclares, L., Garbelli, R., Sola, R.G. *et al.* (2005) Microanatomy of the dysplastic neocortex from epileptic patients. *Brain*, **128** (Pt 1), 158–173.

36. Fauser, S., Huppertz, H.J., Bast, T. *et al.* (2006) Clinical characteristics in focal cortical dysplasia: a retrospective evaluation in a series of 120 patients. *Brain*, **129** (Pt 7), 1907–1916.

37. Kim, D.W., Lee, S.K., Chu, K. *et al.* (2009) Predictors of surgical outcome and pathologic considerations in focal cortical dysplasia. *Neurology*, **72** (3), 211–6.

38. Palmini, A., Andermann, F., Olivier, A. *et al.* (1991) Focal neuronal migration disorders and intractable partial epilepsy: a study of 30 patients. *Ann Neurol*, **30** (6), 741–749.

39. Chapman, K., Wyllie, E., Najm, I. *et al.* (2005) Seizure outcome after epilepsy surgery in patients with normal preoperative MRI. *J Neurol Neurosurg Psychiatry*, **76** (5), 710–713.

40. Mosewich, R.K., So, E.L., O'Brien, T.J. *et al.* (2000) Factors predictive of the outcome of frontal lobe epilepsy surgery. *Epilepsia*, **41** (7), 843–849.

41. Smith, J.R., Lee, M.R., King, D.W. *et al.* (1997) Results of lesional vs. nonlesional frontal lobe epilepsy surgery. *Stereotact Funct Neurosurg*, **69** (1-4, Pt 2), 202–209.

42. Schomer, D.L. and Black, P.M. (2008) A 24-year-old woman with intractable seizures: review of surgery for epilepsy. *J Am Med Assoc*, **300** (21), 2527–2538.

43. Jeha, L.E., Najm, I., Bingaman, W. *et al.* (2007) Surgical outcome and prognostic factors of frontal lobe epilepsy surgery. *Brain*, **130** (Pt 2), 574–584.

44. Kuznicky, R.I., Bilir, E., Gilliam, F. *et al.* (1997) Multimodality MRI in mesial temporal sclerosis: relative sensitivity and specificity. *Neurology*, **49** (3), 774–778.

45. Cascino, G.D., Hopkins, A., and Shorvon, S.D. (eds) (1995) *Epilepsy*, Lippincott Williams & Wilkins, Philadelphia, PA.

46. Malow, B.A., Foldvary-Schaefer, N., Vaughn, B.V. *et al.* (2008) Treating obstructive sleep apnea in adults with epilepsy: a randomized pilot trial. *Neurology*, **71** (8), 572–577.

47. Chen, D.K., Graber, K.D., Anderson, C.T., Fisher, R.S. (2008) Sensitivity and specificity of video alone versus electroencephalography alone for the diagnosis of partial seizures. *Epilepsy Behav*, **13** (1), 115–118.

48. So, E.L. (2006) Value and limitations of seizure semiology in localizing seizure onset. *J Clin Neurophysiol*, **23** (4), 353–357.

49. Curio, G. (2000) Ain't no rhythm fast enough: EEG bands beyond beta. *J Clin Neurophysiol*, **17** (4), 339–340.

50. Vanhatalo, S., Voipio, J., and Kaila, K. (2005) Full-band EEG (FbEEG): an emerging standard in electroencephalography. *Clin Neurophysiol*, **116** (1), 1–8.

51. Jack, C.R. Jr. (1995) Magnetic resonance imaging. Neuroimaging and anatomy. *Neuroimaging Clin N Am*, **5** (4), 597–622.

52. Jack, C.R. Jr. (1996) Magnetic resonance imaging in epilepsy. *Mayo Clin Proc*, **71** (7), 695–711.

53. Berkovic, S. McIntosh A.M., Kalnins R.M. *et al.* (1995) Preoperative MRI predicts outcome of temporal lobectomy: an actuarial analysis. *Neurology*, **45**, 1358–1363.

54. Yun, C.H. Lee, S.K., Lee, S. Y. *et al.* (2006) Prognostic factors in neocortical epilepsy surgery: multivariate analysis. *Epilepsia*, **47** (3), 574–579.

55. Glikmann-Johnston, Y., Saling, M.M., Chen, J. *et al.* (2008) Structural and functional correlates of unilateral mesial temporal lobe spatial memory impairment. *Brain*, **131** (Pt 11), 3006–3018.

56. Kanner, A.M. (2008) Can fMRI replace the Wada test in predicting postsurgical deterioration of verbal memory? *Nat Clin Pract Neurol*, **4** (7), 364–365.

57. Krsek, P. (2009) Incomplete resection of focal cortical dysplasia is the main predictor of poor postsurgical outcome. *Neurology*, **72** (3), 217–23.

58. Carne, R.P., O'Brien, T.J., Kilpatrick, C.J. *et al.* (2007) 'MRI-negative PET-positive' temporal lobe epilepsy (TLE) and mesial TLE differ with quantitative MRI and PET: a case control study. *BMC Neurol*, **7**, 16.

59. Dunn, J.F., Tuor, U.I., Kmech, J. *et al.* (2009) Functional brain mapping at 9.4T using a new MRI-compatible electrode chronically implanted in rats. *Magn Reson Med*, **61** (1), 222–228.

60. Madhavan, D. and Kuzniecky, R. (2007) Temporal lobe surgery in patients with normal MRI. *Curr Opin Neurol*, **20** (2), 203–207.

61. Jack, C.R. Jr., Rydberg, C.H., Krecke, K.N. *et al.* (1996) Mesial temporal sclerosis: diagnosis with fluid-attenuated inversion-recovery versus spin-echo MR imaging. *Radiology*, **199** (2), 367–373 [see comment].

62. Andermann, L.F. Savard, G., Meencke, H.J. *et al.* (1999) Psychosis after resection of ganglioglioma or DNET: evidence for an association. *Epilepsia*, **40** (1), 83–87.

63. Burneo, J.G., Tellez-Zenteno, J., Steven, D.A. *et al.* (2008) Adult-onset epilepsy associated with dysembryoplastic neuroepithelial tumors. *Seizure*, **17** (6), 498–504.

64. Schramm, J. and Aliashkevich, A.F. (2008) Surgery for temporal mediobasal tumors: experience based on a series of 235 patients. *Neurosurgery*, **62** (6, Suppl 3), 1272–1282.

65. Stavrou, I., Baumgartner, C., Frischer, J.M., Trattnig, S., Knosp, E. *et al.* (2008) Long-term seizure control after resection of supratentorial cavernomas: a retrospective single-center study in 53 patients. *Neurosurgery*, **63** (5), 888–896; discussion 897.

66. Dodick, D.W., Cascino, G.D., and Meyer, F.B. (1994) Vascular malformations and intractable epilepsy: outcome after surgical treatment. *Mayo Clin Proc*, **69** (8), 741–745.

67. Kraemer, D.L. and Awad, I.A. (1994) Vascular malformations and epilepsy: clinical considerations and basic mechanisms. *Epilepsia*, **35** (Suppl 6), S30–S43.

68. Lowe, A.J., David, E., Kilpatrick, C.J. *et al.* (2004) Epilepsy surgery for pathologically proven hippocampal sclerosis provides long-term seizure control and improved quality of life. *Epilepsia*, **45** (3), 237–242 [see comment].

69. McIntosh, A.M., Kalnins, R.M., Mitchell, L.A. *et al.* (2004) Temporal lobectomy: long-term seizure outcome, late recurrence and risks for seizure recurrence. *Brain*, **127** (Pt 9), 2018–2030.

70. Jeha, L.E., Najm, I.M., Bingaman, W.E. *et al.* (2006) Predictors of outcome after temporal lobectomy for the treatment of intractable epilepsy. *Neurology*, **66** (12), 1938–1940.

71. Janszky, J., Janszky, I., Schulz, R. *et al.* (2005) Temporal lobe epilepsy with hippocampal sclerosis: predictors for long-term surgical outcome. *Brain*, **128** (Pt 2), 395–404.

72. Quesney, L.F. (2000) Intracranial EEG investigation in neocortical epilepsy. *Adv Neurol*, **84**, 253–274.

73. Carne, R.P., O'Brien, T.J., Kilpatrick, C.J. *et al.* (2004) MRI-negative PET-positive temporal lobe epilepsy: a distinct surgically remediable syndrome. *Brain*, **127** (Pt 10), 2276–2285.

74. O'Brien, T.J., Brinkmann, B.H., Mullan, B.P. *et al.* (1999) Comparative study of 99mTc-ECD and 99mTc-HMPAO for peri-ictal SPECT: qualitative and quantitative analysis. *J Neurol Neurosurg Psychiatry*, **66** (3), 331–339.

75. O'Brien, T.J., So, E.L., Cascino, G.D. *et al.* (2004) Subtraction SPECT coregistered to MRI in focal malformations of cortical development: localization of the epileptogenic zone in epilepsy surgery candidates. *Epilepsia*, **45** (4), 367–376.

76. O'Brien, T.J., So, E.L., Mullan, B.P. *et al.* (2000) Subtraction peri-ictal SPECT is predictive of extratemporal epilepsy surgery outcome. *Neurology*, **55** (11), 1668–1677.

77. O'Brien, T.J., O'Connor, M.K., Mullan, B.P. *et al.* (1998) Subtraction ictal SPECT coregistered to MRI improves clinical usefulness of SPECT in localizing the surgical seizure focus. *Neurology*, **50** (2), 445–454.

78. O'Brien, T.J., So, E.L., Mullan, B.P. *et al.* (1999) Subtraction SPECT co-registered to MRI improves postictal SPECT localization of seizure foci. *Neurology*, **52** (1), 137–146.

79. Knowlton, R.C., Elgavish, R.A., Bartolucci, A. *et al.* (2008) Functional imaging: II. Prediction of epilepsy surgery outcome. *Ann Neurol*, **64** (1), 35–41.

80. Theodore, W.H., Sato, S., Kufta, C.V., Gaillard, W.D., and Kelley, K. (1997) FDG-positron emission tomography and invasive EEG: seizure focus detection and surgical outcome. *Epilepsia*, **38** (1), 81–86.

81. Salamon, N., Salamon, N., Kung, J., Shaw, S.J. *et al.* (2008) FDG-PET/MRI coregistration improves detection of cortical dysplasia in patients with epilepsy. *Neurology*, **71** (20), 1594–1601.

82. Henry, T.R., Babb, T.L., Engel, J., Jr. *et al.* (1994) Hippocampal neuronal loss and regional hypometabolism in temporal lobe epilepsy. *Ann Neurol*, **36** (6), 925–927.

83. Ho, S.S., Berkovic, S.F., Berlangieri, S.U. *et al.* (1995) Comparison of ictal SPECT and interictal PET in the presurgical evaluation of temporal lobe epilepsy. *Ann Neurol*, **37** (6), 738–745.

84. Theodore, W. (ed.) (1996) in *Positron Emission Tomography in the Evaluation of Epilepsy* (eds G.D. Cascino and C.R. Jack Jr.), Butterworth-Heinemann, Boston, pp. 165–175.

85. Spencer, S.S. (1994) The relative contributions of MRI, SPECT, and PET imaging in epilepsy. *Epilepsia*, **35** (Suppl 6), S72–S89.

86. Sata, Y., Sata, Y., Matsuda, K., Mihara, T. *et al.* (2002) Quantitative analysis of benzodiazepine receptor in temporal lobe epilepsy: [(125)I]iomazenil autoradiographic study of surgically resected specimens. *Epilepsia*, **43** (9), 1039–1048.

87. Juhasz, C., Chugani, D.C., Muzik, O. *et al.* (2003) Alpha-methyl-L-tryptophan PET detects epileptogenic cortex in children with intractable epilepsy. *Neurology*, **60** (6), 960–968.

88. Suhy, J., Laxer, K.D., Capizzano, A.A. *et al.* (2002) 1H MRSI predicts surgical outcome in MRI-negative temporal lobe epilepsy. *Neurology*, **58** (5), 821–823.

89. Kuzniecky, R. (1999) Magnetic resonance spectroscopy in focal epilepsy: 31P and 1H spectroscopy. *Rev Neurol (Paris)*, **155** (6–7), 495–498.

90. Vermathen, P., Vermathen, P., Ende, G., Laxer, K.D. *et al.* (1997) Hippocampal N-acetylaspartate in neocortical epilepsy and mesial temporal lobe epilepsy. *Ann Neurol*, **42** (2), 194–199.

91. Duncan, J.S. (1997) Imaging and epilepsy. *Brain*, **120** (Pt 2), 339–377.

92. Duncan, J.S. (1996) Magnetic resonance spectroscopy. *Epilepsia*, **37** (7), 598–605.

93. Cendes, F., Caramanos Z, Andermann F, Dubeau F, and Arnold D.L. (1997) Proton magnetic resonance spectroscopic imaging and magnetic resonance imaging volumetry in the lateralization of temporal lobe epilepsy: a series of 100 patients. *Ann Neurol*, **42** (5), 737–746.

94. Kutsy, R.L., Farrell, D.F., and Ojemann, G.A. (1999) Ictal patterns of neocortical seizures monitored with intracranial electrodes: correlation with surgical outcome. *Epilepsia*, **40** (3), 257–266.

95. Tan, K.M., Britton, J.W., Buchhalter, J.R. *et al.* (2008) Influence of subtraction ictal SPECT on surgical management in focal epilepsy of indeterminate localization: a prospective study. *Epilepsy Res*, **82** (2–3), 190–193.

96. Chang, D.J., Zubal, I.G., Gottschalk, C. *et al.* (2002) Comparison of statistical parametric mapping and SPECT difference imaging in patients with temporal lobe epilepsy. *Epilepsia*, **43** (1), 68–74.

97. Kazemi, N.J., Worrell, G.A., Stead, S.M. *et al.* (2010) Ictal SPECT statistical parametric mapping in temporal lobe epilepsy surgery. *Neurology*, **74** (1), 70–76.

98. Quesney, L.F., Constain, M, Rasmussen, T, Olivier, A, Palmini, A (1992) Presurgical EEG investigation in frontal lobe epilepsy. *Epilepsy Res Suppl*, **5**, 55–69.

99. Theodore, W.H. and Fisher, R.S. (2004) Brain stimulation for epilepsy. *Lancet Neurol*, **3** (2), 111–118.

100. Lee, S.A., Spencer, D.D., and Spencer, S.S. (2000) Intracranial EEG seizure-onset patterns in neocortical epilepsy. *Epilepsia*, **41** (3), 297–307.

101. Wetjen, N.M., Marsh, W.R., Meyer, F.B. *et al.* (2009) Intracranial electroencephalography seizure onset patterns and surgical outcomes in nonlesional extratemporal epilepsy. *J Neurosurg*, **110** (6), 1147–52.

102. Worrell, G., Parish, Landi, Cranstoun, S.D. *et al.* (2004) High Frequency Oscillations and Ictogenesis in Neocortical Epilepsy. *Brain*, **127** (7), 1496–506.

103. Bragin, A., Engel, J., Jr., Wilson, C.L., Fried, I., Buzsaki, G. (1999) High-frequency oscillations in human brain. *Hippocampus*, **9** (2), 137–142.

104. Buzsaki, G. (2004) Large-scale recording of neuronal ensembles. *Nat Neurosci*, **7** (5), 446–451.

105. Bragin, A., Wilson, C.L., Staba, R.J. *et al.* (2002) Interictal high-frequency oscillations (80-500 Hz) in the human epileptic brain: entorhinal cortex. *Ann Neurol*, **52** (4), 407–415.

106. Engel, J. Jr., Bragin, A., Staba, R., Mody, I. (2008) High-frequency oscillations: What is normal and what is not? *Epilepsia*.

107. Worrell, G.A., Gardner, A.B., Stead, S.M. *et al.* (2008) High-frequency oscillations in human temporal lobe: simultaneous microwire and clinical macroelectrode recordings. *Brain*, **131** (Pt 4), 928–937.

108. Jirsch, J.D., Urrestarazu, E., LeVan, P. *et al.* (2006) High-frequency oscillations during human focal seizures. *Brain*, **129** (Pt 6), 1593–1608.

109. Urrestarazu, E., Chander, R., Dubeau, F., Gotman, J. (2007) Interictal high-frequency oscillations (100-500 Hz) in the intracerebral EEG of epileptic patients. *Brain*, **130** (Pt 9), 2354–2366.

110. Sander, J.W., Hart, Y.M., Johnson, A.L., Shorvon, S.D. (1990) National General Practice Study of Epilepsy: newly diagnosed epileptic seizures in a general population. *Lancet*, **336** (8726), 1267–1271.

111. Semah, F., Picot, M.C., Adam, C. *et al.* (1998) Is the underlying cause of epilepsy a major prognostic factor for recurrence? *Neurology*, **51** (5), 1256–1262 [see comment].

112. Wiebe, S., Blume, W.T., Girvin, J.P., and Eliasziw, M. (2001) A randomized, controlled trial of surgery for temporal-lobe epilepsy. *N Engl J Med*, **345** (5), 311–318.

113. Jay, V. and Becker, L.E. (1994) Surgical pathology of epilepsy: a review. *Pediatr Pathol*, **14** (4), 731–750.

114. Cascino, G.D., Trenerry, M.R., So, E.L. *et al.* (1996) Routine EEG and temporal lobe epilepsy: relation to long-term EEG monitoring, quantitative MRI, and operative outcome. *Epilepsia*, **37** (7), 651–656.

115. Pringle, C., Blume, W.T., Munoz, D.G., and Leung, L.S. (1993) Pathogenesis of mesial temporal sclerosis. *Can J Neurol Sci*, **20**, 184–193.

116. O'Brien, T.J., Kilpatrick, C., Murrie, V. *et al.* (1996) Temporal lobe epilepsy caused by mesial temporal sclerosis and temporal neocortical lesions. A clinical and electroencephalographic study of 46 pathologically proven cases. *Brain*, **119** (Pt 6), 2133–2141.

117. Cascino, G., Trenerry, M.R., So, E.L. *et al.* (1996) Routine EEG and temporal lobe epilepsy: relation to long-term EEG monitoring, quantitative MRI, and operative outcome. *Epilepsia*, **37**, 651–656.

118. Trenerry, M.R., Jack C.R. Jr, Ivnik R.J. *et al.* (1993) MRI hippocampal volumes and memory function before and after temporal lobectomy. *Neurology*, **43**, 1800–1805.

119. White, J.R., Matchinsky, D., Beniak, T.E. *et al.* (2002) Predictors of postoperative memory function after left anterior temporal lobectomy. *Epilepsy Behav*, **3** (4), 383–389.

120. Cascino, G.D., Jack, C.R., Jr., Parisi, J.E. *et al.* (1992) MRI in the presurgical evaluation of patients with frontal lobe epilepsy and children with temporal lobe epilepsy: pathologic correlation and prognostic importance. *Epilepsy Res*, **11** (1), 51–59.

121. Diaz-Arrastia, R., Agostini, M.A., Frol, A.B. *et al.* (2000) Neurophysiologic and neuroradiologic features of intractable epilepsy after traumatic brain injury in adults. *Arch Neurol*, **57** (11), 1611–1616.

122. Dunoyer, C., Ragheb, J., Resnick, T. *et al.* (2002) The use of stereotactic radiosurgery to treat intractable childhood partial epilepsy. *Epilepsia*, **43** (3), 292–300.

123. Kraemer, D.L., Griebel, M.L., Lee, N., Friedman, A.H., Radtke, R.A. (1998) Surgical outcome in patients with epilepsy with occult vascular malformations treated with lesionectomy. *Epilepsia*, **39** (6), 600–607.

124. Luhmann, H.J., Raabe, K., Qu, M., Zilles, K. (1998) Characterization of neuronal migration disorders in neocortical structures: extracellular in vitro recordings. *Eur J Neurosci*, **10** (10), 3085–3094.

125. Palmini, A., Gambardella, A., Andermann, F. *et al.* (1995) Intrinsic epileptogenicity of human dysplastic cortex as suggested by corticography and surgical results. *Ann Neurol*, **37**, 476–487.

126. Andermann, F. (2000) Cortical dysplasias and epilepsy: a review of the architectonic, clinical, and seizure patterns. *Adv Neurol*, **84**, 479–496.

127. Kuzniecky, R., Cascino, G., and Jack, C.J. (eds) (1996) Magnetic resonance imaging in cerebral developmental malformations and epilepsy, *Neuroimaging in Epilepsy: Principles and Practice*, Butterworth-Heinemann, Boston, pp. 51–63.

128. Engel, J.J., Van Ness, P., and Rasmussen, T. (1993) Outcome with respect to epileptic seizures, in *Surgical Treatment of the Epilepsies* (ed. J. Engel, Jr.), Raven Press, New York, pp. 609–621.

129. Radhakrishnan, K., So, E.L., Silbert, P.L. *et al.* (1998) Predictors of outcome of anterior temporal lobectomy for intractable epilepsy. A multivariate study. *Neurology*, **51**, 465–471.

130. Holmes, M.D., Born, D.E., Kutsy, R.L. *et al.* (2000) Outcome after surgery in patients with refractory temporal lobe epilepsy and normal MRI. *Seizure*, **9** (6), 407–411.

131. Mosewich, R., So, E.L., O'Brien, T.J. *et al.* (2000) Factors predictive of the outcome of frontal lobe epilepsy surgery. *Epilepsia*, **41**, 843–849.

132. Spencer, S.S., Theodore, W.H., and Berkovic, S.F. (1995) Clinical applications: MRI, SPECT, and PET. *Magn Reson Imaging*, **13** (8), 1119–1124.

133. Jack, C.R. Jr., Mullan, B.P., Sharbrough, F.W. *et al.* (1994) Intractable nonlesional epilepsy of temporal lobe origin: lateralization by interictal SPECT versus MRI. *Neurology*, **44** (5), 829–836.

134. Mosewich, R., So, E.L., O'Brien, T.J. *et al.* (1997) Outcome of lesional vs. nonlesional frontal lobectomy for intractable epilepsy. *Electroencephalogr Clin Neurophysiol*, **103**, 136.

135. Blume, W.T., Ganapathy, G.R., Munoz, D., Lee, D.H. (2004) Indices of resective surgery effectiveness for intractable nonlesional focal epilepsy. *Epilepsia*, **45** (1), 46–53.

136. Wieser, H.G., Ortega, M., Friedman, A., and Yonekawa, Y. (2003) Long-term seizure outcomes following amygdalohippocampectomy. *J Neurosurg*, **98** (4), 751–763.
137. Sylaja, P.N., Radhakrishnan, K., Kesavadas, C., and Sarma, P.S. (2004) Seizure outcome after anterior temporal lobectomy and its predictors in patients with apparent temporal lobe epilepsy and normal MRI. *Epilepsia*, **45** (7), 803–808.
138. Berkovic, S.F., McIntosh A.M., Kalnins R.M. *et al.* (1995) Preoperative MRI predicts outcome of temporal lobectomy: an actuarial analysis. *Neurology*, **45**, 1358–1363.
139. Cohen-Gadol, A.A., Bradley, C.C., Williamson, A. *et al.* (2005) Normal magnetic resonance imaging and medial temporal lobe epilepsy: the clinical syndrome of paradoxical temporal lobe epilepsy. *J Neurosurg*, **102** (5), 902–909 [see comment].
140. Theodore, W., Sato S., Kufta C. *et al.* (1992) Temporal lobectomy for uncontrolled seizures: the role for positron emission tomography. *Ann Neurol*, **32**, 789–794.
141. Bartolomei, F., Hayashi, M., Tamura, M. *et al.* (2008) Long-term efficacy of gamma knife radiosurgery in mesial temporal lobe epilepsy. *Neurology*, **70** (19), 1658–1663.
142. Spencer, S.S. (2008) Gamma knife radiosurgery for refractory medial temporal lobe epilepsy: too little, too late? *Neurology*, **70** (19), 1654–1655.

16 Non-substrate-directed partial epilepsy

Korwyn Williams[1] and Katherine H. Noe[2]

[1]*Department of Pediatrics, University of Arizona College of Medicine, Phoenix, AZ; Division of Neurology, Children's Neuroscience Institute, Phoenix Children's Hospital, Phoenix, AZ, USA*
[2]*Department of Neurology, Division of Epilepsy, Mayo Clinic College of Medicine and Mayo Clinic Arizona, Phoenix, AZ, USA*

16.1 Introduction

Recurrent, unprovoked seizures or epilepsy is seen in approximately 0.5% of the population [1]. Forty percent to 50% of newly diagnosed unprovoked seizures are partial onset [2, 3]. The majority of partial epilepsy can be attributed to an underlying CNS structural lesion or disorders. For newly diagnosed epilepsy, 12–13% of cases are symptomatic partial, 18–29% cryptogenic partial, but only 1–5% idiopathic partial [4–6]. In population-based studies of classification of new onset epilepsy completed since the introduction of widespread use of MRI the incidence of idiopathic partial epilepsy is 1.7–1.8/100 000 person years as compared to 8.4–17.11/100 000 for symptomatic partial epilepsy [3, 6]. The leading sites of onset are frontal, temporal, and central sensorimotor cortex [4].

Classification of seizure type and epilepsy syndrome is useful in determining prognosis and treatment. The idiopathic partial epilepsies (IPEs) are relatively rare, as noted above, but tend to be of childhood onset with relatively benign prognosis. For patients with cryptogenic partial seizures, the absence of a defined underlying structural lesion may add to the challenge faced by patients in understanding and accepting their disorder. Seizures in two-thirds of those with epilepsy are well controlled with medical therapy; however, after two appropriate anticonvulsants have failed, the likelihood of seizure control with further medical therapy is poor [7, 8]. For medically refractory partial epilepsy, surgery may offer the greatest likelihood of seizure freedom. Unfortunately, the process of evaluation for epilepsy surgery in patients with idiopathic partial epilepsy can be particularly challenging, and the outcome for non-substrate-directed epilepsy is less favorable.

16.2 Genetic or IPE syndromes

Most idiopathic focal epilepsies demonstrate complex inheritance patterns, with both mutifactorial genetic and environmental influences, but a small number of single-gene disorders are also recognized in small kindreds (Table 16.1) [9–13]. The pattern of inheritance is autosomal dominant with variable degrees of penetrance in an affected kindred. These epilepsy syndromes usually have defined ages of onset and semiologies, infrequent seizures, relatively high rates of remission, good response to anticonvulsants, and relatively normal neurodevelopment—although learning deficits have been reported in 15% in a recent report [14]. However, some can evolve into refractory epilepsies leading to surgical management [15]. The most commonly encountered IPE is benign childhood epilepsy with centrotemporal spikes (benign rolandic epilepsy), followed by benign occipital epilepsy [4, 6]. The syndromes of autosomal dominant nocturnal frontal lobe epilepsy, familial MTLE, familial lateral TLE, and familial partial epilepsy with variable foci have been described from select pedigrees and affect both children and adults.

16.3 Medically refractory non-substrate-directed partial epilepsy

For those with medically refractory epilepsy, the likelihood of a good surgical outcome improves if a structural abnormality can be detected and completely resected [24–30]. For medically refractory epilepsy with a defined focal MRI abnormality, epilepsy surgery can lead to seizure freedom for 50–70% of patients [31–34]. Even in those with subtle, nonspecific abnormalities on MRI, seizure freedom has been reported in up to 60% [35]. Unfortunately, for refractory epilepsy without MRI abnormalities, seizure-free outcomes tend to be poorer—roughly 40% at

Table 16.1 Selected idiopathic partial epilepsy syndromes

Syndrome	Age of onset	Semiology	Epileptiform activity	Age of remission	Gene or locus
Benign rolandic epilepsy	3–13 years	Sensorimotor oropharyngeal involvement; drooling; anarthria; GTC; usually nocturnal	C-T (unilateral, bilateral, synchronous, asynchronous)	Almost all by 15 years of age	ELP4 [16]; KCNQ2, KCNQ3 [17]
Panayiotopoulos or early-onset occipital epilepsy of childhood	1–14 years (mean age 4–5 years)	Pallor, ictal emesis; impaired consciousness; eye deviation; usually nocturnal; usually infrequent; often prolonged	O (unilateral or bilateral) which attenuate with eye opening—25% may exhibit only extra-occipital discharges	Within 1–2 years; 33–50% will experience only one seizure	SCN1A [18]
Gastaut or late-onset occipital epilepsy of childhood	3–16 years (mean 8 years)	Visual hallucinations, amaurosis, eye deviation, GTC; postictal migraines	O (unilateral or bilateral) which attenuate with eye opening	Within 3–6 years of onset	Unknown
Autosomal dominant nocturnal frontal lobe epilepsy	Childhood (mean age 11 years)	Nocturnal clusters of hyperkinetic with maintained awareness	Often normal, but occasional anterior quadrant abnormalities	Persistent seizures	CHRNA4, CHRNA2, CHRNB2 [19–21]
Familial mesial temporal lobe epilepsy	Adolescence to early adult	Prominent psychic and autonomic features	Interictal often normal	Variable, highly responsive to AEDs	18qter/1q25–q31, 12q23, 4q13.2–q21.3
Familial lateral temporal lobe epilepsy	—	Auditory aura	T-O or normal	—	LGI1 [22]
Familial partial epilepsy with variable foci	Infancy to adult	Variable within family	Often normal, can be multifocal	—	22q11–12 [23]

C-T: centro-temporal; O: occipital; GTC: generalized tonic-clonic; T-O: temporal-occipital.

5–10 year follow-up in a pediatric population [36, 37]. These nonlesional cases constitute 20–30% of the referrals to tertiary epilepsy centers [38]. Many factors contribute to the lower rates of seizure freedom in this population, but the challenge arises in defining the epileptogenic zone in the absence of a clearly defined anatomic target. In the absence of a structural lesion defined by MRI, the use of PET, SPECT, and MEG to supplement localization by EEG becomes increasingly important to determine surgical candidacy.

EEG

The importance of localized EEG findings is demonstrated by a retrospective review of 236 children offered resective surgery. Patil *et al.* reported that 90% of those with MRI abnormalities were offered surgery regardless of EEG results, while when the MRI was normal only 78% with a localizing ictal EEG pattern and 7% without localized EEG findings were offered surgery [39]. *Scott et al.* reported similarly that only three (7.5%) patients from a cohort of 40 adult patients with normal MRI and lack of data concordant with their ictal EEG findings proceeded to surgery (two underwent temporal lobectomy) [40].

Expanded EEG electrode density has the potential to assist with localization in challenging cases. High-density EEG arrays use 256 contacts for source localization to provide a testable hypothesis for intracranial grid implantation in patients without a localizing EEG onset [41, 42]. However, there is no published evidence demonstrating postsurgical outcomes in large numbers of patients with nonlesional epilepsy.

Positron emission tomography (PET)

PET is a noninvasive technology which evaluates cerebral metabolism using different ligands [43]. The most commonly used ligand is [18F]-fluorodeoxyglucose (FDG), but the use of other ligands such as [11C]-flumazenil (FMZ), [11C]-alpha-methyl-tryptophan (AMT), and [18F]-trans-4-fluoro-N-2-[4-(2-methoxyphenyl) piperazin-1-yl]ethyl-N-(2-pyridyl)cyclohexane carboxamide (FCWAY) (a serotonin 1A receptor ligand) has been reported [44–47]. FDG-PET is of greatest proven utility in symptomatic TLE, where it may be localizing 80–100% of the time [32, 43, 48–50].

However, FDG-PET also has utility in the presurgical evaluation of cryptogenic epilepsy. In the absence of localizing information from MRI and EEG, PET can aid surgical decision-making. FDG-PET provided additional information regarding epileptogenic sites in 77% of patients and led to a "major change" in management in 45% following standard MRI and video-EEG evaluation in 113 pediatric patients with temporal and extratemporal epilepsy [51]. FDG-PET changed management in 71% of 110 temporal epilepsy patients following MRI and EEG—in 20%, surgery was based solely on PET results [52].

Salamon and colleagues have reported their use of FDG-PET coregistered with MRI (FDG-PET/MRI) in detecting cortical dysplasia [53]. In the subset of 10 patients with histologically proven cortical dysplasia with normal MR imaging, FDG-PET/MRI identified hypometabolism in 40%. They reported seizure freedom in 80% of their patients and specifically mentioned that persistent seizures were seen only in those with resections limited by eloquent cortex or which would have led to significant neurological disability.

From the standpoint of outcomes, Chung and colleagues reported seizure freedom in 47% of 89 cryptogenic, neocortical epileptic adults and children followed for two years postoperatively; ictal EEG, FDG-PET, and ictal SPECT provided localizing information 71, 44, and 41% of the time, respectively [54]. Seo *et al.* reviewed 27 children with cryptogenic, intractable epilepsy who were followed for at least two years postoperatively—18 (67%) were seizure-free [55]. All had undergone invasive subdural monitoring, ictal SPECT, and FDG-PET. Eighteen (67%) patients had focal hyperperfusion with ictal SPECT. Twenty-one (78%) had hypometabolism of a region or lobe of interest with FDG-PET; of these 90% had either an Engel class I (seizure-free) or II (rare disabling seizures) outcome.

For many of the reports, the utility of FDG-PET in identifying seizure onset zones is difficult to determine as the correlation between the normality of the MR imaging, focality of the PET findings, location of seizure onset zone based on intracranial monitoring, and seizure freedom are not explicitly stated. This issue is addressed more directly in studies comparing the use of FMZ- and FDG-PET in refractory partial epilepsy. FMZ is a benzodiazepine receptor antagonist and loss of FMZ binding in mesial temporal sclerosis is thought to correspond to neuronal cell loss [47, 56]. Several authors have suggested that FMZ-PET is no more likely to lateralize the temporal lobe seizure's onset zone than FDG-PET, and in some cases FMZ may be falsely lateralizing [57, 58].

Other reports presented evidence that FMZ-PET may demonstrate some utility for neocortical epilepsy. Six patients with frontal epilepsy (five with normal MRIs) exhibited FMZ hypometabolism which correlated with seizure onset zones identified with subdural electrode recordings; FDG hypometabolism was seen in only half of the patients [59]. Seven (77%) temporal and extratemporal epilepsy patients (1.5–19 years old) with normal MRI studies had Engel class I outcomes following intracranial monitoring [60]. The extent of unresected FMZ abnormalities and large preoperative FMZ-PET abnormalities independently corresponded with poor outcomes. While FDG-PET abnormalities occurred in the same region, the extent of unresected abnormalities did not correlate with seizure outcomes in this report. In 100 consecutive refractory epilepsy patients, reduced FMZ binding was seen in the epileptogenic lobe based on intracranial monitoring in 8 of 17 (47%) patients with normal MR imaging [58].

Another ligand used for PET evaluation is AMT, a precursor to serotonin, which has been reported to be upregulated in dysplastic epileptogenic tissue. This ligand has been examined in epilepsy presurgical evaluation, primarily for tuberous sclerosis [61, 62]. Only one study has reported surgical outcome using AMT- and FDG-PET, and AMT-PET did not prove to be more sensitive than FDG-PET [63].

SPECT/SISCOM

SISCOM is used for localization of a seizure onset zone for cryptogenic and symptomatic cases. Patients are injected with a radioactive tracer at the time of seizure onset, which then accumulates at cerebral areas of hyperperfusion. A second, interictal SPECT is obtained to determine baseline perfusion characteristics. These two images are subtracted via software and overlaid onto MR images. SISCOM provided localizing information in 88% of 51 consecutive refractory partial epilepsy patients (both symptomatic and cryptogenic) compared to 39% of side-by-side comparison of ictal and interictal scans [64]. Additionally, when SISCOM results were concordant with other studies, 62% of the patients had "excellent" seizure outcomes (no more than nocturnal seizures or nondisabling simple partial seizures). SISCOM results can also significantly impact decision-making: SISCOM changed consensus recommendations in 10/32 (31%) patients with otherwise nonlocalizing studies [65].

Magnetoencephalography

MEG is a noninvasive technique that can complement standard EEG recordings in presurgical evaluations. This technique models the same electromagnetic fields detected with EEG, but MEG offers advantages over EEG such as better spatial resolution and better sensitivity for abnormal activity in sulci permitted by the perpendicular orientation of the magnetic and electric fields [66]. However, several factors limit the availability of MEG, including cost, limited duration of recording, and restriction of the patient's movements during the study.

MEG's sensitivity for abnormal activity (dipole sources) has been reported to be 70–90% for neocortical epilepsy, compared to a 40–50% diagnostic yield with TLE [67–69]. MEG is not simply a more expensive EEG and has been useful in surgical planning. Several authors have reported that MEG led to alterations in surgical planning in more than 20% [70, 71]. Lau et al. reviewed published reports of MEG source imaging (MSI) and seizure outcome which encompassed temporal epilepsy only, extratemporal epilepsy, and combinations of the two in both adults and children [72]. Across the 17 studies reviewed, the average MEG sensitivity was 84% with a 95% confidence interval of 12%, but ranged from 20 to 100% in the individual studies. The specificity ranged from 0 to 100% across the studies, but for the eight non-zero studies, the average specificity was 52% but with a broad confidence interval of 24%. The authors concluded that on the whole MEG can be helpful in localizing a seizure onset zone, but cautioned that its sensitivity and specificity were not consistently high as a primary diagnostic tool.

MEG detects dipole sources, which are derived based on certain mathematical assumptions [73]. "Highly localized" or "densely clustered" dipole sources have been significantly associated with the seizure onset zone identified by intracranial recording and with a seizure-free outcome [71, 74, 75]. Ramachandran Nair *et al.* reported that 36% of 17 pediatric patients with normal or "subtle" MR findings were seizure-free. Of these Engel class I patients, all had highly localized MSI. Those with scattered or bilateral MSI had worse outcomes.

Comparing different modalities

Particularly with nonlesional epilepsy, identification of a seizure onset zone is heavily reliant on investigations adjunctive to the MRI such as PET, MEG, ictal SPECT/SISCOM, and invasive recording. Little research has compared the utility of the techniques compared to each other, in part because not all institutions have access to all of these technologies and not all patients are appropriate candidates for these options.

Won and colleagues reported on 118 consecutive epilepsy patients ranging from 8 to 55 years who underwent resective surgery and were followed for at least 12 months postoperatively [76]. Only 26 of these patients had normal MRI, and not all patients received FDG-PET or SPECT. PET and ictal SPECT correctly lateralized the lesion in 80 and 55% of the cases, respectively; of those with class I or II outcomes, lateralization was correct in 85 and 75%, respectively. No mention was made of localization, a more useful piece of information for surgical planning. Notably, inclusive of all 118 patients, the MRI was concordant with video-EEG, PET, ictal SPECT, and intracranial electrodes 58, 68, 58, and 47% of the time, respectively. The lateralization by these modalities for all of the patients varied depending on whether temporal (80–90% for MRI, PET, ictal SPECT) or extratemporal (40–60%) epilepsy was being evaluated.

Kim *et al.* reviewed their seizure-free pediatric patients (n = 42) who had undergone FDG-PET and SISCOM evaluation [77]. While they did not explicitly state the number of nonlesional epilepsy cases in this cohort, the MRI was concordant with and accurately localized the area of resection 82–84% of the time with all patients with a good outcome. PET correctly localized the epileptic zone in 63% of the extratemporal cases and 73% of temporal epilepsy cases. Similarly, SIS-COM accurately localized the seizure onset zone in 85% of extratemporal epilepsy patients, but only 67% of TLE patients.

Seo *et al.* reviewed 27 pediatric patients who underwent epilepsy surgery for partial seizures, infantile spasms, and Lennox-Gastaut syndrome, had normal or "nonsuspicious" MRI, and two years of follow-up [55]. All had undergone

FDG-PET, ictal and interictal SPECT, and subdural electrodes. Sixty-seven percent were classified as Engel class I. Hypometabolism in the region or lobe identified as the seizure onset zone was detected with PET in 78% of the cases, 90% of whom had an Engel class I or II outcome. Focal hyperperfusion with SPECT at the site of the seizure onset zone identified by the intracranial grids was seen in 67%.

Knowlton *et al.* conducted a prospective observational study of 72 refractory epilepsy surgery patients (children and adults), who underwent intracranial monitoring [78]. Sixty-two proceeded to resective surgery; all had undergone MEG, 51 FDG-PET, and 34 SISCOM. Of the Engel class I patients, MEG accurately localized the seizure onset zone in 75%. In those who underwent both MEG and PET, MEG was accurately localizing in 56% and PET was localizing in 59%; concordance was observed in 25%. In those who underwent both MEG and SISCOM, MEG was accurately localizing in 38% and SISCOM was localizing in 50%; concordance was observed in 19%. In those who underwent all three diagnostic studies, MEG was accurately localizing in 31%, PET was localizing in 54%, and SISCOM was localizing in 62% (concordance was only seen in 3 of 27 patients). The full import of these values is complicated, but the authors concluded that each modality independently has diagnostic and predictive value for postoperative seizure freedom and complements the others. While not sufficiently powered to compare the three modalities collectively, the authors note that localizing SISCOM data had the highest odds ratio for seizure freedom (9.1 vs. 4.4 for MEG and 7.1 for PET). They also noted that SISCOM and MEG were more useful for neocortical epilepsy, while PET was more useful for mesial temporal epilepsy.

Intracranial EEG

Even after the noninvasive diagnostic testing described above, certain hypotheses may need to be tested before proceeding to resection, such as: which of several imaging abnormalities is the seizure onset zone; are the areas localized by the noninvasive tests truly the site of seizure onset; does the seizure onset zone overlap with eloquent cortex. At this time, such questions can only be addressed by the surgical placement of electrodes placed onto the surface or embedded in the substance of the brain.

Several authors have reported on features of seizure onset that predicted postsurgical outcome. Wetjen *et al.* retrospectively reviewed 51 nonlesional, extratemporal epilepsy patients who underwent intracranial EEG monitoring [38]. Ninety percent who underwent resection had sufficient information to review, and of this group, 50% had an Engel class I outcome. Focal, high-frequency (>20 Hz) oscillations at seizure onset were seen in 86% of those with a class I outcome, and 20% of those with a non-excellent outcome. Spencer and colleagues reported that the presence of interictal epileptiform abnormalities outside of the resection zone was associated with poor outcome in 6 of 13 neocortical epilepsy patients [79]. In their review of 22 children with normal, subtle, or nonfocal MRI findings, Ramachandran Nair reported that having five or less adjacent grid contacts involved at seizure onset was associated with seizure freedom (5 of 5), while seizure freedom was seen in only 18% (3 of 17) whose seizure onset zones extended over more than five adjacent electrodes [75].

16.4 Conclusions

Localization-related epilepsy is more common than generalized epilepsy; however, the prognosis for seizure control and remission is variable. Idiopathic or genetic partial-onset epilepsies often have a high likelihood of spontaneous remission, but some epilepsy syndromes are unlikely to remit.

Almost one-third of epilepsy patients do not fully respond to anticonvulsant therapy. Resection of a MRI lesion leads to postoperative seizure freedom in 50–70% of refractory epilepsy patients. For those without a clear lesion on neuroimaging, the likelihood of seizure freedom is 40–50%. The presurgical evaluation for the MRI-negative patients could include PET (FDG, FMZ), SPECT/SISCOM, MEG, and intracranial EEG. No one technology has proven to have better sensitivity or specificity and is not predictive of eventual surgical outcome.

Unfortunately there is no easy protocol to follow in the use of these ancillary technologies. Practical considerations such as availability and cost may supervene over medical decision-making (e.g., temporal versus extratemporal). The evidence-based approach to this decision tree is limited by small numbers, admixture of pediatric and adult cohorts, retrospective series (sometimes collected over years in which practice patterns could have evolved), mixed collections of cryptogenic/symptomatic patients and temporal/extratemporal epilepsy, and no explicit characterization of case complexity.

With these limitations in mind, the report by Knowlton *et al.* prospectively compared these modalities (albeit not every patient received all of the technologies, and the analysis was underpowered in many respects) and noted that the studies were complementary [78]. Less often than might have been expected, the studies were not concordant and did not obviate the need for intracranial EEG. Each localizing study provides a hypothesis, shaped by the history and physical, to be tested with intracranial EEG or nonsurgical management.

As they are more commonly used, the need for more prospective trials to better define the strengths, weaknesses, and indications for these technologies will be helpful in improving surgical outcomes for medically refractory, non-substrate directed epilepsies.

References

1. Hauser, W.A., Annegers, J.F., and Kurland, L.T. (1991) Prevalence of epilepsy in Rochester, Minnesota: 1940–1980. *Epilepsia*, **32** (4), 429–445.

2. Hauser, W.A., Annegers, J.F., and Kurland, L.T. (1993) Incidence of epilepsy and unprovoked seizures in Rochester, Minnesota: 1935–1984. *Epilepsia*, **34** (3), 453–468.

3. Olafsson, E., Ludvigsson, P., Gudmundsson, G. *et al.* (2005) Incidence of unprovoked seizures and epilepsy in Iceland and assessment of the epilepsy syndrome classification: a prospective study. *Lancet Neurol*, **4** (10), 627–634.

4. Manford, M., Hart, Y.M., Sander, J.W., and Shorvon, S.D. (1992) National General Practice Study of Epilepsy (NGPSE): partial seizure patterns in a general population. *Neurology*, **42** (10), 1911–1917.

5. Jallon, P., Loiseau, P., and Loiseau, J. (2001) Newly diagnosed unprovoked epileptic seizures: presentation at diagnosis in CAROLE study. Coordination Active du Reseau Observatoire Longitudinal de l'Epilepsie. *Epilepsia*, **42** (4), 464–475.

6. Loiseau, J., Loiseau, P., Guyot, M. *et al.* (1990) Survey of seizure disorders in the French southwest. I. Incidence of epileptic syndromes. *Epilepsia*, **31** (4), 391–396.

7. Schiller, Y. and Najjar, Y. (2008) Quantifying the response to antiepileptic drugs: effect of past treatment history. *Neurology*, **70** (1), 54–65.

8. Kwan, P. and Brodie, M.J. (2000) Early identification of refractory epilepsy. *N Engl J Med*, **342** (5), 314–319.

9. Shields, W.D. and Snead, O.C. III (2009) Benign epilepsy with centrotemporal spikes. *Epilepsia*, **50** (Suppl 8), 10–15.

10. Tharp, B.R. (2002) Neonatal seizures and syndromes. *Epilepsia*, **43** (Suppl 3), 2–10.

11. Koutroumanidis, M. (2007) Panayiotopoulos syndrome: an important electroclinical example of benign childhood system epilepsy. *Epilepsia*, **48** (6), 1044–1053.

12. Ryvlin, P., Rheims, S., and Risse, G. (2006) Nocturnal frontal lobe epilepsy. *Epilepsia*, **47** (Suppl 2), 83–86.

13. Taylor, I., Scheffer, I.E., and Berkovic, S.F. (2003) Occipital epilepsies: identification of specific and newly recognized syndromes. *Brain*, **126** (Pt 4), 753–769.

14. Fastenau, P.S., Johnson, C.S., Perkins, S.M. *et al.* (2009) Neuropsychological status at seizure onset in children: risk factors for early cognitive deficits. *Neurology*, **73** (7), 526–534.

15. Otsubo, H., Chitoku, S., Ochi, A. *et al.* (2001) Malignant rolandic-sylvian epilepsy in children: diagnosis, treatment, and outcomes. *Neurology*, **57** (4), 590–596.

16. Strug, L.J., Clarke, T., Chiang, T. *et al.* (2009) Centrotemporal sharp wave EEG trait in rolandic epilepsy maps to Elongator Protein Complex 4 (ELP4).*Eur J Hum Genet*, **17** (9), 1171–1181.

17. Hahn, A. and Neubauer, B.A. (2009) Sodium and potassium channel dysfunctions in rare and common idiopathic epilepsy syndromes. *Brain Dev*, **31** (7), 515–520.

18. Livingston, J.H., Cross, J.H., McLellan, A. *et al.* (2009) A novel inherited mutation in the voltage sensor region of SCN1A is associated with Panayiotopoulos syndrome in siblings and generalized epilepsy with febrile seizures plus. *J Child Neurol*, **24** (4), 503–508.

19. Aridon, P., Marini, C., Di Resta, C. *et al.* (2006) Increased sensitivity of the neuronal nicotinic receptor alpha 2 subunit causes familial epilepsy with nocturnal wandering and ictal fear. *Am J Hum Genet*, **79** (2), 342–350.

20. De Fusco, M., Becchetti, A., Patrignani, A. *et al.* (2000) The nicotinic receptor beta 2 subunit is mutant in nocturnal frontal lobe epilepsy. *Nat Genet*, **26** (3), 275–276.

21. Steinlein, O.K., Mulley, J.C., Propping, P. *et al.* (1995) A missense mutation in the neuronal nicotinic acetylcholine receptor alpha 4 subunit is associated with autosomal dominant nocturnal frontal lobe epilepsy. *Nat Genet*, **11** (2), 201–203.

22. Ottman, R., Winawer, M.R., Kalachikov, S. *et al.* (2004) LGI1 mutations in autosomal dominant partial epilepsy with auditory features. *Neurology*, **62** (7), 1120–1126.

23. Berkovic, S.F., Serratosa, J.M., Phillips, H.A. *et al.* (2004) Familial partial epilepsy with variable foci: clinical features and linkage to chromosome 22q12. *Epilepsia*, **45** (9), 1054–1060.

24. Berkovic, S.F., McIntosh, A.M., Kalnins, R.M. *et al.* (1995) Preoperative MRI predicts outcome of temporal lobectomy: an actuarial analysis. *Neurology*, **45** (7), 1358–1363.

25. Jeha, L.E., Najm, I., Bingaman, W. *et al.* (2007) Surgical outcome and prognostic factors of frontal lobe epilepsy surgery. *Brain*, **130** (Pt 2), 574–584.

26. Edwards, J.C., Wyllie, E., Ruggeri, P.M. *et al.* (2000) Seizure outcome after surgery for epilepsy due to malformation of cortical development. *Neurology*, **55** (8), 1110–1114.

27. Kuzniecky, R., Ho, S.S., Martin, R. *et al.* (1999) Temporal lobe developmental malformations and hippocampal sclerosis: epilepsy surgical outcome. *Neurology*, **52** (3), 479–484.

28. Zentner, J., Hufnagel, A., Ostertun, B. *et al.* (1996) Surgical treatment of extratemporal epilepsy: clinical, radiologic, and histopathologic findings in 60 patients. *Epilepsia*, **37** (11), 1072–1080.

29. Clarke, D.B., Olivier, A., Andermann, F., and Fish, D. (1996) Surgical treatment of epilepsy: the problem of lesion/focus incongruence. *Surg Neurol*, **46** (6), 579–585; discussion 85–86.

30. Fish, D., Andermann, F., and Olivier, A. (1991) Complex partial seizures and small posterior temporal or extratemporal structural lesions: surgical management. *Neurology*, **41** (11), 1781–1784.

31. Engel, J. Jr., Wiebe, S., French, J. *et al.* (2003) Practice parameter: temporal lobe and localized neocortical resections for epilepsy: report of the Quality Standards Subcommittee of the American Academy of Neurology, in association with the American Epilepsy Society and the American Association of Neurological Surgeons. *Neurology*, **60** (4), 538–547.

32. Elsharkawy, A.E., Alabbasi, A.H., Pannek, H. *et al.* (2009) Long-term outcome after temporal lobe epilepsy surgery in 434 consecutive adult patients. *J Neurosurg*, **110** (6), 1135–1146.

33. Smyth, M.D., Limbrick, D.D. Jr., Ojemann, J.G. *et al.* (2007) Outcome following surgery for temporal lobe epilepsy with hippocampal involvement in preadolescent children: emphasis on mesial temporal sclerosis. *J Neurosurg*, **106** (Suppl 3), 205–210.

34. Yoon, H.H., Kwon, H.L., Mattson, R.H. *et al.* (2003) Long-term seizure outcome in patients initially seizure-free after resective epilepsy surgery. *Neurology*, **61** (4), 445–450.

35. Bell, M.L., Rao, S., So, E.L. *et al.* (2009) Epilepsy surgery outcomes in temporal lobe epilepsy with a normal MRI. *Epilepsia*, **50** (9), 2053–2060.

36. Jayakar, P., Dunoyer, C., Dean, P. *et al.* (2008) Epilepsy surgery in patients with normal or nonfocal MRI scans: integrative strategies offer long-term seizure relief. *Epilepsia*, **49** (5), 758–764.

37. Chapman, K., Wyllie, E., Najm, I. *et al.* (2005) Seizure outcome after epilepsy surgery in patients with normal preoperative MRI. *J Neurol Neurosurg Psychiatry*, **76** (5), 710–713.

38. Wetjen, N.M., Marsh, W.R., Meyer, F.B. *et al.* (2009) Intracranial electroencephalography seizure onset patterns and surgical outcomes in nonlesional extratemporal epilepsy. *J Neurosurg*, **110** (6), 1147–1152.

39. Patil, S.G., Cross, J.H., Kling Chong, W. *et al.* (2008) Is streamlined evaluation of children for epilepsy surgery possible? *Epilepsia*, **49** (8), 1340–1347.

40. Scott, C.A., Fish, D.R., Smith, S.J. *et al.* (1999) Presurgical evaluation of patients with epilepsy and normal MRI: role of scalp video-EEG telemetry. *J Neurol Neurosurg Psychiatry*, **66** (1), 69–71.

41. Thompson, P., Rae, J., Weber, L. *et al.* (2008) Long-term seizure monitoring using a 256 contact dense array system. *Am J Electroneurodiagnostic Technol*, **48** (2), 93–106.

42. Holmes, M.D., Brown, M., Tucker, D.M. *et al.* (2008) Localization of extratemporal seizure with noninvasive dense-array EEG. Comparison with intracranial recordings. *Pediatr Neurosurg*, **44** (6), 474–479.

43. Asenbaum, S. and Baumgartner, C. (2001) Nuclear medicine in the preoperative evaluation of epilepsy. *Nucl Med Commun*, **22** (7), 835–840.

44. Manno, E.M., Sperling, M.R., Ding, X. *et al.* (1994) Predictors of outcome after anterior temporal lobectomy: positron emission tomography. *Neurology*, **44** (12), 2331–2336.

45. Kuhl, D.E., Engel, J. Jr., Phelps, M.E., and Selin, C. (1980) Epileptic patterns of local cerebral metabolism and perfusion in humans determined by emission computed tomography of 18FDG and 13NH3. *Ann Neurol*, **8** (4), 348–360.

46. Goffin, K., Dedeurwaerdere, S., Van Laere, K., and Van Paesschen, W. (2008) Neuronuclear assessment of patients with epilepsy. *Semin Nucl Med*, **38** (4), 227–239.

47. Mauguiere, F. and Ryvlin, P. (2004) The role of PET in presurgical assessment of partial epilepsies. *Epileptic Disord*, **6** (3), 193–215.

48. Henry, T.R., Mazziotta, J.C., and Engel, J. Jr. (1993) Interictal metabolic anatomy of mesial temporal lobe epilepsy. *Arch Neurol*, **50** (6), 582–589.

49. Salanova, V., Markand, O., Worth, R. *et al.* (1998) FDG-PET and MRI in temporal lobe epilepsy: relationship to febrile seizures, hippocampal sclerosis and outcome. *Acta Neurol Scand*, **97** (3), 146–153.

50. Hwang, S.I., Kim, J.H., Park, S.W. *et al.* (2001) Comparative analysis of MR imaging, positron emission tomography, and ictal single-photon emission CT in patients with neocortical epilepsy. *AJNR Am J Neuroradiol*, **22** (5), 937–946.

51. Ollenberger, G.P., Byrne, A.J., Berlangieri, S.U. *et al.* (2005) Assessment of the role of FDG PET in the diagnosis and management of children with refractory epilepsy. *Eur J Nucl Med Mol Imaging*, **32** (11), 1311–1316.

52. Uijl, S.G., Leijten, F.S., Arends, J.B. *et al.* (2007) The added value of [18F]-fluoro-D-deoxyglucose positron emission tomography in screening for temporal lobe epilepsy surgery. *Epilepsia*, **48** (11), 2121–2129.

53. Salamon, N., Kung, J., Shaw, S.J. *et al.* (2008) FDG-PET/MRI coregistration improves detection of cortical dysplasia in patients with epilepsy. *Neurology*, **71** (20), 1594–1601.

54. Lee, S.K., Lee, S.Y., Kim, K.K. *et al.* (2005) Surgical outcome and prognostic factors of cryptogenic neocortical epilepsy. *Ann Neurol*, **58** (4), 525–532.

55. Seo, J.H., Noh, B.H., Lee, J.S. *et al.* (2009) Outcome of surgical treatment in non-lesional intractable childhood epilepsy. *Seizure*, **18** (9), 625–629.

56. Burdette, D.E., Sakurai, S.Y., Henry, T.R. *et al.* (1995) Temporal lobe central benzodiazepine binding in unilateral mesial temporal lobe epilepsy. *Neurology*, **45** (5), 934–941.

57. Koepp, M.J., Hammers, A., Labbe, C. *et al.* (2000) 11C-flumazenil PET in patients with refractory temporal lobe epilepsy and normal MRI. *Neurology*, **54** (2), 332–339.

58. Ryvlin, P., Bouvard, S., Le Bars, D. *et al.* (1998) Clinical utility of flumazenil-PET versus [18F]fluorodeoxyglucose-PET and MRI in refractory partial epilepsy. A prospective study in 100 patients. *Brain*, **121** (Pt 11), 2067–2081.

59. Savic, I., Thorell, J.O., and Roland, P. (1995) [11C]flumazenil positron emission tomography visualizes frontal epileptogenic regions. *Epilepsia*, **36** (12), 1225–1232.

60. Juhasz, C., Chugani, D.C., Muzik, O. *et al.* (2000) Electroclinical correlates of flumaze-nil and fluorodeoxyglucose PET abnormalities in lesional epilepsy. *Neurology*, **55** (6), 825–835.

61. Kagawa, K., Chugani, D.C., Asano, E. *et al.* (2005) Epilepsy surgery outcome in children with tuberous sclerosis complex evaluated with alpha-[11C]methyl-L-tryptophan positron emission tomography (PET). *J Child Neurol*, **20** (5), 429–438.

62. Fedi, M., Reutens, D., Okazawa, H. *et al.* (2001) Localizing value of alpha-methyl-L-tryptophan PET in intractable epilepsy of neocortical origin. *Neurology*, **57** (9), 1629–1636.

63. Juhasz, C., Chugani, D.C., Muzik, O. *et al.* (2003) Alpha-methyl-L-tryptophan PET detects epileptogenic cortex in children with intractable epilepsy. *Neurology*, **60** (6), 960–968.

64. O'Brien, T.J., So, E.L., Mullan, B.P. *et al.* (1998) Subtraction ictal SPECT co-registered to MRI improves clinical usefulness of SPECT in localizing the surgical seizure focus. *Neurology*, **50** (2), 445–454.

65. Tan, K.M., Britton, J.W., Buchhalter, J.R. *et al.* (2008) Influence of subtraction ictal SPECT on surgical management in focal epilepsy of indeterminate localization: a prospective study. *Epilepsy Res*, **82** (2–3), 190–193.

66. Baumgartner, C., Pataraia, E., Lindinger, G., and Deecke, L. (2000) Magnetoencephalog-raphy in focal epilepsy. *Epilepsia*, **41** (Suppl 3), S39–S47.

67. Knowlton, R.C., Laxer, K.D., Aminoff, M.J. *et al.* (1997) Magnetoencephalography in partial epilepsy: clinical yield and localization accuracy. *Ann Neurol*, **42** (4), 622–631.

68. Baumgartner, C., Pataraia, E., Lindinger, G., and Deecke, L. (2000) Neuromagnetic record-ings in temporal lobe epilepsy. *J Clin Neurophysiol*, **17** (2), 177–189.

69. Park, H., Nakasato N., Iwasaki, M. *et al.* (eds.) (2002) Detectability of convexity spikes by conventional EEG and helmet MEG. *Biomag 2002: Proceedings of the Thirteenth Interna-tional Conference on Biomagnetism,* Jena, Germany, VDE Verlag GMBH, Berlin, Germany.

70. Sutherling, W.W., Mamelak, A.N., Thyerlei, D. *et al.* (2008) Influence of magnetic source imaging for planning intracranial EEG in epilepsy. *Neurology*, **71** (13), 990–996.

71. Knowlton, R.C., Razdan, S.N., Limdi, N. *et al.* (2009) Effect of epilepsy magnetic source imaging on intracranial electrode placement. *Ann Neurol*, **65** (6), 716–723.

72. Lau, M., Yam, D., and Burneo, J.G. (2008) A systematic review on MEG and its use in the presurgical evaluation of localization-related epilepsy. *Epilepsy Res*, **79** (2–3), 97–104.

73. Knowlton, R.C. and Shih, J. (2004) Magnetoencephalography in epilepsy. *Epilepsia*, **45** (Suppl 4), 61–71.

74. Mamelak, A.N., Lopez, N., Akhtari, M., and Sutherling, W.W. (2002) Magnetoencephalography-directed surgery in patients with neocortical epilepsy. *J Neurosurg*, **97** (4), 865–873.

75. Ramachandran Nair, R., Otsubo, H., Shroff, M.M. *et al.* (2007) MEG predicts outcome following surgery for intractable epilepsy in children with normal or nonfocal MRI findings. *Epilepsia*, **48** (1), 149–157.

76. Won, H.J., Chang, K.H., Cheon, J.E. *et al.* (1999) Comparison of MR imaging with PET and ictal SPECT in 118 patients with intractable epilepsy. *AJNR Am J Neuroradiol*, **20** (4), 593–599.

77. Kim, J.T., Bai, S.J., Choi, K.O. *et al.* (2009) Comparison of various imaging modalities in localization of epileptogenic lesion using epilepsy surgery outcome in pediatric patients. *Seizure,* **18** (7), 504–510.

78. Knowlton, R.C., Elgavish, R.A., Bartolucci, A. *et al.* (2008) Functional imaging: II. Pre-diction of epilepsy surgery outcome. *Ann Neurol*, **64** (1), 35–41.

79. Bautista, R.E., Cobbs, M.A., Spencer, D.D., and Spencer, S.S. (1999) Prediction of surgical outcome by interictal epileptiform abnormalities during intracranial EEG monitoring in patients with extrahippocampal seizures. *Epilepsia*, **40** (7), 880–890.

17 Surgical treatment

Cheolsu Shin

Department of Neurology, Division of Epilepsy, Mayo Clinic, Rochester, MN, USA

17.1 Introduction

Surgery for epilepsy has been around for almost a century. Many of the functional neuroanatomic correlations have come through the practices related to epilepsy surgery from the days of Wilder Penfield. Nevertheless, the surgical option was more for lesional cases with tumors, malformations, and other gliotic processes. It was made much more widely applicable through developments in neuroimaging, MRI, neurophysiologic monitoring, and video-EEG monitoring. Still, in the early days of epilepsy surgery, the surgical option was viewed as the last resort option, as practitioners and patients alike had an inherent fear of "brain surgery." More recently, due to favorable success rates in certain subgroups of patients and increasing realization of the severity of the medical and psychosocial burdens of refractory epileptic condition, epilepsy surgery has become much more widely available and has become a readily accessible option in most communities in the United States and the developed countries. Long-term follow-up of patients undergoing epilepsy surgery also demonstrated long-lasting seizure freedom in many patients [1].

This chapter will provide an overview of various aspects of epilepsy surgery for different types of epileptic conditions. Obviously the subject is too vast to cover in any detail as many reviews and books have been written on the subject [2, 3].

Adult Epilepsy, First Edition. Edited by Gregory D. Cascino and Joseph I. Sirven.
© 2011 John Wiley & Sons, Ltd. Published 2011 by John Wiley & Sons, Ltd.

The perspective presented here is from the practice of the Mayo Clinic's Comprehensive Epilepsy Program, but would be applicable in most tertiary epilepsy surgical programs.

17.2   The process of presurgical evaluation

Timing of surgical evaluation

The decision to consider surgery may come at any time in the course of epilepsy evaluation and care. In general, if medical therapy fails to provide satisfactory clinical and psychosocial outcome, then the surgical option should be considered. Nowadays with many excellent medications available to control the seizures with more tolerable side-effect profiles, one may have more monotherapies and combination therapies to try over time. However, if two or three effective monotherapies in sufficient doses fail, then the likelihood of successful medical management becomes quite low and it may be time to consider the surgical option. It is also important to note that not doing surgery is not necessarily risk-free, as intractable epileptic conditions have morbidity and mortality such as sudden unexplained death in epilepsy (SUDEP) [4]. Obviously, if the epileptic seizure occurs in the setting of other intracranial processes that would require surgery on its own merit for diagnosis or therapy, then the surgical option would be considered very early. Brain tumors, arteriovenous malformations, abscesses, or indeterminate lesions in need of diagnosis may need surgical intervention apart from epilepsy consideration, but the presence of an epileptic condition may modify the surgical approach.

In the most ideal situation, epilepsy surgery may be curative. Surgically remediable situations may provide a chance for the cure of the epileptic condition, implying the possibility of discontinuing the antiseizure medication therapy eventually. There are also situations where surgery may be palliative, in that it may modify some aspects of the seizure condition to improve the clinical situation. Seizure frequency or severity may improve, or certain types of disabling seizure may be eliminated without affecting other types. Lastly, there are now deep brain stimulation therapy options, either responsive or duty-cycle (scheduled repetitive) stimulation. The extracranial stimulation device, vagus nerve stimulator (VNS), is also to be considered a surgical option, in that it is not a medication or a dietary modification.

Noninvasive monitoring

Once a decision is made to consider the surgical option, we begin the phase of presurgical evaluation. This involves initial evaluation in the clinic by an epilepsy specialist who would take careful history, including different seizure types, to make sure there is no evidence for a multifocal epileptic condition, which makes curative surgery much less feasible. High-resolution imaging with MRI is essential to look for potential epileptogenic lesions. The next step is the electrophysiologic correlation of epileptic focus by continuous video-EEG monitoring, where the ictal onset zone can be localized using scalp EEG monitoring. This step also verifies that the intractable seizures are indeed a surgically approachable condition and not a primary generalized epilepsy. Occasionally, nonepileptic behavioral spells may masquerade as intractable epilepsy, even in patients who also have an epileptic condition.

Functional imaging may also be useful to help localize the focus. These include ictal SPECT scan with subtraction of the interictal SPECT scan co-registered on MRI (SISCOM) [5]. Interictal PET scan using 2-DG may also be useful to seek hypometabolic epileptic focus [6]. Other radioligands, flumazenil or AMT (alpha-methyl-tryptophan) may also be helpful in certain circumstances [7]. MR spectroscopy and MEG may also provide additional information. Other functional studies may include intracarotid amytal study (Wada test) to lateralize language and to assess memory processing. Neuropsychometric testing can identify any cognitive deficits that may be lateralizing or localizing and can also serve as a baseline for comparison postoperatively.

Once these studies are completed, it may be best to reassess the situation. An interdisciplinary team approach works the best, such as in an epilepsy surgical conference where all the data are discussed with the participation of epileptologists, neurosurgeons, neuroradiologists, and neuropsychologists. This works especially well for complex and challenging cases.

In simpler situations where an epileptogenic lesion is identified in neuroimaging and electrophysiologic localization is consistent, then surgery could be done in a straightforward fashion to remove the lesion. Obviously, the neurosurgical expertise is critical in tackling surgery in delicate or eloquent areas of cortex. Further refinements, such as stereotaxic MRI guidance, intraoperative MRI, functional MRI, intraoperative functional mapping in awake patients, and intraoperative electrocorticography (ECoG) require highly trained and experienced teamwork, involving neurosurgery, neurophysiology, and neuroradiology.

17.3 Intracranial monitoring

If the consensus of the epilepsy surgical conference discussion is to refine the localization further with intracranial monitoring, the primary epileptologist, and the neurosurgeon will counsel the patient and the family in preparation for the phase II evaluation. Some patients choose not to pursue surgery, if they feel that the risk of intracranial monitoring may not be worth the potential likelihood of seizure freedom. In these instances, palliative procedures such as brain stimulation protocol may be considered as well as other nonsurgical options.

First surgery, usually with stereotaxic guidance (frame or frameless), implants the electrodes onto the cortical surface, using combinations of grids (8×8, 4×6, etc.), and strips (eight or four contact straight or eight contact T). Deeper structures, such as amygdala and hippocampus, require the use of the depth electrodes with stereotaxic guidance. Functional imaging data can be co-registered onto the stereotaxic representation to refine electrode placements over or near critical functional areas. Dura is approximated over the electrode set up and the wires from the electrodes are then tunneled through the skin to the outside to be then connected to the amplifiers for recording. Reference electrodes may be placed on the mastoids or an extra four contact strip electrode can be secured into the subgaleal space outside the skull for stable recording. Skull bone flap can be stored sterilely until the second surgery so that the volume of the implanted electrode hardware would not pose significant mass effect.

Once the electrodes are implanted and ECoG recordings are satisfactory, imaging with a high-resolution spiral CT scan allows verification of the location of the electrodes to correlate with ictal electrophysiology. Co-registration of these electrode images onto the 3D rendering of the cortex along with functional imaging data may also help with the interpretation and correlation of the information gathered. Verifying the localization of the electrodes by imaging after the implantation is important for accurate interpretation of the ECoG data, as the electrode tips need to be close to the area of your target.

With the intracranial electrode recording, it is important that the ECoG onset of the seizure is prior to the clinical onset. In many cases, the ECoG onset is characterized by fast activity that may be of low amplitude. One must be careful to look at the recordings at a reasonable sensitivity. Frequently, due to the large number of electrodes implanted, the reviewing station's monitor screen may not have sufficient resolution to show these low-amplitude signals. In that situation, you must examine subgroups of electrodes to insure that a low-amplitude fast activity is correctly identified. If the electrographic onset is after the clinical onset, then one must assume that the seizure onset zone is not close to where the electrodes are recording. That is not a situation where resection can be confidently recommended.

Once the ECoG localization of the seizure onset zone is determined, the next step would be to consider functional mapping, if the area is near the functional cortex. It is usually done after a sufficient number of seizures are recorded for confident localization of the epileptic focus to be resected, and after the anti-seizure medications are restarted, so that the stimulus train does not easily trigger the seizure afterdischarge, which would not allow the assignment of the observed functional change to the electrode pair being stimulated. It is useful to have a map of the electrode set up with markings for seizure onset zones, that is, the resection zones, and for the eloquent cortical areas, to guide the surgical resection margin. Additionally, vascular and gyral anatomy may further modify the resection margin intraoperatively. In cases where the functional zone is very close to the resection margin, the neurosurgeons may elect to perform resection with the patient awake to clinically monitor the function as the resection is carried out. This is a complex approach that requires the right kind of patient preparation and a well-organized operating room team of surgeons, anesthesiologists, electro-physiologists, and neuropsychologists. Obviously, if the seizure localization is not possible, or if the resection would entail unacceptable risk of functional loss, then the electrode set up is removed without any resection.

Postoperative care of the patient is also important in that the antiseizure medications have to be continued and if oral intake is compromised, parenteral option should be considered to maintain a reasonable AED level to prevent perioperative seizures. Patients obviously will have a severe headache from the craniotomy and resection, along with usual post-anesthesia difficulties. Periorbital swelling from the edema migrating from the scalp can be quite disconcerting, although quite transient.

Patients are then followed up approximately three months after surgery, usu-ally with an EEG sleep and awake, and a visit with the neurosurgeon and the epileptologist. Postoperative MRI may not be necessary, unless neoplasm or vascular malformations were resected. If the patient is seizure-free and the EEG appears favorable, then the antiseizure medication regimen can be simplified and gradually lowered over the next couple of years. Many seizure-free patients choose to remain on a single medication at a low dose for many years, rather than discontinuing altogether.

17.4   Surgical procedures

Temporal lobectomy

Temporal lobectomy is the most frequent surgical intervention for intractable epilepsy, since complex partial seizures of temporal lobe onset are the most resistant and disabling epileptic condition. It is also one of the most effective surgeries for long-term seizure-free outcome [1]. Most frequently, mesial tempo-ral sclerosis is the underlying pathology and extensive mesial resection to include amygdala and the anterior and middle portion of the hippocampus is carried out with relatively modest resection of the lateral temporal neocortex.

In experienced hands, the standard anterior temporal lobectomy is of very low risk, but the extent of the posterior resection toward the tail of the hippocampus may be somewhat variable. The more posterior the resection, the more complete quadrantanopsia may result due to the interruption of the Meyer's loop of the optic radiation that courses through the temporal lobe. The lateral neocortical resection margin is determined in part through the intraoperative ECoG defining the area of interictal epileptiform activity and in part anatomically regarding the arteriovenous anatomy, such as the vein of Labbé.

In cases where the MRI demonstrates hippocampal atrophy with T2 signal change, the surgical outcome is excellent. Reasons for failure may be speculated as residual atrophic hippocampus, usually the tail of the hippocampus that is beyond safe surgical resection margin or other epileptogenic zones, since the pathogenetic mechanisms of mesial temporal sclerosis may actually involve other brain structures, including the contralateral hippocampus [8].

In nonlesional temporal lobe onset seizures, one could still consider surgical resection without intracranial monitoring, if ancillary studies are supportive [9]. These include FDG-PET that demonstrates ipsilateral hypometabolism of the temporal lobe with the electrographic onset, as well as MR spectroscopy showing asymmetry [6]. If there are questions regarding the potential for lateral cortical versus mesial temporal onset from scalp EEG monitoring, then one may have to proceed to phase II evaluation with electrodes both mesially and laterally [10]. This could be done with stereotaxic depth electrode into the hippocampal region and temporal craniotomy for lateral neocortical grids and strips, including subtemporal strips into the inferior mesial temporal region. One may also use single temporal craniotomy to implant grids, along with orthogonal depth electrodes into the mesial structures using frameless stereotaxic guidance.

Although the risk is considered quite low for nondominant, usually right, temporal lobectomy, that is not always the case for dominant, usually left, temporal lobectomy. As the verbal memory processing occurs with involvement of the hippocampal circuitry, resection of the mesial hippocampus and the associated connections of the adjacent structures in the standard anterior temporal lobectomy may impact on the verbal memory processing. An intracarotid amobarbital study (Wada test) may provide some measure of risk prediction, but it is not a highly predictive test. Although some centers do not offer surgery if the risk is considered high, many centers including the Mayo Clinic offer surgery to the fully informed patients. Other measures also are predictive of the risk, such as a normal volume and normal T2 signal hippocampus being associated with higher risk of verbal memory deficit postoperatively. Ultimate satisfaction from the temporal lobectomy depends heavily on seizure-free outcome, so that the verbal memory deficit may be tolerated in that situation and the patient is more functional postoperatively. The least favorable outcome would be in patients who are not seizure-free postoperatively and also have verbal memory decline.

Extratemporal lobe resections

Unlike the temporal lobe where well-defined hippocampal functional anatomy predisposes to epileptogenesis and well-defined surgical resection can be done, other neocortical regions have more diffuse and ill-defined gyral anatomy that is not easily resectable on anatomic demarcations. Unless there are abnormal imaging lesions, this is an area of epilepsy surgery that is the most difficult and likely the least effective in terms of seizure-free outcome. This continues to be the most challenging aspect of the surgical approach to medically intractable epilepsy over many decades, despite significant advances in neuroimaging. High-resolution MR imaging, possible through higher magnet strength scanners, has revealed subtle lesions that are epileptogenic. Other MR imaging sequences such as double inversion recovery (DIR) sequence may accentuate the presence of cortical dysplasia. Functional imaging such as FDG-PET has not been that helpful in extratemporal cases, although different radioligands such as flumazenil or alpha-methyl tryptophan may still prove to be more useful [7].

On the other hand, SISCOM has provided significant localizing information in many cases of nonlesional extratemporal cases [5]. Although it does not always localize the epileptogenic focus precisely, it provides reasonable guidance to the phase II evaluation with intracranial monitoring. Both hyperperfusion and hypoperfusion imaging may be useful. Actual performance of the ictal radioisotope tracer injection requires coordination of many personnel, including the ready availability of the radioisotope tracer, rapid recognition and detection of the seizure onset, and access to nuclear medicine to perform the scan. A sufficient number of seizures need to be recorded initially to demonstrate the recognizable pattern of the habitual seizures, both semiologically and electrographically. Once the ictal SPECT scan is completed, then at least 24 hours later the interictal SPECT scan is done. This allows for the decay of the radioactivity from the ictal scan and for the vascular pathophysiology to recover from the ictal hyperperfusion. The usual protocol is to restart the antiepileptic medication at the full dose and also to supplement with intravenous lorazepam every 6 hours to prevent further seizure occurrences during the 24 hours preceding the interictal radioisotope tracer injection.

Lesionectomy

If the lesion is thought to be highly epileptogenic, such as cavernous hemangioma, dysembryoplastic neuro epithelial tumor (DNET), and so on, then one could consider lesionectomy, even in eloquent areas, as long as there is good scalp EEG monitoring correlation in terms of seizure onset [11]. However, if the lesion is large or multiple, then additional localizing information will be necessary, including the intracranial monitoring. In this situation, functional neuroimaging may also be useful such as PET scan with specific ligands or SISCOM study to guide the implantation of the electrodes intracranially.

Dual or multiple pathology

Bilateral hippocampal atrophy

The pathogenetic processes that cause hippocampal atrophy may frequently be diffuse and cause bilateral damage [8]. Many times, the significant damage occurs mostly unilaterally with epileptic focus ipsilateral to the apparent damage. However, some may have significant atrophy of both hippocampi. In this situation, obvious concern is that both hippocampi may be epileptogenic and therefore not amenable to resection. Indeed, this may be a situation where deep brain stimulation may be a more attractive option. Additional concern is that the resection of one hippocampus may leave the patient with a hippocampus on the other side that is atrophic and nonfunctional in terms of memory processing. Despite these concerns, the seizure-free outcome is possible, if all the seizures arise from one side to be resected [12]. Hippocampal volume measurement can be useful to determine which hippocampus is smaller, but ultimately intracranial monitoring with bilateral hippocampal depth electrodes may be necessary [13].

Lesion plus hippocampal atrophy

In cases where the lesion is present in the temporal lobe, especially mesially, then standard anterior temporal lobectomy including the lesion may be a simpler approach. If the lesion is outside of the temporal lobe and there is hippocampal atrophy, then it may be difficult to determine the focus of the seizures, and intracranial monitoring may be necessary. One may consider a staged surgery, based upon noninvasive studies, to do lesionectomy first and then, if necessary, consider temporal lobectomy, or vice versa.

Multiple lesions (e.g., tubers)

In tuberosclerosis, usually the intracranial tubers are quite numerous so that it is difficult to determine which tuber may be epileptogenic. If one can identify and resect the epileptogenic tuber, then reasonable long-term seizure-free outcome is possible. A PET scan using special ligand, AMT, may identify which tuber may be epileptogenic, but usually intracranial monitoring is necessary to determine the focus [14].

Corpus callosotomy

In cases of multifocal or generalized seizures where the falls from the seizure are life-threatening or injurious, corpus callosotomy may offer a palliative option to prevent the falls and also to improve seizure control [15]. Some would advocate trying VNS first. Morbidity of complete corpus callosotomy led to changes in surgical practice to first try anterior two-thirds callosotomy. Postoperative abulia may be quite disabling for many patients, although most recover in a few days to weeks. If anterior two-thirds callosotomy is not effective, then completion of callosotomy can be considered. Mixed language dominance may pose a higher risk of language dysfunction postoperatively. Partial onset seizures may actually be more poorly controlled postoperatively and should be considered in the risk assessment.

Hemispherectomy

This surgical approach seems quite drastic and indeed this is usually in the setting of catastrophic hemispheric refractory epileptic condition, such as Rasmussen's encephalitis with progressive hemispheric atrophy with epileptic encephalopathy [16]. The efficacy can be quite satisfactory in terms of seizure control and the resulting spastic hemiparesis is usually well tolerated as most patients already have significant hemiparetic process. Original anatomic hemispherectomy was frequently associated with complication of superficial hemosiderosis and therefore, nowadays, functional hemispherectomy is done where frontal and occipital lobe is not resected, but disconnected by corpus callosal section.

Vagus nerve stimulator (VNS)

The mechanism of action of the VNS is not clearly delineated, but the effectiveness could be likened to the trial of a new medication in that it is effective in about half the patients to reduce the seizure burden by half [17]. The left vagus nerve is stimulated, since in most patients the right vagus nerve controls the cardiac function. The most common side effect is the hoarseness of voice that occurs due to the stimulation of the recurrent laryngeal nerve within the vagus nerve. Otherwise, the stimulation is well tolerated. A magnet device can be used to trigger extra stimulation train to attempt to abort or shorten the seizure. There may be also some degree of mood improvement, which led to its use in refractory depression.

Deep brain stimulation

Two different stimulation paradigms are being considered for approval by the FDA after the clinical trials. Anterior thalamic stimulation is a duty-cycle stimulation where a set pattern of stimulation is applied continuously, suppressing the seizure occurrences [18]. Responsive neurostimulation system (RNS) is an as-needed stimulation paradigm, where the device is programmed to detect the onset of the seizure from the electrodes near the seizure focus and then deliver the stimulus train that arrests the seizure evolution. In patients without a good resective surgical option, these stimulation protocols may be useful, but in most cases, these are palliative measures [19].

Stereotactic radiosurgery (Gamma-Knife)

This relatively new "surgical" approach is used in many intracranial lesional cases such as arteriovenous malformation and tumors of small to moderate sizes, unrelated to epilepsy. In these lesional cases associated with epilepsy, the results appear favorable. For hypothalamic hamartoma, classically associated with gelastic epilepsy, radiosurgery may be a very reasonable option to consider, as the regular craniotomy approach in the hypothalamus is not without risk [20].

In mesial temporal lobe epilepsy, stereotactic radiosurgery is being investigated for its efficacy and safety in comparison to the standard craniotomy approach. It may be advantageous for the elderly or patients with higher risk for general anesthesia and craniotomy. In addition, it would allow preservation of brain parenchyma that is usually sacrificed during the craniotomy approach. This could potentially reduce the likelihood of verbal memory decline from dominant temporal lobe surgery. Preliminary data appear favorable, but further clinical trial will be necessary to validate the approach.

17.5 Conclusion

Epilepsy surgery is no longer the last resort option for many patients with medically intractable epilepsy. Advances in anatomic neuroimaging have improved detection of lesions amenable to highly effective epilepsy surgery. The surgical option then may be considered earlier in the clinical management of epilepsy, balancing the risk of surgery with risk of ineffective medical therapy. There are many different situations amenable to the surgical option and a comprehensive epilepsy surgical center is the best option to evaluate the complex processes involved in performing epilepsy surgery. New surgical therapy options such as brain stimulation and stereotaxic radiosurgery may also provide additional avenues for improvement in the management of patients with medically refractory epilepsy.

References

1. Cohen-Gadol, A.A., Wilhelmi, B.G., Collignon, F. *et al.* (2006) Long-term outcome of epilepsy surgery among 399 patients with nonlesional seizure foci including mesial temporal lobe sclerosis. *J Neurosurg*, **104**, 513–524.
2. Cascino, G.D. (2004) Surgical treatment for epilepsy. *Epilepsy Res*, **60**, 179–186.
3. Luders, H.O. and Comair, Y.G. (eds.) (2001) *Epilepsy Surgery*, 2nd edn, Lippincott Williams & Wilkins, Philadelphia, PA.
4. So, E.L., Bainbridge, J., Buchhalter, J.R. *et al.* (2009) Report of the American Epilepsy Society and the Epilepsy Foundation joint task force on sudden unexplained death in epilepsy. *Epilepsia*, **50**, 917–922.
5. O'Brien, T.J., So, E.L., Mullan, B.P. *et al.* (1998) Subtraction ictal SPECT co-registered to MRI improves clinical usefulness of SPECT in localizing the surgical seizure focus. *Neurology*, **50**, 445–454.
6. Salamon, N., Kung, J., Shaw, S.J. *et al.* (2008) FDG-PET/MRI co-registration improves detection of cortical dysplasia in patients with epilepsy. *Neurology*, **71**, 1594–1601.
7. Kagawa, K., Chugani, D.C., Asano, E. *et al.* (2005) Epilepsy surgery outcome in children with tuberous sclerosis complex evaluated with alpha-[11C]methyl-L-tryptophan positron emission tomography (PET). *J Child Neurol*, **20**, 429–438.
8. Madden, M. and Sutula, T. (2009) Beyond hippocampal sclerosis: the rewired hippocampus in temporal lobe epilepsy. *Neurology*, **73**, 1008–1009.

9. Bell, M.L., Rao, S., So, E.L. *et al.* (2009) Epilepsy surgery outcomes in temporal lobe epilepsy with a normal MRI. *Epilepsia*, **50**, 2053–2060.

10. Madhavan, D. and Kuzniecky, R. (2007) Temporal lobe surgery in patients with normal MRI. *Curr Opin Neurol*, **20**, 203–207.

11. Cascino, G.D., Kelly, P.J., Sharbrough, F.W. *et al.* (1992) Long-term follow-up of stereotactic lesionectomy in partial epilepsy: predictive factors and electroencephalographic results. *Epilepsia*, **33**, 639–644.

12. Sirven, J.I., Malamut, B.L., Liporace, J.D. *et al.* (1997) Outcome after temporal lobectomy in bilateral temporal lobe epilepsy. *Ann Neurol*, **42**, 873–878.

13. Spencer, S. and Huh, L. (2008) Outcomes of epilepsy surgery in adults and children. *Lancet Neurol*, **7**, 525–537.

14. Jansen, F.E., van Huffelen, A.C., Algra, A. *et al.* (2007) Epilepsy surgery in tuberous sclerosis: a systematic review. *Epilepsia*, **48**, 1477–1484.

15. Rahimi, S.Y., Park, Y.D., Witcher, M.R. *et al.* (2007) Corpus callosotomy for treatment of pediatric epilepsy in the modern era. *Pediatr Neurosurg*, **43**, 202–208.

16. Jonas, R., Nguyen, S., Hu, B. *et al.* (2004) Cerebral hemispherectomy: hospital course, seizure, developmental, language, and motor outcomes. *Neurology*, **62**, 1712–1721.

17. Uthman, B.M. (2000) Vagus nerve stimulation for seizures. *Arch Med Res*, **31**, 300–303.

18. Kerrigan, J.F., Litt, B., Fisher, R.S. *et al.* (2004) Electrical stimulation of the anterior nucleus of the thalamus for the treatment of intractable epilepsy. *Epilepsia*, **45**, 346–354.

19. Morrell, M. (2006) Brain stimulation for epilepsy: can scheduled or responsive neurostimulation stop seizures? *Curr Opin Neurol*, **19**, 164–168.

20. Yang, I. and Barbaro, N.M. (2007) Advances in the radiosurgical treatment of epilepsy. *Epilepsy Curr*, **7**, 31–35.

Index

Note: page numbers in *italics* refer to figures; those in **bold** to tables.

Adult Epilepsy, First Edition. Edited by Gregory D. Cascino and Joseph I. Sirven.
© 2011 John Wiley & Sons, Ltd. Published 2011 by John Wiley & Sons, Ltd.

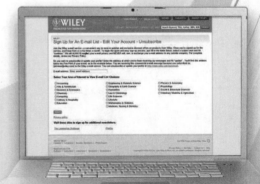
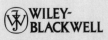